W9-BNH-700

For anyone concerned about lowering their
cholesterol or high blood pressure . . . for anyone
who's been told by their doctor thay have or may be
at risk for heart disease . . .

Here is the one-stop resource for good heart health.

THE HEALTHY HEART FOOD COUNTER
is a one-of-a-kind guide that lists thousands of everyday,
take-out, and chain-restaurant foods, giving reliable
counts of fat, cholesterol, sodium, and calories—and
giving you a personalized program for customizing
your diet to fit your health needs. Preventing and
managing heart disease has never been easier; let
America's nutrition experts put you on the road
to improved heart health—today!

ANNETTE B. NATOW, Ph.D., R.D., CDN, and JO-ANN
HESLIN, M.A., R.D., CDN, are the authors of twenty-eight
books on nutrition, including two college textbooks. Both
are former faculty members of Adelphi University and
the State University of New York, Downstate Medical
Center. They are editors of the *Journal of Nutrition for
the Elderly,* and serve as editorial board members for
Environmental Nutrition Newsletter. For more information on
other books by Annette B. Natow and Jo-Ann Heslin, go to
www.thenutritionexperts.com

Books by Annette B. Natow and Jo-Ann Heslin

Published by POCKET BOOKS

THE
HEALTHY HEART
FOOD COUNTER

Annette B. Natow, Ph.D., R.D.
and **Jo-Ann Heslin, M.A., R.D.**

POCKET BOOKS

New York London Toronto Sydney Singapore

The sale of this book without its cover is unauthorized. If you purchased this book without a cover, you should be aware that it was reported to the publisher as "unsold and destroyed." Neither the author nor the publisher has received payment for the sale of this "stripped book."

An *Original* Publication of POCKET BOOKS

 POCKET BOOKS, a division of Simon & Schuster, Inc.
1230 Avenue of the Americas, New York, NY 10020

Copyright © 2002 by Annette Natow and Jo-Ann Heslin

All rights reserved, including the right to reproduce
this book or portions thereof in any form whatsoever.
For information address Pocket Books, 1230 Avenue
of the Americas, New York, NY 10020

ISBN: 0-7434-2684-3

First Pocket Books printing September 2002

10 9 8 7 6 5 4

POCKET and colophon are registered trademarks of
Simon & Schuster, Inc.

For information regarding special discounts for bulk purchases,
please contact Simon & Schuster Special Sales at 1-800-456-6798
or business@simonandschuster.com

Front cover photo by Eric Jacobson/Getty Images

Printed in the U.S.A.

The authors and publisher of this book are not physicians and are not licensed to give medical advice. The information in this book has been collected for the convenience of the reader. The nutrient values for prepared foods are subject to change and might currently vary from listings herein, which are based on research conducted prior to Fall 2001. Such information does not constitute a recommendation or endorsement of any individual, institution or product, nor is it intended as a substitute for personalized consultation with your physician. The authors and publisher disclaim any liability arising directly or indirectly from the use of this book.

To our families who support us through every project:
Harry, Allen, Irene, Sarah, Meryl, Laura, Marty,
George, Emily, Steven, Joe, Kristen, Brian and Karen.

Acknowledgments

Without the tireless cooperation of Steven Natow, M.D., and Stephen Llano, *The Healthy Heart Food Counter* would never have been completed. Our thanks to all the food manufacturers and processors who shared product information. A special thanks to our most supportive agent, Nancy Trichter, and our editor, Micki Nuding.

The values in this book are based on research conducted prior to Fall 2001. Manufacturers' ingredients are subject to change, so current values may vary from those listed in the book. If the serving size on the package label is different from that listed in this counter, use the nutrition information provided as a guide. If the nutrition information listed in the Nutrition Facts panel is different from the information in this counter, assume that the product has been recently reformulated.

"There is no magic diet for any disease . . ."

"In sickness even more than in health, every person is a law unto himself and all rules must be modified according to the requirement of the individual."

MARY SWARTZ ROSE, PH.D.
Feeding the Family
The Macmillan Company, 1919

Contents

What Is Your Risk?

Heart disease is still the #1 killer in the U.S.

The Third National Health Examination Survey (NHANES III), 1994, found that 1 in 5 men and women have some type of heart disease.

The following 5 questions will help you determine your risk for heart disease. The questions are slightly different for men and women. The men's section starts below. The women's questions begin on page 3.

Estimated 10-Year Risk for Heart Disease*

For Men

For each of the following questions, write down the point value that best describes you.

1. Your age:

Age in Years	Points
20–34	-9
35–39	-4
40–44	0
45–49	3
50–54	6
55–59	8
60–64	10
65–69	11
70–74	12
75–79	13

Points _____

*Adapted from the Executive Summary of the Third Report of the National Cholesterol Education Program (NCEP), Expert Panel on Detection, Evaluation and Treatment of High Blood Cholesterol in Adults (Adults Treatment Panel III), National Heart, Lung and Blood Institute, 2001.

2. Your total cholesterol:

Total Cholesterol	Age 20–39	Age 40–49	Age 50–59	Age 60–69	Age 70–79
Less than 160	0	0	0	0	0
160 to 199	4	3	2	1	0
200 to 239	7	5	3	1	0
240 to 279	9	6	4	2	1
Greater than or equal to 280	11	8	5	3	1

Points _____

3. Do you smoke?

	Age 20–39	Age 40–49	Age 50–59	Age 60–69	Age 70–79
Nonsmoker	0	0	0	0	0
Smoker	8	5	3	1	1

Points _____

4. Your HDLs (high density lipoproteins) are:

HDLs	Points
Greater than or equal to 60	-1
50 to 59	0
40 to 49	1
Less than 40	2

Points _____

5. Your blood pressure is:

Systolic Blood Pressure	If Untreated	If Treated
Less than 120	0	0
120 to 129	0	1
130 to 139	1	2
140 to 159	1	2
Greater than 160	2	3

Points _____

Your 10-Year Risk For Heart Disease Is:

Point Total	10-Year Risk
Less than 0	Less than 1%
0	1%
1	1%
2	1%
3	1%
4	1%
5	2%
6	2%
7	3%
8	4%
9	5%
10	6%
11	8%
12	10%
13	12%
14	16%
15	20%
16	25%
More than or equal to 17	More than or equal to 30%

Total Points _____   % of Risk _____

For Women

For each of the following questions, write down the point value that best describes you.

1. Your age:

Age in Years	Points
20–34	-7
35–39	-3
40–44	0
45–49	3
50–54	6
55–59	8
60–64	10
65–69	12
70–74	14
75–79	16

Points _____

2. Your total cholesterol:

Total Cholesterol	Age 20–39	Age 40–49	Age 50–59	Age 60–69	Age 70–79
Less than 160	0	0	0	0	0
160 to 199	4	3	2	1	1
200 to 239	8	6	4	2	1
240 to 279	11	8	5	3	2
Greater than or equal to 280	13	10	7	4	2

Points _____

3. Do you smoke?

	Age 20–39	Age 40–49	Age 50–59	Age 60–69	Age 70–79
Nonsmoker	0	0	0	0	0
Smoker	9	7	4	2	1

Points _____

4. Your HDLs (high density lipoproteins) are:

HDLs	Points
Greater than or equal to 60	-1
50 to 59	0
40 to 49	1
Less than 40	2

Points _____

5. Your blood pressure is:

Systolic Blood Pressure	If Untreated	If Treated
Less than 120	0	0
120 to 129	1	3
130 to 139	2	4
140 to 159	3	5
Greater than 160	4	6

Your 10-Year Risk For Heart Disease Is:

Point Total	10-Year Risk
Less than 9	Less than 1%
9	1%
10	1%
11	1%
12	1%
13	2%
14	2%
15	3%
16	4%
17	5%
18	6%
19	8%
20	11%
21	14%
22	17%
23	22%
24	27%
Greater than or equal to 25	Greater than or equal to 30%

Total Points _____ % of Risk _____

The Numbers Stay Up

Heart disease (diseases of the heart and blood vessels) kills more people than cancer, diabetes, accidents, AIDS, or infectious diseases and causes about 40% of all deaths. Yearly, a million lives are lost as a result. One person dies from heart disease every 33 seconds. And more than 150,000 of these deaths occur in people under age 65.

While the death rate from heart disease has gone down in the U.S. over the last fifty years, the rate of sudden death from heart disease in 15- to 34-year-olds has gone up. Experts believe risk factors, such as being overweight, put younger people at as much risk as older people. As younger people get fatter, the incidence of heart disease starts earlier.

Surveys show that two-thirds of women think that cancer is their greatest health risk. They're wrong. Cancer kills about 250,000 women a year while heart disease (heart attack and stroke) kills twice as many—more than half a million a year.

Most people think that heart disease is more of a man's problem than it is a woman's. This is in spite of the fact that after they've had a heart attack, 44% of women die during the following year compared to 27% of men. The reason for this may be that women wait too long to go to the hospital once they develop symptoms.

Both women and men can have similar heart attack symptoms—tightness or pain in the chest, jaws, arms and shoulders, and shortness of breath. But many times for women, heart attack symptoms may appear as flu, nausea, even back pain, and the symptoms may occur only during exercise.

You Should Know:

Research at Harvard Medical School shows that hair loss is a good indicator of a man's tendency to have heart trouble. Men with a lot of hair have the lowest risk of heart disease while men with severe balding have a 36% higher than normal risk. And receding hairlines predict a 9% greater risk. Incorporating heart-healthy activities into your life can reduce these risks.

What Is Heart Disease?

The heart muscle needs a constant supply of oxygen and nutrients that are carried by the blood through the arteries. Heart disease is the narrowing of these arteries to the point that they no longer supply enough blood to the heart. This is called atherosclerosis. It can take years for plaque deposits in the arteries to build up. Smoking, eating high fat foods, having high blood pressure, too much stress, and too little exercise can speed up this plaque buildup. Infections, like bronchitis, inflamed sinuses and even urinary tract infections, cause inflammation in the body that increase your risk for developing plaque.

Angina (chest pain) happens when too little blood reaches the heart. A heart attack (myocardial infarction or MI) occurs when the blood supply to the heart is completely cut off because an artery is totally blocked. A stroke happens when the arteries supplying blood to the brain become clogged. It has been estimated that there will be more than one million strokes a year by 2010. Walking 30 minutes a day can reduce the risk of stroke by about 40%.

You Should Know:

Warning Signs for Heart Attack or Stroke*

Heart attack: Pressure; squeezing or pain in the center of the chest lasting more than a few minutes; pain spreading to the shoulders, neck or arms; chest discomfort with light-headedness; fainting, sweating, nausea or shortness of breath.

Stroke: Sudden numbness or weakness of the face, arm or leg, especially on one side of the body; sudden confusion, trouble speaking or understanding; sudden trouble seeing in one or both eyes; sudden trouble walking, dizziness, loss of balance or coordination; sudden severe headache with no known cause.

*According to the American Heart Association

Take Prevention to Heart—
Identify Your Risk Factors

Take the following health risks quiz. While you cannot change your age or your genes, many other risk factors can be changed.

Your Health Risks Quiz

Circle the answer that best applies to you. You may not know the answers to every question. That's okay; just skip the ones you don't know and go on. (For scoring purposes, not every question has 3 options.)

FAMILY HISTORY

1. One or more close blood relatives (parents, grandparents, siblings) has had a heart attack or stroke.
   A. No family history of heart attack or stroke
   B. After age 55
   C. Before age 55

2. One or more close blood relatives has high blood pressure.
   A. No family history of high blood pressure
   C. One or more family members has been treated for high blood pressure

3. One or more close blood relatives has been treated for diabetes.
   A. No family history of diabetes
   B. After age 60
   C. Before age 60

4. One or more close blood relatives is overweight.
   A. No family members are overweight
   B. Few family members are overweight
   C. Many family members are overweight

PERSONAL HISTORY

5a. (for men only) Your age is
    A. Younger than 45
    C. Older than 45

5b. (for women only) Your age is
    A. Younger than 55
    C. Older than 55

6. Have you had a heart attack or stroke?
    A. No
    C. Yes

7. Do you have high blood pressure?
    A. No
    C. Yes

8. Do you have diabetes?
    A. No
    B. Yes, and the condition is controlled
    C. Yes, but the condition is not well controlled

9. Are you overweight?
    A. No
    B. Less than 20 pounds over my target weight
    C. More than 20 pounds over my target weight

10. Your total cholesterol is:
    A. Below 200 mg/dl
    B. 200 to 239 mg/dl
    C. 240 mg/dl or higher

11. Your HDL (high density lipoprotein) level is:
    A. More than 60 mg/dl
    B. Between 41 to 59 mg/dl
    C. Less than 40 mg/dl

12. Your LDL (low density lipoprotein) level is:
    A. Below 130 mg/dl
    B. 130 to 159 mg/dl
    C. 160 mg/dl or higher

13. Your triglyceride level is:
    A. Less than 150 mg/dl
    B. 150 to 199 mg/dl
    C. Over 200 mg/dl

14. Your blood pressure is:
    A. Less than 130/85 mm Hg
    B. Between 131/86 to 139/89 mm Hg
    C. 140/90 mm Hg or higher

15. Do you smoke?
    A. Never smoked or quit more than 4 years ago
    B. Less than 1 pack a day or quit 2 to 4 years ago
    C. One or more packs a day

16. Do you exercise:
    A. 30 minutes 3 or more times a week
    B. 30 minutes once or twice a week
    C. Occasionally or not at all

17. How does stress affect you?
    A. You are easygoing and seldom rushed or irritable
    B. You are sometimes impatient, rushed or irritable
    C. You are easily angered, often mistrustful, rushed, impatient and irritable

18. You practice other good health habits like wearing seat belts, eating fruits and vegetables, and using sunscreen.
    A. All the time
    B. Most of the time
    C. Rarely or never

Rating Your Health Risks

Add up the number of As, Bs and Cs you've circled and write them below.

A answers _____   B answers _____   C answers _____

"A" answers signal the least risk. "B" answers signal moderate risk. And "C" answers indicate the most risk.

1, 2, 3, 4—Your family history can alert you to the health problems that exist in your family. While it is not written in stone that you'll have the same health history as your relatives, you do run a greater risk of similar problems. When close relatives have had a heart attack or stroke before age 55, have been treated for high blood pressure or diabetes, and are overweight, you have been put on notice. It's time to make those lifestyle changes that can help you prevent or postpone similar health problems.

5a, 5b—Age is a risk factor you cannot control, but simply getting older does increase your risk for heart disease. After age 45, men are at a greater risk for heart problems than when they were younger. Women do not usually develop heart disease until they reach 55—ten years after the time when men start to be affected. Women over 55, or who have passed menopause, or who have had their ovaries removed and do not take estrogen, are at an increased risk for heart disease. According to Carlos Ayers, director of vascular medicine and preventive cardiology at the University of Virginia Medical Center, "Women fear breast cancer and cervical cancer, but while they fear all these, they die of heart disease."

6—If you've had a heart attack or stroke, it's important that you follow your doctor's advice carefully. You can make a positive impact on your treatment by making lifestyle changes that reduce health risks. If you are still smoking, resolve to stop. If you are overweight, losing as little as 5 to 10 pounds makes you look and feel better. Explore exercise options with your doctor or health practitioner—another positive lifestyle change.

7—One in 4 American adults has high blood pressure— 140/90 or higher. At these levels, there is an increased risk for heart disease. For more on high blood pressure, see page 30.

8—Sixteen million Americans have diabetes, and one third of them do not know it. From 1990 to 1998, the incidence of diabetes rose 33%. Eighty percent of people with Type 2 diabetes, the most common kind, are overweight. Symptoms — increased thirst, frequent urination, slow-healing cuts and bruises, blurred vision—develop gradually. But many people have no symptoms at all; the condition is often discovered during a routine physical. Heart disease is the leading complication and cause of death among people with diabetes; they are also at a much greater risk for stroke.

9—Being overweight puts you at a greater risk of developing heart disease, high blood pressure, and stroke. Compared to normal-weight people, those who are overweight have heart attacks almost 4 years earlier. People who are obese have heart attacks more than 8 years earlier. Although some body fat is needed for storing energy and insulating the body, too much interferes with your health. Fat deposits around the belly are a risk factor. A waist measurement of more than 40 inches in males or 35 inches in females is too high. A small weight loss in the area of 10 to 20 pounds can be enough to reduce risks.

10—The higher your cholesterol, the greater your risk for heart disease and stroke. Many large population studies show that lowering cholesterol reduces the risk of heart disease. A cholesterol value of less than 200 is desirable. A cholesterol level of 200 to 239 is considered borderline-high and values over this amount are too high and put you at greater risk. For more on cholesterol, see page 27.

11—HDL (high density lipoprotein) is known as "good cholesterol" because it helps the body get rid of cholesterol. HDLs take cholesterol away from the artery walls and carry it to the liver where it's removed from the body. People who have high levels of HDLs (over 60) have reduced risk of heart disease and stroke. Levels of HDLs under 40 are considered too low. Every 1% increase in HDLs reduces the risk of heart disease by 2 to 3%. Losing weight, exercising and moderate intake of alcohol raise HDLs. Being overweight, inactive and smoking cigarettes reduces HDLs. Your risk of heart disease goes down as your HDLs go up.

12—LDL (low density lipoprotein) is often referred to as "bad cholesterol" because it is the source of buildup in the arteries. LDL levels of less than 100 are considered best. Levels of 130 to 159 are borderline high and levels over 160 are too high. LDLs tend to go up as people get older. A decrease of 1 milligram of LDLs can decrease heart disease risk by 1 to 2%. Eating foods low in saturated fats and cholesterol, increasing activity and losing weight, if needed, will help reduce LDLs in most people. But some people are not able to lower LDL levels through diet and lifestyle changes alone. They may need medicine as well. The statin family of drugs—like Zocor, Lipitor, Mevacor, Pravachol—are considered effective. They are currently used by more than 13 million Americans. Your risk for heart disease goes down as your LDLs go down.

13—Almost all the fats in foods are triglycerides; the fat in our bodies is too. High levels of triglycerides in the blood are a risk factor for heart disease. Being overweight, inactive, smoking cigarettes, drinking too much alcohol, and eating too many carbohydrates—particularly sugar—are some of the causes of high triglycerides. Normal triglycerides are less than 150. Borderline-high triglycerides are 150 to 199, and levels over 200 are considered too high. Lowering triglycerides lowers your risk for heart disease.

14—Healthy blood pressure values are 120/80 or even a little less. As people get older, their risk for high blood pressure goes up. By age 75, about 41% of men and 54% of women have high blood pressure. The role of salt in high blood pressure has been controversial. But recent studies show that eating less salt (no more than one teaspoon a day) reduces blood pressure. You can help lower your blood pressure by eating more fruits and vegetables, losing weight if you are overweight, limiting the amount of alcohol you drink, not smoking, getting enough potassium, calcium and magnesium, and trying relaxation techniques. For more on high blood pressure, see page 30.

15—Forty-seven million Americans smoke—nearly a quarter of the adult population. Twenty-eight percent of men and 23% of women smoke. Smoking kills 400,000 people a year. One out of 5 deaths from heart disease is due to smoking— 20% of all heart disease deaths. The risk of heart disease goes up with the number of cigarettes smoked each day. When you live or work around people who smoke, your risk increases as well. There is no safe level of smoking. A study done on women who smoked only 1 to 4 cigarettes a day showed that they still had a higher risk for heart disease than nonsmokers. Certainly, quitting is worthwhile. One year after you stop smoking, your risk of heart disease drops by half. In 15 years, you have the same risk as a nonsmoker.

16—You should try to include 30 minutes of moderate exercise into your daily routine. You can do this in 10-minute segments throughout the day. Exercising doesn't mean you have to become a marathon runner. The "no pain, no gain" approach to exercise is outdated. Middle-aged women can lower their heart disease risk simply by walking for at least 1 hour a week, regardless of pace. Take the stairs instead of an elevator. Walk to the mailbox or post office. Make a walking date with a friend a couple of times a week. Leave your car at the far end of the parking lot. Every step you take lowers your risk for heart disease. When you have just a few dishes to clean, wash them by hand. Use hand power instead of electric appliances. Put down the TV remote control, get up to change the channel instead. Avoiding exercise is a risk factor equivalent to smoking, high cholesterol, or high blood pressure. Keep moving—studies show that exercise alone can reduce the risk of heart attack and stroke by 50%.

17—People who are quick to anger are two and a half times more likely than calmer people to have a heart attack. Dr. Janice E. Williams, a cardiovascular epidemiologist with the Centers for Disease Control and Prevention says, "What we're finding is that the risk for heart attacks associated with anger is comparable to that of smoking and high cholesterol." Laughter that reduces stress may also reduce your risk for heart disease. People with good friends or close families tend to have lower blood pressure.

18—When you practice good health habits like wearing seat belts, eating fruits and vegetables, and using sunscreen, you increase your chances for good health. People who practice these good health habits practice others, too—eating only when they're hungry, exercising, having good friends and being a good friend. Think about adding more good health habits to your lifestyle.

You Should Know:

Although many find change to be threatening, Benjamin Franklin had the right idea when he said "When you're finished changing, you're finished."

Protect Your Heart

The Healthy Heart Food Counter will help you make lifestyle changes to reduce your risk of heart disease. This book will make it simple and easy for you to follow your doctor's advice.

What has your doctor told you to do?

_____ Lose weight

_____ Eat less fat

_____ Lower your cholesterol

_____ Eat less salt

Are you confused about how to get started? The good news is that when you lose some weight—even as little as 5 to 10 pounds—you reduce your cholesterol and your blood pressure goes down. So let's start with calories.

Calories

The bathroom scale shows heart disease risk. When you see the numbers going up, you know it's time to do something about it. Weighing too much puts you at a greater risk for heart attack, stroke, high blood pressure, high cholesterol, high triglycerides and other serious problems.

Everything you eat and drink, except water, contains calories. While your body needs calories to work, when you eat too many, the extra is stored as fat. Americans are eating almost 300 calories more a day than they did 20 years ago and most are not active. More calories and less activity equals more weight gain. And 61% of American adults and 25% of American children are overweight.

Calories are calories, whether you get them from an apple or a candy bar. It doesn't matter if the food is high in carbohydrates, protein or fat, the calories still can add up. While it's true that fat has more calories than protein and carbohydrates, most foods are combinations, so when you eat a meal or snack you usually get all three. The end result is the same—when you take in more calories than you need, you gain weight.

How many calories should you have each day? It's easy to figure it out once you decide the best weight for you.

What do you weigh? _____

What do you want to weigh? _____

How much do you need to lose? _____

Targeting your calorie zone:

1. Select the calorie factor that best describes you:

    _____ 20 = Very active men

    _____ 15 = Moderately active men or very active women

    _____ 13 = Inactive men, moderately active women, and all people over age 55

    _____ 10 = Inactive women, repeat dieters, and seriously overweight people

2. Find your target calorie zone:

    The weight you are aiming for × calorie factor = target calorie zone

    130 (weight you are aiming for) × 13 (for a moderately active woman) = 1600 calories a day

Your target calorie zone: _____

In the example shown, if your target weight is 130 and you are a moderately active woman, your target calorie zone would be 1600 to 1700 calories a day. Eating that number of calories will help you reach the weight you want.

Track your calories for one day. Include everything you eat and drink to get the most realistic account of what you eat during a typical day. You'll find the calorie values for over 12,000 foods in *The Healthy Heart Food Counter*.

Daily Calorie Record

Your target calorie zone _____

Food Eaten	Amount	Calories
Breakfast		
Lunch		
Dinner		
Snacks		

Total _____

How many calories did you eat on the sample day? What is your calorie zone? If you ate more calories than you need, you should reduce your calories to your target weight.

For more information on how to lose weight, look for one of our other books: *Get Skinny the Smart Way.*

Fat

When you eat a lot of fat, your calorie intake goes up and you get fatter. That puts you at risk for a heart attack, high blood pressure and other serious health problems. Experts recommend keeping your total daily fat intake to no more than 30 to 35% of your calories and your saturated fat intake to 7 to 10% of your daily calories. It makes sense to eat less saturated fats and moderate amounts of other fats. One way to accomplish this is to choose natural liquid vegetable oils like olive, corn, canola or peanut. And to eat fish a couple of times a week for the healthy fish oils they contain.

How much fat should you eat each day? If you are an average weight, moderately active adult, simply divide your weight in half.

$$130 \text{ pounds} \div 2 = 65 \text{ grams of fat a day}$$

By dividing your weight in half, you get a quick benchmark for the number of fat grams to eat each day.

If you are overweight, you can use the same method but use the weight you'd like to be, not your current weight, to get the number of fat grams for the day.

To help you keep track of the fat you eat, *The Healthy Heart Food Counter* lists the fat grams in over 12,000 foods.

Rate Your Fat Intake

The following quiz will help you recognize where the fats in your food are hiding.

1. I eat meat almost every day.   YES   NO

2. I eat bacon or sausage.   YES   NO

3. I use butter or margarine.   YES   NO

4. I drink coffee or tea with cream.   YES   NO

5. I think a salad without dressing is like eating grass.   YES   NO

6. I eat out a few times a week.   YES   NO

7. I eat take-out foods often.   YES   NO

8. I eat vegetables with butter or cheese sauce.   YES   NO

9. I eat few fruits and vegetables.   YES   NO

10. I often eat fried foods.   YES   NO

11. I use mayonnaise.   YES   NO

12. I eat sour cream, cream cheese or gravy.   YES   NO

13. I eat cheese almost every day.   YES   NO

14. I drink regular milk.   YES   NO

15. I use oil in cooking.   YES   NO

16. I eat ice cream.   YES   NO

17. I eat cookies and cakes.   YES   NO

Every "yes" answer is a signal that you are eating too much fat and that there are better food choices you can make.

1—It's better to alternate meat with chicken, fish or vegetarian meals. When you eat meat, buy lean cuts like flank steak and pork loin and keep portions small (about 4 ounces). Be adventurous; many who enjoy eating meat for dinner are surprised to find that they can be just as happy with bean, pasta, or tofu dishes.

2—Bacon and sausage are fine occasionally. Keep portions small and try Canadian bacon, turkey sausage, turkey bacon, or veggie links for a lower fat choice.

3—It's healthy to limit the amount of butter or margarine you use to a teaspoon a serving. Instead of butter, try a little jelly or honey on bread. On potatoes or vegetables, try butter spray or sprinkles.

4—Try using whole milk or lowfat evaporated milk instead of cream.

5—You don't have to learn to enjoy grass. There are many lowfat dressings available—or you can try flavored vinegar or lemon juice on your salad.

6—While restaurants may offer some low calorie, lowfat choices, the most popular selections are fries, cheeseburgers, wraps, fried chicken and fried fish. Choose grilled or broiled chicken with the skin removed, use mustard or ketchup instead of creamy dressings, have pizza without meat toppings, and order small portions of fries most of the time.

7—Take-out foods are higher in fat than most foods you eat at home. To keep fat low, order plain foods and ask for toppings on the side. Switch from fried to grilled.

8—Look for lower fat versions of your favorite vegetables. Or stick with plain and try a drizzle of lowfat salad dressing as a topper.

9—Most people don't eat enough fruits and vegetables. If you're not a fresh fruit fan, try some fruits canned in their own juice. Fruit sauces are available in many flavors too. If you don't like cooked vegetables, try ready-to-eat choices like baby carrots, celery sticks, green beans, peas, broccoli florets and mixed salads.

10—Fried foods are very high in fat but they can be enjoyed now and then. Most of the time stick with grilled, steamed, broiled or roasted.

11—Try a reduced calorie mayonnaise—plenty of flavor and less fat.

12—Reduced fat sour cream or cream cheese can replace regular. Small servings of gravy can add flavor with less fat; au jus is also very low in fat.

13—If you enjoy cheese, eat small portions less often; try different reduced fat versions. A tablespoon of grated cheese offers a lot of flavor with less fat.

14—First try 2% milk; it has a rich taste and less fat. Then try 1% or skim; every change reduces fat.

15—Using oil in cooking is fine as long as you use smaller amounts. Try measuring out an amount instead of pouring it into the pan. Cooking sprays are a better lower fat choice.

16—Try eating lowfat ice cream, frozen yogurt, sorbet, sherbet and ices instead of ice cream.

17—Cookies and cakes have a lot of hidden fat. They can be enjoyed once in a while in reasonable portions. Choose graham crackers, angel food cake, raisin and sugar wafer cookies instead—all lower in fat.

You Should Know:

Go Easy on Heavy Meals

Watch out for big meals. Doctors from Brigham and Women's Hospital in Boston found that a heavy meal quadruples the ordinary risk of a heart attack in the 2 hours immediately following eating. After 3 hours, the extra risk is almost gone.

Know Your Fats

Fats come in various forms. Some are more likely to increase your risk for heart disease. Others may lower it.

Saturated fat is solid at room temperature. A stick of butter, high in saturated fat, remains solid at room temperature. When you eat a lot of saturated fats, your cholesterol goes up. Research has shown that not all saturated fats raise cholesterol. While that's true, the foods we eat never contain only one type of saturated fat. Foods often have some saturated fats that raise cholesterol and some that don't. The best overall advice is to eat less saturated fats.

Foods high in saturated fats include bacon, beef, veal, pork, sausage, butter, cheese, chocolate, coconut, cream, ice cream, deli meats, hot dogs, whipped cream and whole milk.

Polyunsaturated fats are liquid at room temperature and help to lower cholesterol. But research suggests that eating too much polyunsaturated fat may not be good for you either. High intakes reduce beneficial HDLs, can cause gallbladder disease, and depress the immune system. Eating less saturated fat lowers cholesterol more than substituting polyunsaturated fat for saturated fat.

Polyunsaturated fats are in many foods but their major source is vegetable oils—corn oil, cottonseed oil, sesame oil, soybean oil, sunflower oil. Other rich sources are bluefish, tuna, salmon, whitefish, rainbow trout, mayonnaise, walnuts, wheat germ, and soft margarine.

Omega-3 fatty acids are a form of polyunsaturated fat that is found mostly in fish oils. Research suggests that fish oil may help lower the risk of heart attacks and stroke. These fats lower the risk by making blood less sticky and less likely to form blood clots. Omega-3 fatty acids also reduce high levels of triglycerides and lower blood pressure.

Good sources of Omega-3 fatty acids include Atlantic salmon, Atlantic herring, whitefish, bluefin tuna, sardines, Atlantic mackerel and sockeye salmon.

The American Heart Association has advised that everyone should eat at least two servings of fish a week in order to lower their risk of heart disease.

Monounsaturated fats are liquid at room temperature but become cloudy when refrigerated. These fats may help lower cholesterol. Studies show that in Mediterranean countries where people eat a lot of monounsaturated fat—mainly from olive oil—cholesterol levels are lower and so is the incidence of heart disease. But don't take this as license to eat a lot of this type of fat. Too much fat of any kind can pile on pounds, putting you at a greater risk for heart disease.

Foods high in monounsaturated fats include almonds, cashews, macadamia nuts, pine nuts, pistachio nuts, peanuts, peanut butter, canola oil, olive oil, sesame oil, chicken fat, and soybean oil.

Trans fatty acids make up 4 to 7% of the fat eaten in the U.S. When liquid oils are hardened to make margarine and solid shortenings, some of the unsaturated fat is turned into trans fats, which can raise cholesterol and lower HDLs. On food labels, these hardened oils are called "partially hydrogenated" or "hydrogenated vegetable oils." Two-thirds of the soybean oil in the U.S. is hydrogenated. Trans fats are not formed during cooking.

You Should Know:

In a study of trans fats, researchers in the Netherlands found that when subjects eating a lot of trans fats were stressed, their blood vessels did not expand or contract normally, putting them at a greater risk of heart disease.

Large amounts of trans fats increase the risk of heart disease the same way that saturated fat does. Margarine is a major source of trans fats, followed by cakes, cookies, crackers, pastries and restaurant French fries. Trans fats are used in baked products to extend their shelf life. Softer margarines contain fewer trans fats—there are even some brands that are completely free of them.

What has your doctor recommended? A lowfat diet.

A low fat diet means that 30 to 35% of your daily calories come from fat. How do you translate this into how much fat you can eat in one day? On page 17, you figured out your calorie zone, which is the number of calories you can eat each day to either lose weight or maintain your weight. Find that number on the table Upper Limit of Grams of Fat Each Day. In the column to the right you will see the number of fat grams for your calorie level. The list gives you the upper limit of fat grams you should be eating each day.

Upper Limit of Grams of Fat Each Day

Calories	Grams of Fat
1200	40
1300	43
1400	47
1500	50
1600	53
1700	57
1800	60
1900	63
2000	67
2100	70
2200	73
2300	77
2400	80
2500	83
2600	87
2700	90
2800	93

Your goal is to lower your total fat intake at the same time that you choose foods with vegetable oils more often and choose foods with dairy or animal fat less often. This will lower your total fat and saturated fat intake for the day.

To help you keep track of the fat, *The Healthy Heart Food Counter* gives you the fat grams in over 12,000 foods.

Cholesterol

Studies found that for every 1% decrease in cholesterol, risk for heart disease drops as much as 3 to 4%.

What exactly is cholesterol? It's a waxy, fatlike substance that is part of every cell in your body. You need cholesterol to function; in fact, the brain is particularly high in cholesterol. The body uses cholesterol to make many hormones, vitamin D, bile (that helps fat digestion), and sebum (fats that keep your skin soft). It takes only a small amount of cholesterol to meet your needs. When there is too much cholesterol in the blood, the excess is deposited in your arteries, narrowing and clogging them, and interfering with blood flow. Heart attack or stroke can be the result.

We get some cholesterol every time we eat animal foods: meat, poultry, fish, eggs, milk, yogurt, cheese and butter. All foods that come from animals have cholesterol. Foods that grow in the ground—fruits and vegetables—don't. Cholesterol is also made naturally in the body. Most people make three times as much cholesterol as they get from food.

In May 2001, the U.S. National Cholesterol Education Program (NCEP) published their newest set of guidelines for the treatment of high cholesterol in adults. The NCEP recommends no more than 200 milligrams of cholesterol a day and that all adults age 20 or over have their cholesterol levels checked every five years. People with higher than normal cholesterol (above 200) need to be checked more often.

Cholesterol in the blood is reduced by losing weight, exercising, eating less fat and cholesterol, and eating more fiber from whole grains, vegetables and fruit. Lowfat, high-carbohydrate diets (which are low in sugars) have been recommended to lower cholesterol and reduce the risk for heart disease.

What is a healthy cholesterol level? NCEP guidelines recommend that a cholesterol value of 200 or less is best. But that's not all. The total cholesterol number is mainly the sum of two different types of cholesterol—LDLs (low density lipoproteins) and HDLs (high density lipoproteins). It is healthier to have low LDLs (less than 100) and higher HDLs (more than 60). Eating less cholesterol and less saturated fat helps to improve this ratio. As more research is done, it has been found that the ratio of total cholesterol to HDL cholesterol is a better predictor of the risk for heart disease than either one of these by itself.

Add Up Your Cholesterol

Now it's your turn to track your cholesterol intake for one day. Include everything you eat and drink to get the most realistic account of a typical day. You'll find cholesterol values for over 12,000 foods in *The Healthy Heart Food Counter,* beginning on page 46. Experts recommend no more than 200 mg a day. If your total is more than this, consider switching to food choices that are lower in cholesterol.

Daily Cholesterol Record

Aim for 200 milligrams a day.

Food Eaten	Amount	Cholesterol
Breakfast		
Lunch		
Dinner		
Snacks		

Total _____

What has your doctor recommended? A low cholesterol diet.

Are you confused about what this means? A low cholesterol diet is one that has no more than 200 mg of cholesterol a day. Plant foods have no cholesterol—choose more of these. Animal foods, (meat, milk, cheese, fish, poultry) have cholesterol—eat these less often and eat smaller portions.

There may be times when you want to eat more than 200 mg of cholesterol. For example, if you go out for a steak dinner, a 1-pound steak has between 300–400 mg of cholesterol, almost double the recommended intake. You can enjoy this occasional steak dinner by compensating and lowering your cholesterol intake over the next day or two. It just takes a little planning.

You Should Know:

What About Eggs?

The tide has turned—people are now eating more eggs. In fact, research shows no association between the consumption of 1 egg a day and the risk of heart disease in nondiabetic men and women. The American Heart Association, which formerly recommended no more than 3 or 4 eggs a week, has raised its suggested egg intake to up to 7 a week.

Salt—Sodium and High Blood Pressure (Hypertension)

One out of every 4 American adults (almost 50 million people) have high blood pressure—half of these will have a heart attack. Two-thirds of heart attack victims have a blood pressure higher than 160/95. High blood pressure also increases the risk of stroke and, in half of the people who have a stroke, their blood pressure is higher than 160/95. More men than women have high blood pressure before the age of 55. But after 55, the risks are reversed and more women than men have high blood pressure. According to Dr. Rose Marie Robertson, president of the American Heart

Association, "Of fifty million Americans with high blood pressure, only half are being treated, and only half of that half receive proper treatment."

Normal blood pressure is 120/80. The first number, 120 (systolic), is pressure when the heart contracts. The second number, 80 (diastolic), is the pressure between heartbeats. When the numbers go up, so does the risk for heart disease. The Joint National Committee on Prevention, Detection, Evaluation and Treatment says that to lower the risk of heart disease, optimal blood pressure should be lower than 120/80. High normal is 131–139/86–89. High blood pressure (hypertension) is more than 140/90.

Weight loss of as little as 5 to 10% of a person's actual weight can reduce blood pressure, as does eating a diet high in fiber, fruits and vegetables. Population studies suggest that diets rich in oatmeal or other fiber-rich foods (bran, beans, whole wheat bread and crackers) lower blood pressure and reduce the risk of heart disease.

You Should Know:

High blood pressure is bad for a woman's bones. Women with high blood pressure have bones that are less dense and they also lose more calcium in their urine. Regular exercise and cutting back on salt can lower their blood pressure.

Salt—sodium

Eating too much salt raises blood pressure in most people. Ten to 15% of all people, and 50% of those with high blood pressure, are salt sensitive. African Americans, people with diabetes, and older adults may be more salt-sensitive than others. Too much salt can make your body retain fluid, which causes the heart and kidneys to work harder.

What's the difference between salt and sodium? It's easy to confuse the two. Sometimes the terms are used interchangeably. Salt is actually a mixture of two minerals—sodium and chloride. In a teaspoon of salt (which equals 5,000 milligrams), 2,000 are sodium and the other 3,000 are chloride. Sodium without the chloride is found in many ingredients, like sodium bicarbonate (baking soda), sodium benzoate, sodium sulfite and other food additives. There's also sodium in many medications. The sodium in these plus the sodium in table salt add up.

To lower your intake, don't put salt on the table and use less when cooking.

What about salt substitutes? These are reduced-sodium or "lite" salts in which some of the sodium is replaced by the mineral potassium. They can help you adjust to using less salt. Try salt-free herb and spice blends, and cook with fresh or dried herbs, lemon or lime juice, and seasoned vinegars for added flavor.

You Should Know:

Sea salt and kosher salt are different from table salt in taste and texture, but they have the same amount of sodium as regular salt.

Are you getting too much salt?

Americans do eat too much salt. They average 2 to 3 teaspoons a day. The amount of salt you actually need is less than a quarter of a teaspoon, though it's close to impossible to keep your intake that low. Salt is in almost everything you eat—milk, meat, vegetables, bread—and about 10% of the salt we eat is naturally present in food. Fifteen percent is added during cooking and at the table. The rest is in packaged, processed and ready-to-eat foods. In fact, most of your salt (75%) comes from prepared foods you get at the supermarket, eat at restaurants, or take-out.

Does eating a lot of salt cause high blood pressure?

Many studies around the world have shown that in places where little salt is used, blood pressure does not increase with age as it does in the U.S. Reducing salt can lower high blood pressure in people who have it and even, to a lesser extent, in people who have normal blood pressure. Because of time demands, Americans buy a lot of ready-to-eat processed foods and often eat out. These kinds of foods are much higher in salt.

When your body accumulates more salt than is needed, the excess passes out in the urine, pulling calcium along with it. This can weaken bones and also set the stage for kidney stones.

You can wean yourself off a high salt diet by changing some of the things you eat. Babies are not born with a preference for salt, but by the time they are toddlers, children prefer salted foods to unsalted ones. This preference can be unlearned, it just takes a little time. You'll find that within two months of eating less salt, foods begin to taste saltier to you. And the salty foods—chips, salted pretzels, nuts, olives, deli meats, soy sauce—taste too salty. While you're eating foods that are lower in salt, be sure to eat more fruits and vegetables. They are rich in potassium and calcium, two minerals that protect against high blood pressure.

You Should Know:

About Potassium

Studies show that high intakes of the mineral potassium can lower blood pressure. They also show that one or two extra servings a day of potassium-rich fruit or vegetables can help decrease deaths from stroke. Dried apricots, avocados, bananas, dried beans, broccoli, cantaloupe, mushrooms, orange juice, white potatoes, sweet potatoes, tomatoes, dried plums (prunes) and watermelon are all high in potassium and low in salt.

Lower Salt Choices

Buy Often	Buy Less Often
Fresh fruit	Fruit-filled pastries
Frozen fruit	Fruit pie
Canned fruit	Dried fruit
Fresh vegetables	Canned vegetables, pickled vegetables
Cabbage	Coleslaw, sauerkraut
Cucumbers	Pickles, olives
Frozen vegetables	Frozen vegetables in sauce
Plain bread, hard rolls, bagels, wraps	Muffins, biscuits, scones
Unsalted crackers	Regular crackers
Puffed wheat or rice, shredded wheat, low-salt cereals	Ready-to-eat cereals
Hot cereal	Instant hot cereal
Baldy (unsalted) pretzels	Salted pretzels
Rice cakes, matzo, breadsticks	Cheese crackers, salted crackers
Pasta	Cheese filled pasta
Plain rice, plain couscous	Rice mixes, couscous mixes
Snack-size yogurt	Instant pudding
Unsalted butter and margarine	Salted butter and margarine
Fresh meat	Seasoned meats, ready-to-eat meats, frankfurters, ham, deli meats, Canadian bacon, bacon
Frozen meat	Frozen seasoned meat, meat with sauce or gravy, frozen sausage
Fresh poultry	Seasoned, breaded, smoked, ready-to-eat, stuffed poultry
Frozen poultry	Frozen seasoned, fried, and battered poultry, poultry with gravy
Fresh fish	Breaded, stuffed, smoked, pickled or canned fish
Frozen fish	Frozen breaded, battered, sauced or lemon, buttered fish
Salsa, fresh chili peppers, fresh onions, fresh garlic	Ketchup, garlic salt, onion salt
Seasoned pepper	Lemon pepper

Buy Often	Buy Less Often
Lite salt soy sauce	Regular soy sauce
Unsalted potato chips	Regular potato chips
Unsalted nuts	Salted nuts
Canned chicken or beef broth, no salt added	Regular chicken or beef broth, bouillon cubes
Mustard	Relish
Lemon juice, flavored vinegars	Salad dressing

You Should Know:

Some people mistakenly believe that ocean fish raised in salty water contain more salt than freshwater fish. There actually is very little difference in the amount of salt. Ocean fish have gill cells that excrete excess salt back into the sea while freshwater fish have gill cells that extract salt from the water. So you can enjoy all fresh fish without worrying about eating too much salt.

Add up your sodium

Now it's your turn to track your salt intake for one day. Include everything you eat and drink to see what you eat on a typical day. You can't count salt but you can count sodium, which is listed on food labels. You'll find sodium values for over 12,000 foods in *The Healthy Heart Food Counter,* beginning on page 46. Experts recommend no more than 2,400 mg of sodium a day. If your total is more than this, consider switching to lower salt choices.

What has your doctor recommended? A low sodium diet.

A low sodium diet includes no more than 2,400 mg of sodium a day. You'll be surprised by how many foods this amount of sodium allows you to enjoy.

Daily Sodium Record

Aim for 2400 milligrams or less a day

Food eaten	Amount	Sodium
Breakfast		
Lunch		
Dinner		
Snacks		

Total _____

The DASH diet

Dietary **A**pproaches to **S**top **H**ypertension was released by the National Institutes of Health in January 2001. Researchers showed the Dash diet is effective in both controlling and lowering blood pressure. It includes lowfat and fat free dairy products, fish, beans, poultry and lean meats. The Dash diet limits salt to 2,400 mg a day and is also rich in fruits, vegetables and grain products.

What About Stress?

A study of almost 13,000 people found that those who were frequently angry were two and a half times more likely to have heart attacks or suffer from sudden cardiac deaths than calmer people. Stress, which also raises blood pressure, is cumulative and takes its toll over the years. You owe it to yourself to reduce stress, especially anger, whenever you can.

How to Reduce Stress in Your Life

* Get enough sleep to recharge your body.
* Find exercise that you enjoy and do it often—walking, bicycling, running, dancing, gardening.
* Learn relaxation techniques like meditation, tai chi, and yoga.
* Laugh a lot— read funny books, see funny films; laughter can help prevent heart disease.
* Listen to music—sing or hum along.
* Cultivate close friendships; find people you can confide in and count on.
* Don't use food to relax—it doesn't work.
* Don't smoke to relax—it increases health risks.
* Avoid stimulants—caffeine, tobacco and drugs.

- Change is inevitable—accept it rather than wasting energy fighting it.
- Say no to requests that interfere with your personal time.
- Eat well.

What About Homocysteine?

Homocysteine, a protein made in the body, is normally found in low levels in the blood. High blood levels of homocysteine are an important risk factor for heart attack, stroke, and blood clots. Some medical conditions like kidney disease can raise homocysteine, as does a diet high in protein and low in carbohydrates. Studies show that high homocysteine levels are just as important as high cholesterol in predicting heart disease.

Three "B" vitamins—folic acid, B6, and B12—lower homocysteine. Surveys of the U.S. population show that most people do not get enough folic acid. Since 1998, the Food and Drug Administration (FDA) has required manufacturers to enrich non-whole grain products—bread, rolls, farina, corn grits, rice, pasta, and noodles—with folic acid. Dark green leafy vegetables, beans, strawberries, oranges, and liver are good sources of folic acid and vitamin B6. Meat, fish, eggs and milk are good sources of vitamin B12. Most multivitamin supplements have the recommended daily allowance of all three vitamins.

Folic acid supplements increase blood levels of folic acid, which reduces homocysteine. But taking large doses of folic acid can cover up a vitamin B12 deficiency. This may be dangerous. It is not wise to take more than 1 mg of folic acid daily (more than two times the amount in most daily supplements).

What About Alcohol?

Many studies show that drinking moderate amounts of alcohol lowers the risk of heart disease. It increases blood levels of HDLs (the good cholesterol), lowers blood pressure, reduces narrowing of the arteries, and lowers the risk of blood clots. Another benefit of moderate alcohol use may be lowered risk of heart failure in older adults.

Research shows that moderate wine drinkers live longer than those who don't drink and those who drink heavily. Heavy drinking, more than 3 drinks a day, increases the risk of heart problems including high blood pressure, some types of stroke, and heart muscle disease.

What is a moderate amount of alcohol? The U.S. Dietary Guidelines recommend no more than 2 drinks a day for men and 1 drink for women. One drink is equal to:

5 ounces of wine
1½ ounces of spirits
12 ounces of beer

There are more than 60 studies that show a relationship between moderate alcohol consumption and reduced heart disease. A few suggest that wine may be more of a health promoter than beer or spirits. Wine drinkers tend to be thinner, to exercise more, and to have alcohol with meals. One explanation for the lower risk of heart disease among the French is an increased intake of wine, especially red wine.

But Ira Goldberg, M.D., a member of the American Heart Association's Nutrition Committee and professor of medicine at Columbia University says, "If you want to reduce your risk of heart disease, talk to your doctor about lowering your cholesterol and blood pressure, controlling your weight, getting enough exercise and following a healthy diet. There is no proof that drinking wine or any other alcoholic beverage can replace these effective conventional measures."

Using the Counter Section of
The Healthy Heart Food Counter

The Healthy Heart Food Counter lists the calories, fat, cholesterol and sodium content of over 12,000 foods. Now you can check and compare the values in your favorite foods and, when necessary, choose substitutes before you go out to shop or eat. This will help you make the right choices when you are deciding what to buy.

The counter section of the book is divided into two parts: Part 1, Brand Name, Nonbranded and Take-Out Foods, and Part 2, Restaurant Chains.

In Part 1, all foods are listed alphabetically from abalone to zucchini. For each category, you will first find nonbranded (generic) foods listed in alphabetical order, followed by an alphabetical listing of brand name foods. The nonbranded listing will help you to determine calorie, fat, cholesterol, and sodium values for foods when you aren't able to find your favorite brand listed. They will also help you to evaluate store brands. Large categories are often divided into subcategories, such as canned, fresh, frozen, and ready-to-eat, to make it easier to find what you're looking for.

Because we all eat out so often, there are over 450 take-out foods listed in Part 1. These are found in the take-out subcategory in many categories throughout this section. Look there for foods you take-out or order in a store or restaurant because these foods are not nutrition-labeled.

In some cases, foods are grouped by category. For example, chow mein is found under the category Asian Food. Other group categories include:

Asian Food   Page 48
>   includes all types of Asian foods
>   except egg rolls and sushi, which
>   are found in separate categories

Deli Meats/Cold Cuts   Page 175
>   includes all sandwich meats
>   except chicken, ham and turkey,
>   which are found in separate
>   categories

Dinner   Page 176
>   includes all frozen dinners by
>   brand name

Liquor/Liqueur   Page 230
>   includes all alcoholic beverages
>   except beer, champagne and
>   wine

Nutrition Supplements   Page 245
>   includes all meal replacers and
>   diet drinks, except energy bars,
>   energy drinks, and sports drinks,
>   which are found in separate
>   categories

Sandwiches   Page 300
>   includes popular sandwich
>   choices

Spanish Food   Page 324
>   includes all types of Spanish and
>   Mexican foods

In Part 2, Restaurant Chains, there are 69 national and regional restaurant, doughnut, ice cream and candy chains listed.

Definitions

as prep (as prepared)—refers to food that has been prepared according to package directions.

lean and fat—describes meat with some fat on its edges that is not cut away before cooking or poultry prepared with skin and fat as purchased.

lean only—refers to lean meat that is trimmed of all visible fat or poultry without skin.

shelf stable—refers to prepared products found on the supermarket shelf that are ready-to-eat or be heated and do not require refrigeration.

take-out—describes prepared dishes that you purchase ready-to-eat; those included serve as a guide to the calorie, fat, cholesterol and sodium values of similar products you may purchase.

Abbreviations

avg	=	average
diam	=	diameter
fl	=	fluid
frzn	=	frozen
g	=	gram
in	=	inch
lb	=	pound
lg	=	large
med	=	medium
mg	=	milligram
oz	=	ounce
pkg	=	package
pt	=	pint
prep	=	prepared
qt	=	quart
reg	=	regular
sec	=	second
serv	=	serving
sm	=	small
sq	=	square
tbsp	=	tablespoon
tr	=	trace
tsp	=	teaspoon
w/	=	with
w/o	=	without
<	=	less than

Equivalent Measures

1 tablespoon	=	3 teaspoons
4 tablespoons	=	¼ cup
8 tablespoons	=	½ cup
12 tablespoons	=	¾ cup
16 tablespoons	=	1 cup
1000 milligrams	=	1 gram
28 grams	=	1 ounce

Liquid Measurements

2 tablespoons	=	1 ounce
¼ cup	=	2 ounces
½ cup	=	4 ounces
¾ cup	=	6 ounces
1 cup	=	8 ounces
2 cups	=	1 pint
4 cups	=	1 quart

Dry Measurements

4 ounces	=	¼ pound
8 ounces	=	½ pound
12 ounces	=	¾ pound
16 ounces	=	1 pound

Notes

Fat values are given in grams (g).

Cholesterol and sodium values are given in milligrams (mg).

tr (trace) = less than 1 gram of fat or less than 1 milligram of cholesterol or sodium.

Discrepancies in figures are due to rounding, product reformulation and reevaluation. Labeling law allows rounding of values. Because much of the data is analysis data obtained directly from manufacturers, not from labels, in some cases our values may not be exactly the same as label information because they have not been rounded.

Part 1

**Brand Name,
Nonbranded (Generic)
and Take-Out Foods**

FOOD	PORTION	CALS	FAT	CHOL	SOD
ABALONE					
fresh fried	3 oz	161	6	80	502
ACEROLA					
fresh	1	2	tr	0	0
ACEROLA JUICE					
juice	1 cup	51	1	0	7
ADZUKI BEANS					
canned sweetened	1 cup	702	tr	0	646
dried cooked	1 cup	294	tr	0	18
yokan sliced	3 slices (1/4 in)	112	tr	0	36
Eden					
Organic	1/2 cup (4.6 oz)	110	0	0	10
ALE					
(*see* BEER AND ALE, MALT)					
ALFALFA					
(*see also* SPROUTS)					
sprouts	1 tbsp	1	tr	0	0
ALLSPICE					
ground	1 tsp	5	tr	0	1
ALMONDS					
almond butter w/ salt	1 tbsp	101	9	0	75
almond butter w/o salt	1 tbsp	101	10	0	2
almond meal	1 oz	116	5	0	2
almond paste	1 oz	127	8	0	3
jordan almonds	10 (1.4 oz)	190	7	0	0
Lance					
Smoked	1 pkg (0.8 oz)	130	10	0	125
AMARANTH					
(*see also* CEREAL, COOKIES)					
uncooked	1 cup (6.8 oz)	729	13	0	41
ANISE					
seed	1 tsp	7	tr	0	tr
ANTELOPE					
roasted	3 oz	127	2	107	46
APPLE					
canned					
sliced sweetened	1 cup	136	1	0	7
Del Monte					
Fruit Pleasures Pie Spiced Apples	1/2 cup (4 oz)	70	0	0	10
Luck's					
Fried Apples	1/2 cup (4.7 oz)	130	0	0	0
dried					
cooked w/o sugar	1/2 cup	172	tr	0	26
rings	10	155	tr	0	56
fresh					
apple	1	81	tr	0	1
w/o skin sliced	1 cup	62	tr	0	0

FOOD	PORTION	CALS	FAT	CHOL	SOD
Cool Cut					
Apples & Caramel Dip	1 pkg (4.25 oz)	180	5	5	80
Tastee					
Candy Apple	1 (3 oz)	160	5	0	20
Caramel Apple	1 (3 oz)	160	5	0	20
frozen					
Stouffer's					
Escalloped	1 cup (6 oz)	180	3	0	70
take-out					
baked	1 (5.3 oz)	126	tr	0	1
baked no sugar	1 (5.9 oz)	82	1	0	6
APPLE JUICE					
Apple & Eve					
Cider	8 oz	110	0	0	10
Everfresh					
Apple Juice	1 can (8 oz)	110	0	0	10
Hansen's					
Junior Juice 100%	1 box (4.23 oz)	60	0	0	0
Mott's					
100% Juice	1 box (8 oz)	120	0	0	15
Nantucket Nectars					
100% Pressed	8 oz	100	0	0	10
NutraBalance					
Plus Fibre	1 pkg (8 oz)	120	0	0	8
Ocean Spray					
100% Juice	8 oz	110	0	0	35
Swiss Miss					
Hot Apple Cider Mix	1 serv	84	tr	0	58
Hot Apple Cider Mix Low Calorie	1 serv	14	0	0	78
Tropicana					
Season's Best	8 oz	110	0	0	25
Veryfine					
100% Juice	1 bottle (10 oz)	150	0	0	20
Juice-Ups	8 oz	120	0	0	35
White House					
Juice	8 oz	120	0	0	25
APPLESAUCE					
Mott's					
Single-Serve Cinnamon	1 pkg (4 oz)	100	0	0	0
Single-Serve Natural	1 pkg (4 oz)	50	0	0	0
Single-Serve Original	1 pkg (4 oz)	100	0	0	0
White House					
Applesauce	1/2 cup (4.4 oz)	90	0	0	15
Chunky	1/2 cup (4.4 oz)	90	0	0	15
Cinnamon	1/2 cup (4.5 oz)	100	0	0	15
Natural Plus	1/2 cup (4.4 oz)	70	0	0	15

FOOD	PORTION	CALS	FAT	CHOL	SOD
APRICOT JUICE					
nectar	1 cup	141	tr	0	9
APRICOTS					
canned					
halves heavy syrup pack w/ skin	1 cup (9.1 oz)	214	tr	0	10
halves water pack w/ skin	1 cup (8.5 oz)	65	tr	0	7
water pack w/ skin	3 halves	22	tr	0	2
dried					
halves	10	83	tr	0	3
halves cooked w/o sugar	1/2 cup	106	tr	0	4
fresh					
apricots	3	51	tr	0	1
ARROWHEAD					
fresh boiled	1 med (1/3 oz)	9	tr	0	2
ARROWROOT					
flour	1 cup (4.5 oz)	457	tr	0	3
ARTICHOKE					
canned					
Progresso					
Hearts	2 pieces (2.9 oz)	30	0	0	240
Hearts Marinated	2 pieces (1.1 oz)	170	5	0	110
fresh					
boiled	1 med (4 oz)	60	tr	0	114
hearts cooked	1/2 cup	42	tr	0	80
frozen					
cooked	1 pkg (9 oz)	108	1	0	127
ARUGULA					
raw	1/2 cup	2	tr	0	3
ASIAN FOOD					
(*see also* DINNER, EGG ROLLS, PASTA, SUSHI)					
canned					
Chun King					
Beef Pepper Oriental BiPack	1 cup (8.8 oz)	98	2	14	865
Chow Mein Beef BiPack	1 cup (8.6 oz)	78	1	6	718
Chow Mein Chicken BiPack	1 cup (8.8 oz)	98	3	6	1123
Chow Mein Pork BiPack	1 cup (8.6 oz)	78	2	10	1183
Hot & Spicy Chicken BiPack	1 cup (8.6 oz)	98	3	19	857
Sweet & Sour Chicken BiPack	1 cup (8.9 oz)	161	2	25	687
La Choy					
Beef Pepper Oriental BiPack	1 cup (8.8 oz)	98	2	14	865
Chow Mein Beef BiPack	1 cup (8.6 oz)	78	1	6	718
Chow Mein Chicken BiPack	1 cup (8.9 oz)	98	3	6	1123
Chow Mein Shrimp BiPack	1 cup (8.6 oz)	52	1	4	965
Main Entree Chow Mein Chicken	1 cup (9.3 oz)	80	4	9	1325
Oriental Beef w/ Noodles BiPack	1 cup (8.8 oz)	156	3	17	896

FOOD	PORTION	CALS	FAT	CHOL	SOD
Oriental Chicken w/ Noodles BiPack	1 cup (8.7 oz)	154	4	23	1100
Sweet & Sour Chicken BiPack	1 cup (8.9 oz)	161	2	25	687
Teriyaki Chicken BiPack	1 cup (8.6 oz)	109	3	20	1230
fresh					
wonton wrappers	1	23	tr	1	46
frozen					
Birds Eye					
Easy Recipe Meal Starter Oriental Stir Fry as prep	1 serv	280	8	69	336
Easy Recipe Meal Starter Spicy Asian	1 serv	280	8	69	336
Easy Recipe Meal Starter Teriyaki Stir Fry as prep	1 serv	280	8	69	336
Green Giant					
Create A Meal LoMein Stir Fry as prep	1 1/4 cups (10 oz)	320	70	60	980
Create A Meal Sweet & Sour Stir Fry as prep	1 1/4 cups (10 oz)	290	7	60	460
Create A Meal Szechuan Stir Fry as prep	1 1/4 cups (10 oz)	340	15	60	1280
Create A Meal Teriyaki Stir Fry as prep	1 1/4 cups (10 oz)	240	6	55	940
La Choy					
Beef Pepper Oriental	1 cup (7.1 oz)	151	1	10	714
Chow Mein Vegetable	1 cup (8.9 oz)	108	2	0	1135
Lean Cuisine					
Everyday Favorites Oriental Style Dumplings	1 pkg (9 oz)	300	6	20	520
Everyday Favorites Teriyaki Stir Fry	1 pkg (10 oz)	290	4	20	590
Stouffer's					
Chicken Chow Mein w/ Rice	1 pkg (10.6 oz)	260	5	25	1090
Tyson					
Chicken Fried Rice Kit w/ Sauce	1 pkg (14 oz)	440	6	30	1810
Weight Watchers					
Smart Ones Chicken Chow Mein	1 pkg (9 oz)	200	2	25	570
Smart Ones Hunan Style Rice & Vegetables	1 pkg (10.34 oz)	280	0	0	630
Smart Ones King Pao Noodles & Vegetables	1 pkg (10 oz)	250	8	5	650
Smart Ones Spicy Szechaun Style Vegetables & Chicken	1 pkg (9 oz)	220	2	10	730

FOOD	PORTION	CALS	FAT	CHOL	SOD
take-out					
buddha's delight w/ cellophane noodles fat choi jai	1 serv (7.6 oz)	211	4	tr	772
cha siu bao steamed buns w/ chicken filling	1 (2.3 oz)	160	3	15	300
chicken teriyaki	3/4 cup	399	27	92	2190
chicken teriyaki w/ rice	1 serv (11 oz)	430	6	25	1210
chop suey w/ beef & pork	1 cup	300	17	68	1053
chop suey w/ pork	1 cup	375	29	62	1378
chow mein chicken	1 cup	255	10	75	718
chow mein pork	1 cup	425	24	89	1673
chow mein shrimp	1 cup	221	10	55	1658
chow mein vegetable	1 serv (8 oz)	90	3	0	1010
filipino chicken adobo	1 serv (15 oz)	555	26	116	468
phad thai	1 serv (9.2 oz)	232	9	0	426
sesame seed paste bun	1 (2.5 oz)	220	6	0	53
shrimp chips	1 1/4 cups (1 oz)	140	6	0	240
shu mai chicken & vegetable dumplings	6 (3.6 oz)	160	5	35	910
sweet & sour pork	1 serv (8 oz)	250	8	30	1500
sweet red bean bun	1 (2.5 oz)	130	1	0	95
szechuan chicken w/ lo mein	1 cup (5.3 oz)	190	1	5	560
wonton fried	1/2 cup (1 oz)	111	8	31	147
wonton soup	1 cup	205	3	89	322
ASPARAGUS					
canned					
Green Giant					
Cut Spears	1/2 cup (4.2 oz)	20	0	0	420
Cut Spears 50% Less Sodium	1/2 cup (4.2 oz)	20	0	0	210
Extra Long Spears	4.5 oz	20	0	0	400
Spears	4.5 oz	20	0	0	450
LeSueur					
Spears Extra Large	4.5 oz	20	0	0	440
fresh					
cooked	4 spears	14	tr	0	7
frozen					
cooked	4 spears	17	tr	0	2
Green Giant					
Harvest Fresh Cuts	2/3 cup (3 oz)	25	0	0	85
AVOCADO					
fresh	1	324	31	0	21
fresh mashed	1 cup	370	35	0	24
take-out					
guacamole	1 serv (2.2 oz)	105	10	0	187
BACON					
(*see also* BACON SUBSTITUTES)					

FOOD	PORTION	CALS	FAT	CHOL	SOD
Armour					
Star cooked	1 strip	38	3	6	185
Black Label					
Center Cut cooked	3 slices (0.5 oz)	70	6	15	260
Cooked	2 slices (0.5 oz)	80	7	15	330
Low Salt cooked	2 slices (0.5 oz)	80	7	15	230
Health Is Wealth					
Uncured Sliced	2 slices (0.5 oz)	70	7	10	380
Hormel					
Bacon Bits	1 tbsp (7 g)	30	2	5	250
Bacon Pieces	1 tbsp (7 g)	25	2	10	180
Microwave cooked	2 slices (0.5 oz)	70	5	15	230
Old Smokehouse					
Cooked	2 slices (0.5 oz)	80	7	15	280
Oscar Mayer					
Bacon Bits	1 tbsp (0.2 oz)	25	2	5	220
Bacon Pieces	1 tbsp (0.2 oz)	25	2	5	170
Center Cut cooked	2 slices (0.4 oz)	70	5	15	270
Cooked	2 slices (0.5 oz)	70	6	15	290
Lower Sodium cooked	2 slices (0.5 oz)	70	5	15	200
Thick Cut cooked	1 slice (0.4 oz)	60	5	10	250
Range Brand					
Cooked	2 slices (0.7 oz)	100	9	20	460
Ready Crisp					
Fully Cooked	3 slices (0.5 oz)	70	6	15	270
Red Label					
Cooked	2 slices (0.5 oz)	80	7	15	330
BACON SUBSTITUTES					
Bac-Os					
Chips or Bits	1 1/2 tbsp (7 g)	30	2	0	120
Lightlife					
Fakin' Bacon Bits	1 tsp	45	1	0	25
Smart Bacon	2 strips (0.8 oz)	45	2	0	360
Louis Rich					
Turkey Bacon	1 slice (0.5 oz)	35	3	15	180
Morningstar Farms					
Breakfast Strips	2 (0.5 oz)	60	5	0	220
Worthington					
Stripples	2 strips (0.5 oz)	60	5	0	220
BAGEL					
fresh					
plain toasted	1 (3 1/2 in)	195	1	0	379
Pepperidge Farm					
Plain	1 (3.5 oz)	290	1	0	480
Thomas'					
Everything	1 (3.6 oz)	300	4	0	510
Multi-Grain	1 (3.6 oz)	280	2	0	460
Plain	1 (3.6 oz)	280	2	0	530

FOOD	PORTION	CALS	FAT	CHOL	SOD
Uncle B's					
Plain	1 (2.8 oz)	210	1	0	310
Wonder					
Blueberry	1 (3 oz)	210	1	0	450
Cinnamon Raisin	1 (3 oz)	210	1	0	360
Onion	1 (3 oz)	210	1	0	340
Plain	1 (3 oz)	210	1	0	350
Rye	1 (3 oz)	220	1	0	520
Wheat	1 (3 oz)	210	1	0	350
frozen					
Amy's Organic					
Cinnamon Raisin	1 (3.5 oz)	240	2	0	480
Plain	1 (3.5 oz)	230	2	0	490
Poppy Seed	1 (3.5 oz)	230	2	0	480
Sesame	1 (3.5 oz)	240	2	0	480
Otis Spunkmeyer					
Barnstormin' Blueberry	1 (3.6 oz)	250	3	0	390
Barnstormin' Cinnamon Raisin	1 (3.6 oz)	230	2	0	370
Barnstormin' Onion	1 (3.6 oz)	230	2	0	370
Barnstormin' Plain	1 (3.6 oz)	240	3	0	390
Sara Lee					
Blueberry	1 (2.8 oz)	210	1	0	230
Cinnamon Raisin	1 (2.8 oz)	220	1	0	320
Egg	1 (2.8 oz)	210	1	0	460
Oat Bran	1 (2.8 oz)	210	1	0	570
Onion	1 (2.8 oz)	210	0	0	540
Plain	1 (2.8 oz)	210	1	0	500
Poppy Seed	1 (2.8 oz)	210	1	0	570
Sesame Seed	1 (2.8 oz)	210	2	0	530
BAKING POWDER					
baking powder	1 tsp	2	0	0	488
low sodium	1 tsp	5	0	0	4
Calumet					
Baking Powder	1/4 tsp (1 g)	0	0	0	100
BAKING SODA					
baking soda	1 tsp	0	0	0	1259
BALSAM PEAR					
leafy tips cooked	1/2 cup	10	tr	0	4
pods cooked	1/2 cup	12	tr	0	4
BAMBOO SHOOTS					
fresh cooked	1/2 cup	15	tr	0	5
Chun King					
Bamboo Shoots	2 tbsp (0.8 oz)	3	tr.	0	0
La Choy					
Bamboo Shoots	2 tbsp (0.8 oz)	3	tr	0	0
BANANA					
banana chips	1 oz	147	10	0	2

FOOD	PORTION	CALS	FAT	CHOL	SOD
fresh	1	105	tr	0	1
fresh mashed	1 cup	207	1	0	2
powder	1 tbsp	21	tr	0	0
Rainforest Farms					
Slices Dried	5 slices (1.3 oz)	60	0	0	10
BARBECUE SAUCE					
(*see also* SAUCE)					
House Of Tsang					
Hong Kong	1 tbsp (0.6 oz)	10	0	0	150
Hunt's					
Bold Hickory	2 tbsp (1.2 oz)	47	tr	0	283
Bold Original	2 tbsp (1.2 oz)	46	tr	0	315
Hickory & Brown Sugar	2 tbsp (1.3 oz)	75	tr	0	382
Honey Hickory	2 tbsp (1.2 oz)	54	tr	0	411
Honey Mustard	2 tbsp (1.2 oz)	48	tr	0	450
Hot & Spicy	2 tbsp (1.2 oz)	48	tr	0	450
Light Original	2 tbsp (1.2 oz)	23	tr	0	169
Mesquite	2 tbsp (1.2 oz)	40	tr	0	361
Mild	2 tbsp (1.2 oz)	41	tr	0	381
Mild Dijon	2 tbsp (1.2 oz)	39	tr	0	400
Open Range Original	2 tbsp (1.2 oz)	39	tr	0	333
Open Range Premier	2 tbsp (1.3 oz)	56	tr	0	415
Open Range Smokey	2 tbsp (1.2 oz)	37	tr	0	423
Original	2 tbsp (1.2 oz)	40	tr	0	410
Teriyaki	2 tbsp (1.2 oz)	46	tr	0	351
Kraft					
Char-Grill	2 tbsp (1.3 oz)	60	0	0	460
Extra Rich Original	2 tbsp (1.2 oz)	50	0	0	440
Hickory Smoke	2 tbsp (1.2 oz)	40	0	0	420
Hickory Smoke Onion Bits	2 tbsp (1.2 oz)	45	0	0	360
Honey	2 tbsp (1.3 oz)	50	0	0	360
Honey Hickory	2 tbsp (1.3 oz)	60	0	0	370
Honey Mustard	2 tbsp (1.3 oz)	60	0	0	300
Hot	2 tbsp (1.2 oz)	40	0	0	520
Hot Hickory Smoke	2 tbsp (1.2 oz)	40	0	0	380
Kansas City Style	2 tbsp (1.2 oz)	50	0	0	310
Mesquite Smoke	2 tbsp (1.2 oz)	40	0	0	420
Molasses	2 tbsp (1.3 oz)	70	0	0	390
Onion Bits	2 tbsp (1.2 oz)	45	0	0	360
Original	2 tbsp (1.2 oz)	40	0	0	420
Roasted Garlic	2 tbsp (1.2 oz)	50	0	0	360
Spicy Honey	2 tbsp (1.3 oz)	60	0	0	360
Teriyaki	2 tbsp (1.3 oz)	60	1	0	440
Thick'N Spicy Brown Sugar	2 tbsp (1.2 oz)	60	0	0	350
Thick'N Spicy Hickory Bacon	2 tbsp (1.2 oz)	60	1	0	570
Thick'N Spicy Hickory Smoke	2 tbsp (1.2 oz)	50	0	0	450
Thick'N Spicy Honey	2 tbsp (1.3 oz)	60	0	0	360

FOOD	PORTION	CALS	FAT	CHOL	SOD
Kraft (cont.)					
Thick'N Spicy Honey Mustard	2 tbsp (1.3 oz)	60	0	0	310
Thick'N Spicy Kansas City Style	2 tbsp (1.3 oz)	60	0	0	310
Thick'N Spicy Mesquite Smoke	2 tbsp (1.2 oz)	50	0	0	440
McIlhenny					
Sauce	2 tbsp (1.1 oz)	70	5	0	290
BARLEY					
flour	1 cup (5.2 oz)	511	2	0	6
malt flour	1 cup (5.7 oz)	585	3	0	18
pearled cooked	1 cup (5.5 oz)	193	1	0	5
BASIL					
fresh chopped	2 tbsp	1	tr	0	0
ground	1 tsp	4	tr	0	tr
leaves fresh	5	1	tr	0	0
BASS					
sea cooked	3 oz	105	2	45	74
striped baked	3 oz	105	3	87	75
BAY LEAF					
crumbled	1 tsp	2	tr	0	tr
BEAN SPROUTS					
(*see* ALFALFA, SPROUTS)					
BEANS					
(*see also individual names*)					
canned					
B&M					
Barbeque Baked Beans	1/2 cup (4.6 oz)	210	1	0	570
Bush's					
Barbecue	1/2 cup (4.6 oz)	150	1	0	510
Vegetarian	1/2 cup (4.6 oz)	130	0	0	550
Chi-Chi's					
Refried	1/2 cup (4.2 oz)	100	1	0	580
Refried Beans Fat Free	1/2 cup (4.2 oz)	120	0	0	570
Refried Beans Vegetarian	1/2 cup (4.2 oz)	100	1	0	580
Eden					
Organic Baked w/ Sweet Sorghum & Organic Mustard	1/2 cup (4.6 oz)	150	0	0	130
Gebhardt					
Chili	1/2 cup (4.6 oz)	134	1	0	630
Refried Jalapeno	1/2 cup (4.5 oz)	105	3	1	380
Refried No Fat	1/2 cup (4.5 oz)	92	tr	0	480
Refried Traditional	1/2 cup (4.5 oz)	109	3	1	497
Refried Vegetarian	1/2 cup (4.5 oz)	118	2	tr	550
Green Giant					
Pork And Beans w/ Tomato Sauce	1/2 cup (4.5 oz)	120	1	0	490

FOOD	PORTION	CALS	FAT	CHOL	SOD
Spicy Chili	1/2 cup (4.5 oz)	110	1	0	490
Three Bean Salad	1/2 cup (4.2 oz)	90	0	0	490
Health Valley					
Honey Baked	1/2 cup	110	0	0	135
Honey Baked No Salt	1/2 cup	110	0	0	25
Hormel					
Beans & Wieners	1 can (7.5 oz)	290	12	50	1310
Hunt's					
Big John's Beans & Fixin's	1/2 cup (4.7 oz)	127	4	3	590
Homestyle Country Kettle	1/2 cup (4.6 oz)	152	2	1	425
Homestyle Special Recipe	1/2 cup (4.7 oz)	185	3	1	687
Mix & Serve	1/2 cup (4.7 oz)	125	3	1	575
Pork & Beans	1/2 cup (4.5 oz)	130	1	tr	516
Kid's Kitchen					
Microwave Meals Beans & Wieners	1 cup (7.5 oz)	310	13	45	760
Open Range					
Ranch	1/2 cup (4.4 oz)	124	3	1	628
Rosarita					
3 Bean Recipe Bacon & Jalapeno	1/2 cup (4.6 oz)	117	2	1	543
3 Bean Recipe Chiles & Chicken	1/2 cup (4.6 oz)	115	1	1	517
3 Bean Recipe Chiles & Chorizo	1/2 cup (4.6 oz)	111	2	1	591
3 Bean Recipe Onions & Peppers	1/2 cup (4.6 oz)	104	1	1	539
Fiesta Beans Bacon & Jalapenos	1/2 cup (4.6 oz)	117	2	1	543
Fiesta Beans Chicken & Chiles	1/2 cup (4.6 oz)	115	1	1	517
Fiesta Beans Chiles & Chorizo	1/2 cup (4.6 oz)	110	2	1	591
Fiesta Beans Onions & Peppers	1/2 cup (4.6 oz)	104	1	1	539
Refried Bacon	1/2 cup (4.5 oz)	116	3	1	489
Refried Green Chile	1/2 cup (4.5 oz)	110	3	1	495
Refried Low Fat Black	1/2 cup (4.5 oz)	107	1	0	569
Refried Nacho Cheese	1/2 cup (4.5 oz)	108	2	2	574
Refried No Fat	1/2 cup (4.5 oz)	120	0	0	570
Refried No Fat Green Chiles & Lime	1/2 cup (4.5 oz)	101	tr	0	565
Refried No Fat w/ Zesty Salsa	1/2 cup (4.5 oz)	105	tr	0	599
Refried Onion	1/2 cup (4.5 oz)	114	3	1	508
Refried Spicy	1/2 cup (4.5 oz)	118	3	0	574
Refried Traditional	1/2 cup (4.5 oz)	108	1	0	510
Refried Vegetarian	1/2 cup (4.5 oz)	237	5	tr	1101

FOOD	PORTION	CALS	FAT	CHOL	SOD
S&W					
Barbecue Beans Ranch Recipe	1/2 cup (4.5 oz)	100	2	0	640
Taco Bell					
Home Originals Fat Free Refried Beans	1/2 cup (4.6 oz)	110	0	0	460
Home Originals Fat Free Refried Beans w/ Mild Chilies	1/2 cup (4.5 oz)	110	0	0	480
Home Originals Refried Beans	1/2 cup (4.7 oz)	140	3	0	530
Van Camp					
Baked Fat Free	1/2 cup (4.6 oz)	132	tr	0	505
Baked Original	1/2 cup (4.7 oz)	143	1	1	535
Baked Southern Style Sauteed Onion	1/2 cup (4.8 oz)	145	1	1	555
Baked Sweet Hickory & Bacon	1 can (4.8 oz)	143	1	tr	471
Beanee Weenee BBQ	1 cup (7.7 oz)	290	12	35	970
Beanee Weenee Baked	1 cup (9.1 oz)	410	14	40	1210
Beanee Weenee Microwave	1 cup (7.5 oz)	260	11	35	1020
Beanee Weenee Original	1 cup (9.1 oz)	320	14	40	1240
Beanee Weenee Zestful	1 cup (7.7 oz)	300	12	35	1030
Brown Sugar	1/2 cup (4.6 oz)	170	3	5	410
Pork And Beans	1/2 cup (4.6 oz)	110	2	0	490
Vegetarian	1/2 cup (4.6 oz)	110	1	0	400
frozen					
Natural Touch					
Nine Bean Loaf	1 in slice (3 oz)	160	8	<5	350
mix					
Melting Pot					
Terrazza Napoli Mixed Beans	1 cup	200	2	<5	460
take-out					
baked beans	1/2 cup	190	6	6	532
barbecue beans	3.5 oz	120	tr	0	460
four bean salad	3.5 oz	100	tr	0	280
three bean salad	3/4 cup	230	11	0	500
BEEF					
(*see also* BEEF DISHES, VEAL)					
canned					
Armour					
Chopped Beef	2 oz	170	15	40	810
Corned Beef	2 oz	120	7	50	490
Potted Meat	1 can (3 oz)	120	7	75	750
Tripe	3 oz	90	2	125	100

FOOD	PORTION	CALS	FAT	CHOL	SOD
Hormel					
Corned Beef	2 oz	120	7	50	490
Cubed Beef	1/2 cup (4.9 oz)	130	3	60	600
Potted Meat	4 tbsp (2 oz)	100	8	50	610
Treet					
Luncheon Loaf	2 oz	130	11	50	740
Luncheon Loaf 50% Less Fat	2 oz	110	8	45	750
dried					
Armour					
Sliced	7 slices (1 oz)	60	2	25	1370
Hormel					
Pillow Pack	10 slices (1 oz)	45	1	20	1010
fresh					
bottom round lean & fat trim 0 in Choice roasted	3 oz	172	8	66	56
bottom round lean & fat trim 0 in Select braised	3 oz	171	6	82	43
bottom round lean & fat trim 0 in Select roasted	3 oz	150	24	66	56
bottom round lean & fat trim 0 in braised	3 oz	193	26	82	43
bottom round lean & fat trim 1/4 in Choice braised	3 oz	241	15	81	42
bottom round lean & fat trim 1/4 in Choice roasted	3 oz	221	14	68	53
bottom round lean & fat trim 1/4 in Select braised	3 oz	220	13	81	42
bottom round lean & fat trim 1/4 in Select roasted	3 oz	199	11	68	54
brisket flat half lean & fat trim 0 in braised	3 oz	183	8	81	53
brisket flat half lean & fat trim 1/4 in braised	3 oz	309	24	81	48
brisket point half lean & fat trim 0 in braised	3 oz	304	24	78	57
brisket point half lean & fat trim 1/4 in braised	3 oz	343	29	79	55
brisket whole lean & fat trim 0 in braised	3 oz	247	17	79	55
brisket whole lean & fat trim 1/4 in braised	3 oz	327	27	80	52
chuck arm pot roast lean & fat trim 0 in braised	3 oz	238	14	85	53
chuck arm pot roast lean & fat trim 1/4 in braised	3 oz	282	20	85	51
chuck blade roast lean & fat trim 0 in braised	3 oz	284	21	88	56

FOOD	PORTION	CALS	FAT	CHOL	SOD
chuck blade roast lean & fat trim 1/4 in braised	3 oz	293	22	88	55
corned beef brisket cooked	3 oz	213	16	83	964
eye of round lean & fat trim 0 in Choice roasted	3 oz	153	5	59	53
eye of round lean & fat trim 0 in Select roasted	3 oz	137	4	59	53
eye of round lean & fat trim 1/4 in Choice roasted	3 oz	205	12	62	50
eye of round lean & fat trim 1/4 in Select roasted	3 oz	184	10	61	51
flank lean & fat trim 0 in braised	3 oz	224	14	62	60
flank lean & fat trim 0 in broiled	3 oz	192	11	58	69
ground extra lean broiled medium	3 oz	217	14	71	59
ground extra lean broiled well done	3 oz	225	14	84	70
ground extra lean fried medium	3 oz	216	14	69	59
ground extra lean fried well done	3 oz	224	14	79	69
ground extra lean raw	4 oz	265	19	78	75
ground lean broiled medium	3 oz	231	16	74	65
ground lean broiled well done	3 oz	238	15	86	76
ground regular broiled medium	3 oz	246	18	76	70
ground regular broiled well done	3 oz	248	17	86	79
ground low-fat w/ carrageenan raw	4 oz	160	7	53	70
porterhouse steak lean & fat trim 1/4 in Choice broiled	3 oz	260	19	70	52
rib eye small end lean & fat trim 0 in Choice broiled	3 oz	261	19	70	54
rib large end lean & fat trim 0 in roasted	3 oz	300	24	72	55
rib large end lean & fat trim 1/4 in broiled	3 oz	295	24	69	54
rib large end lean & fat trim 1/4 in roasted	3 oz	310	25	72	54
rib small end lean & fat trim 0 in broiled	3 oz	252	18	70	54
rib small end lean & fat trim 1/4 in broiled	3 oz	285	22	71	53

FOOD	PORTION	CALS	FAT	CHOL	SOD
rib small end lean & fat trim 1/4 in roasted	3 oz	295	24	71	53
rib whole lean & fat trim 1/4 in Choice broiled	3 oz	306	25	70	53
rib whole lean & fat trim 1/4 in Choice roasted	3 oz	320	27	72	53
rib whole lean & fat trim 1/4 in Prime roasted	3 oz	348	30	72	54
rib whole lean & fat trim 1/4 in Select broiled	3 oz	274	21	69	54
rib whole lean & fat trim 1/4 in Select roasted	3 oz	286	23	71	54
shank crosscut lean & fat trim 1/4 in Choice simmered	3 oz	224	12	68	52
short loin top loin lean & fat trim 0 in Choice broiled	3 oz	193	10	65	57
short loin top loin lean & fat trim 0 in Choice broiled	1 steak (5.4 oz)	353	19	119	104
short loin top loin lean & fat trim 0 in Select broiled	1 steak (5.4 oz)	309	14	119	104
short loin top loin lean & fat trim 1/4 in Choice braised	3 oz	253	18	68	54
short loin top loin lean & fat trim 1/4 in Choice broiled	1 steak (6.3 oz)	536	38	143	114
short loin top loin lean & fat trim 1/4 in Prime broiled	1 steak (6.3 oz)	582	43	143	114
short loin top loin lean & fat trim 1/4 in Select broiled	1 steak (6.3 oz)	473	31	140	114
short loin top loin lean only trim 0 in Choice broiled	1 steak (5.2 oz)	311	14	113	101
short loin top loin lean only trim 1/4 in Choice broiled	1 steak (5.2 oz)	314	15	112	100
shortribs lean & fat Choice braised	3 oz	400	36	80	43
t-bone steak lean & fat trim 1/4 in Choice broiled	3 oz	253	18	70	52
t-bone steak lean only trim 1/4 in Choice broiled	3 oz	182	9	68	56
tenderloin lean & fat trim 0 in Select broiled	3 oz	194	11	72	52
tenderloin lean & fat trim 1/4 in Choice broiled	3 oz	259	19	73	50
tenderloin lean & fat trim 1/4 in Choice roasted	3 oz	288	22	73	55
tenderloin lean & fat trim 1/4 in Choice broiled	3 oz	208	12	72	52
tenderloin lean & fat trim 1/4 in Prime broiled	3 oz	270	20	73	50

FOOD	PORTION	CALS	FAT	CHOL	SOD
tenderloin lean & fat trim 1/4 in Select roasted	3 oz	275	21	73	48
tip round lean & fat trim 0 in Choice roasted	3 oz	170	8	69	54
tip round lean & fat trim 0 in Select roasted	3 oz	158	6	69	55
tip round lean & fat trim 1/4 in Choice roasted	3 oz	210	13	70	53
tip round lean & fat trim 1/4 in Prime roasted	3 oz	233	15	70	53
tip round lean & fat trim 1/4 in Select roasted	3 oz	191	10	70	53
top round lean & fat trim 0 in Choice braised	3 oz	184	6	77	38
top round lean & fat trim 0 in Select braised	3 oz	170	5	77	38
top round lean & fat trim 1/4 in Choice braised	3 oz	221	11	77	38
top round lean & fat trim 1/4 in Choice broiled	3 oz	190	9	72	51
top round lean & fat trim 1/4 in Choice fried	3 oz	235	13	82	58
top round lean & fat trim 1/4 in Prime broiled	3 oz	195	9	72	51
top round lean & fat trim 1/4 in Select braised	3 oz	199	8	77	38
top round lean & fat trim 1/4 in Select braised	3 oz	175	7	72	51
top sirloin lean & fat trim 0 in Choice broiled	3 oz	194	10	76	55
top sirloin lean & fat trim 0 in Select broiled	3 oz	166	6	76	55
top sirloin lean & fat trim 1/4 in Choice broiled	3 oz	228	14	76	53
top sirloin lean & fat trim 1/4 in Choice fried	3 oz	277	19	83	59
top sirloin lean & fat trim 1/4 in Select broiled	3 oz	208	12	76	54
tripe raw	4 oz	111	4	107	52
Laura's Lean					
Eye Of Round	4 oz	140	4	60	40
Flank Steak	4 oz	140	5	50	45
Ground 92% Lean	4 oz	160	9	60	70
Ground Round 94% Lean	4 oz	140	5	60	50
Ribeye Steak	4 oz	140	5	60	40
Sirloin Tip Round	4 oz	120	3	65	50
Sirloin Top Butt	4 oz	140	5	60	45

FOOD	PORTION	CALS	FAT	CHOL	SOD
Strip Steak	4 oz	140	4	55	45
Tenderloins	4 oz	140	6	65	45
Top Round	4 oz	130	3	55	45
Maverick Ranch					
Ground Round Extra Lean	4 oz	130	4	60	65
Organic Valley					
Extra Lean Ground	3 oz	130	6	55	55
Extra Lean Patties	1 (3.2 oz)	130	6	60	55
ready-to-eat					
Alpine Lace					
Roast Beef 97% Fat Free	2 oz	70	2	40	200
Boar's Head					
Corned Beef Brisket	2 oz	80	4	40	460
Eye Round Pepper Seasoned	2 oz	90	3	40	130
Italian Style Oven Roasted Top Round	2 oz	80	2	40	350
Roast Beef Cajun	2 oz	80	3	35	200
Top Round Deluxe	2 oz	90	3	30	80
Top Round Oven Roasted No Salt Added	2 oz	90	3	30	40
Jordan's					
Healthy Trim 97% Fat Free Roast Beef Medium	1 slice (1 oz)	30	1	20	130
Healthy Trim 97% Fat Free Roast Beef Rare	1 slice (1 oz)	30	1	20	130
Tyson					
Beef Strips Seasoned	1 serv (3 oz)	140	6	55	420
BEEF DISHES					
canned					
Armour					
Corned Beef Hash	1 cup (8.3 oz)	440	30	100	840
Corned Beef Hash w/ Peppers & Onions	1 cup (8.3 oz)	270	30	100	1220
Roast Beef Hash	1 cup (8.4 oz)	400	25	95	1460
Roast Beef In Gravy	1/2 cup (4.6 oz)	150	4	75	640
Stew	1 cup (8.6 oz)	220	12	30	1250
Dinty Moore					
Meatball Stew	1 cup (8.4 oz)	250	15	40	1120
Sliced Potatoes & Beef	1 can (7.5 oz)	230	9	35	1080
Stew	1 cup (8.2 oz)	230	14	40	950
Hormel					
Beef Goulash	1 can (7.5 oz)	230	11	50	1040
Roast Beef With Gravy	2 oz	60	2	30	280
Mary Kitchen					
Corned Beef Hash	1 cup (8.3 oz)	410	27	80	1020
Corned Beef Hash 50% Reduced Fat	1 cup (8.3 oz)	280	12	65	1070

FOOD	PORTION	CALS	FAT	CHOL	SOD
Mary Kitchen (cont.)					
Roast Beef Hash	1 cup (8.3 oz)	390	24	70	790
Roast Turkey Hash	1 can (14.9 oz)	420	11	110	1800
Sausage Hash	1 cup (8.3 oz)	410	27	85	1020
mix					
Hamburger Helper					
BBQ Beef as prep	1 cup	320	10	55	760
Beef Pasta as prep	1 cup	270	10	50	910
Beef Romanoff as prep	1 cup	280	10	50	890
Beef Stew as prep	1 cup	260	10	50	760
Beef Taco as prep	1 cup	280	10	50	960
Beef Teriyaki as prep	1 cup	290	10	50	990
Cheddar & Broccoli as prep	1 cup	350	15	60	830
Cheddar Melt as prep	1 cup	310	12	55	890
Cheddar'n Bacon as prep	1 cup	330	15	65	980
Cheeseburger Macaroni	1 cup	360	16	65	940
Cheesy Hashbrowns as prep	1 cup	400	19	60	530
Cheesy Italian as prep	1 cup	320	14	60	920
Cheesy Shells as prep	1 cup	330	15	60	840
Chili Macaroni as prep	1 cup	290	10	55	870
Fettuccine Alfredo as prep	1 cup	300	13	55	860
Four Cheese Lasagne as prep	1 cup	330	14	55	860
Italian Parmesan w/ Rigatoni as prep	1 cup	300	11	50	870
Lasagne as prep	1 cup	270	10	50	1000
Meat Loaf as prep	1/6 loaf	270	14	110	580
Meaty Spaghetti & Cheese as prep	1 cup	290	10	50	970
Mushroom & Wild Rice as prep	1 cup	310	12	55	880
Nacho Cheese as prep	1 cup	320	13	55	930
Pizza Pasta w/ Cheese Topping as prep	1 cup	280	10	50	750
Pizzabake as prep	1/6 pie	270	10	45	720
Potatoes Au Gratin as prep	1 cup	280	13	55	730
Potatoes Stroganoff as prep	1 cup	250	11	50	870
Reduced Sodium Cheddar Spirals as prep	1 cup	300	13	55	590
Reduced Sodium Italian Herb as prep	1 cup	270	10	50	630
Reduced Sodium Southwestern Beef as prep	1 cup	300	10	50	620
Rice Oriental as prep	1 cup	280	10	50	990
Salisbury as prep	1 cup	270	10	50	790
Spaghetti as prep	1 cup	270	10	50	940
Stroganoff as prep	1 cup	320	13	55	830
Swedish Meatballs as prep	1 cup	290	14	55	780

FOOD	PORTION	CALS	FAT	CHOL	SOD
Three Cheeses as prep	1 cup	340	15	55	830
Zesty Italian as prep	1 cup	300	10	50	580
Zesty Mexican as prep	1 cup	280	10	50	690
shelf-stable					
Dinty Moore					
Microwave Cup Corned Beef Hash	1 pkg (7.5 oz)	350	22	60	850
Microwave Cup Hearty Burger Stew	1 pkg (7.5 oz)	240	13	40	930
Microwave Cup Stew	1 pkg (7.5 oz)	190	10	40	900
Hormel					
Microcup Meals Stew	1 cup (7.5 oz)	190	10	35	900
Lunch Bucket					
Beef Stew	1 pkg (7.5 oz)	170	9	25	810
take-out					
beef bourguignon	1 serv (7 oz)	254	16	128	212
bulgoghi korean grilled beef	1 serv (5.2 oz)	256	15	67	834
greek moussaka	1 serv (8.5 oz)	450	33	179	763
shepherds pie	1 serv (7 oz)	282	16	70	840
stew w/ vegetables	1 cup	220	11	71	292
stroganoff	3/4 cup	260	19	69	503
swiss steak	4.6 oz	214	9	61	139
BEEFALO					
roasted	3 oz	160	5	49	70
BEER AND ALE					
beer light	12 oz can	100	0	0	10
beer regular	12 oz can	146	0	0	19
BEET JUICE					
juice	3 1/2 oz	36	0	0	200
BEETS					
canned					
Green Giant					
Harvard	1/3 cup (3.1 oz)	60	0	0	270
Sliced	1/2 cup (4.2 oz)	35	0	0	260
Sliced No Salt Added	1/2 cup (4.2 oz)	35	0	0	60
Whole	1/2 cup (4.2 oz)	35	0	0	260
LeSueur					
Baby Whole	1/2 cup (4.3 oz)	35	0	0	260
fresh					
greens cooked	1/2 cup	20	tr	0	173
sliced cooked	1/2 cup (3 oz)	38	tr	0	65
whole cooked	2 (3.5 oz)	44	tr	0	77
BEVERAGES					

(*see* BEER AND ALE, CHAMPAGNE, COFFEE, DRINK MIXERS, ENERGY DRINKS, FRUIT DRINKS, ICED TEA, LIQUOR/LIQUEUR, MALT, MILKSHAKE, SODA, SPORTS DRINKS, TEA/HERBAL TEA, WATER, WINE, WINE COOLER)

FOOD	PORTION	CALS	FAT	CHOL	SOD
BISCUIT					
mix					
Bisquick					
Original Sweet	1/4 cup (1.4 oz)	170	4	0	260
Reduced Fat	1/3 cup (1.4 oz)	150	3	0	460
Gold Medal					
Biscuits	2	180	6	0	480
refrigerated					
1869 Brand					
Buttermilk	1 (1.1 oz)	100	5	0	320
Hungry Jack					
Butter Tastin' Flaky	1 (1.2 oz)	100	5	0	350
Cinnamon & Sugar	1 (1.2 oz)	110	4	0	280
Flaky	1 (1.2 oz)	100	5	0	360
Flaky Buttermilk	1 (1.2 oz)	100	5	0	360
Pillsbury					
Big Country Butter Tastin'	1 (1.2 oz)	100	4	0	360
Big Country Buttermilk	1 (1.2 oz)	100	4	0	360
Big Country Southern Style	1 (1.2 oz)	100	4	0	360
Buttermilk	1 (2.2 oz)	150	2	0	540
Country	1 (2.2 oz)	150	2	0	540
Grands Blueberry	1 (2.1 oz)	210	9	0	510
Grands Butter Tastin'	1 (2.1 oz)	200	10	0	620
Grands Buttermilk	1 (2.1 oz)	200	10	0	620
Grands Buttermilk Reduced Fat	1 (2.1 oz)	190	7	0	620
Grands Extra Rich	1 (2.1 oz)	220	12	0	580
Grands Flaky	1 (2.1 oz)	200	9	0	580
Grands Golden Corn	1 (1.2 oz)	210	10	0	600
Grands HomeStyle	1 (2.1 oz)	210	10	0	620
Grands Southern Style	1 (2.1 oz)	200	10	0	620
Southern Style Flakey	1 (1.2 oz)	100	5	0	360
Tender Layer Buttermilk	1 (2.2 oz)	160	5	0	520
take-out					
buttermilk	1 (2 oz)	212	10	2	348
plain	1 (35 g)	276	34	5	584
tea biscuit	1 (3 oz)	210	3	0	370
w/ egg	1 (4.8 oz)	316	20	233	654
w/ egg & bacon	1 (5.2 oz)	458	31	353	999
w/ egg & ham	1 (6.7 oz)	442	27	300	1382
w/ egg & sausage	1 (6.3 oz)	581	39	302	1141
w/ egg & steak	1 (5.2 oz)	410	28	272	888
w/ egg cheese & bacon	1 (5.1 oz)	477	31	261	1260
w/ ham	1 (4 oz)	386	18	25	1433
w/ sausage	1 (4.4 oz)	485	32	35	1071
w/ steak	1 (4.9 oz)	455	26	25	795
BISON					
roasted	3 oz	122	2	70	48

FOOD	PORTION	CALS	FAT	CHOL	SOD
BLACK BEANS					
canned					
Eden					
Organic	1/2 cup (4.6 oz)	100	0	0	15
Organic w/ Ginger & Lemon	1/2 cup (4.6 oz)	120	0	0	200
Green Giant					
Black Beans	1/2 cup (4.5 oz)	50	0	0	400
Progresso					
Black Beans	1/2 cup (4.6 oz)	110	1	0	400
dried					
cooked	1 cup	227	1	0	1
BLACKBERRIES					
canned in heavy syrup	1/2 cup	118	tr	0	3
fresh	1/2 cup	37	tr	0	0
unsweetened frozen	1 cup	97	1	0	2
BLACKBERRY JUICE					
Kool-Aid					
Scary Blackberry Ghoul-Aid Drink as prep w/ sugar	1 serv (8 oz)	100	0	0	0
BLACKEYE PEAS					
canned					
Green Giant					
Blackeye Peas	1/2 cup (4.4 oz)	90	0	0	250
dried					
cooked	1 cup	198	1	0	6
frozen					
Birds Eye					
Blackeye Peas	1/2 cup (2.8 oz)	110	1	0	10
BLINTZE					
take-out					
cheese	1 (2.7 oz)	160	9	65	240
BLUEBERRIES					
canned in heavy syrup	1 cup	225	1	0	9
fresh	1 cup	82	1	0	9
unsweetened frozen	1 cup	78	1	0	1
Sonoma					
Dried	1/4 cup (1.3 oz)	140	0	0	0
BLUEFIN					
fillet baked	4.1 oz	186	6	88	90
BLUEFISH					
fresh baked	3 oz	135	5	64	65
BORAGE					
fresh chopped cooked	3 1/2 oz	25	1	0	88
BOTTLED WATER					
(*see* WATER)					
BOYSENBERRIES					
in heavy syrup	1 cup	226	tr	0	9
unsweetened frozen	1 cup	66	tr	0	2

FOOD	PORTION	CALS	FAT	CHOL	SOD
BRAINS					
beef pan-fried	3 oz	167	13	1696	134
beef simmered	3 oz	136	11	1746	102
lamb braised	3 oz	124	9	1737	114
lamb fried	3 oz	232	19	2128	133
pork braised	3 oz	117	8	2169	77
veal braised	3 oz	115	8	2635	133
veal fried	3 oz	181	14	1802	150
Armour					
Pork Brains in Milk Gravy	2/3 cup (5.5 oz)	150	5	3500	550
BRAN					
corn	1 cup (2.7 oz)	170	1	0	5
oat	1/2 cup (1.6 oz)	116	3	0	2
oat cooked	1/2 cup (3.8 oz)	44	1	0	1
rice	1/2 cup (2.1 oz)	187	12	0	3
wheat	1/2 cup (2 oz)	63	1	0	1
BRAZIL NUTS					
dried unblanched	1 oz	186	19	0	0
BREAD					
(*see also* BAGEL, BISCUIT, BREADSTICK, CROISSANT, ENGLISH MUFFIN, MUFFIN, ROLL, SCONE)					
frozen					
New York					
Garlic	1 slice (2 oz)	190	8	0	390
Garlic Reduced Fat	1 slice (2 oz)	160	4	0	340
Texas Garlic Toast	1 in slice (1.4 oz)	160	9	0	260
Pepperidge Farm					
Garlic	1 slice (1.8 oz)	170	10	30	270
Garlic Sourdough 30% Reduced Fat	1 slice (1.8 oz)	170	7	5	310
Monterey Jack Jalapeno Cheese	1 slice (2 oz)	145	11	41	279
Mozzarella Garlic Cheese	1 slice (2 oz)	201	10	40	280
ready-to-eat					
baguette whole wheat	2 oz	140	0	0	360
egg	1 slice (1.4 oz)	115	2	20	197
french	1 slice (1 oz)	78	1	0	172
italian	1 slice (1 oz)	81	1	0	175
navajo fry	1 (5 in diam)	296	9	0	625
pita	1 reg (2 oz)	165	1	0	322
pita	1 sm (1 oz)	78	tr	0	152
pita whole wheat	1 reg (2 oz)	170	2	0	340
pita whole wheat	1 sm (1 oz)	76	1	0	151
pumpernickel	1 slice	80	1	0	215
raisin	1 slice	71	1	0	101
rye	1 slice	83	1	0	211
seven grain	1 slice	65	1	0	127
sourdough	1 slice (1 oz)	78	1	0	172

FOOD	PORTION	CALS	FAT	CHOL	SOD
vienna	1 slice (1 oz)	78	1	0	172
white	1 slice	67	1	0	135
white cubed	1 cup	80	1	0	154
white toasted	1 slice	67	1	0	136
Arnold					
Country Buttermilk	1 slice (1.3 oz)	110	2	0	180
Country Wheat	1 slice (1.3 oz)	100	2	0	190
Bread Du Jour					
French	3 in slice (2 oz)	140	1	0	310
Damascus					
Pita	1 (2 oz)	130	0	0	150
Pita Whole Wheat	1 (2 oz)	160	0	0	230
Wraps Honey Wheat	1/2 wrap (2 oz)	130	0	0	150
Wraps Plain	1/2 wrap (2 oz)	130	0	0	150
Wraps Spinach	1 (2 oz)	280	0	0	460
Wraps Tomato	1 12-inch (4 oz)	240	0	0	440
La Mexicana					
Wraps Chocolate	1 (1.3 oz)	120	3	0	360
Wraps Southwestern Mild Chili	1 (1.3 oz)	120	4	0	360
Wraps Spinach	1 (1.3 oz)	120	4	0	360
Wraps Tomato Basil	1 (1.3 oz)	120	4	0	360
Milton's					
Healthy Multi-Grain	1 slice (1.4 oz)	110	1	0	150
Pepperidge Farm					
Apple Cinammon	1 slice (1 oz)	80	2	0	120
Deli Swirl Rye & Pump	1 slice (1.1 oz)	80	1	0	220
Natural Whole Grain Whole Wheat	1 slice (1.2 oz)	90	1	0	135
Sandwich Pocket Wheat	1 (2 oz)	160	1	0	260
Sandwich Pocket White	1 (2 oz)	150	1	0	290
Swirl Cinnamon	1 slice (1 oz)	90	3	0	110
Swirl Raisin Cinnamon	1 slice (1 oz)	80	2	0	105
Stroehmann					
100% Whole Wheat	1 slice (1.3 oz)	90	1	0	180
D'Italiano Italian No Seeds	1 slice (1 oz)	80	1	0	170
D'Italiano Italian Seeded	1 slice (1 oz)	80	1	0	170
Family White	1 slice (0.8 oz)	65	1	0	135
Homestyle Split Top Wheat	1 slice (0.8 oz)	60	0	0	110
Homestyle Split Top White	1 slice (0.8 oz)	65	1	0	110
Honey Cracked Wheat	1 slice (1.2 oz)	80	1	0	170
King White	1 slice (0.8 oz)	65	1	0	135
Potato	1 slice (1.2 oz)	100	2	0	170
Ranch White	1 slice (0.8 oz)	65	1	0	135
Rye	1 slice (1.1 oz)	80	1	0	180
Rye w/ Caraway	1 slice (1.1 oz)	80	1	0	170
Twelve Grain	1 slice (1.2 oz)	90	1	0	140

FOOD	PORTION	CALS	FAT	CHOL	SOD
Valley Lahvosh					
Valley Wraps	1 (1 oz)	100	1	0	125
ZA					
Pit-Za Hearty Multi-Grain	1/9 bread (2 oz)	130	2	0	210
Pit-Za Salt-Free Garlic Whole Wheat	1/9 bread (2 oz)	150	1	0	10
refrigerated					
Pillsbury					
Crusty French Loaf	1/5 loaf (2.2 oz)	150	2	0	390
Grands Wheat	1 (2.1 oz)	200	8	0	600
take-out					
chapatis as prep w/ fat	1 bread (1.6 oz)	95	2	3	180
focaccia onion	1 piece (4.6 oz)	282	10	0	536
focaccia rosemary	1 piece (3.5 oz)	251	7	0	535
focaccia tomato olive	1 piece (4.7 oz)	270	8	0	683
garlic bread	2 slices (2 oz)	190	8	0	290
irish soda bread	1 slice (2 oz)	174	3	11	239
naan	1 bread (3.5 oz)	286	9	46	546
paratha	1 bread (2.1 oz)	201	10	27	268
BREAD COATING					
Mrs. Dash					
Crispy Coating	2 tbsp (0.6 oz)	65	1	0	3
Oven Fry					
Extra Crispy For Chicken	1/8 pkg (0.5 oz)	60	1	0	420
Extra Crispy For Pork	1/8 pkg (0.5 oz)	60	2	0	340
Shake 'N Bake					
Buffalo Wings	1/10 pkg (0.4 oz)	40	1	0	300
Classic Italian Chicken or Pork	1/8 pkg (0.4 oz)	40	1	0	270
Country Mild Recipe	1/8 pkg (0.3 oz)	35	2	0	240
Glazes Barbecue Chicken or Pork	1/8 pkg (0.4 oz)	45	1	0	410
Glazes Honey Mustard Chicken or Pork	1/8 pkg (0.4 oz)	45	1	0	300
Glazes Tangy Honey Chicken or Pork	1/8 pkg (0.4 oz)	45	1	0	300
Home Style Flour Recipe For Chicken	1/8 pkg (0.4 oz)	40	1	0	470
Hot & Spicy Chicken or Pork	1/8 pkg (0.4 oz)	40	1	0	170
Original For Chicken	1/8 pkg (0.4 oz)	40	1	0	220
Original For Fish	1/4 pkg (0.7 oz)	80	2	0	350
Original For Pork	1/8 pkg (0.4 oz)	45	1	0	230
BREAD MACHINE MIX					
Fleischmann's					
Apple Cinnamon	1/8 loaf	160	1	0	160
Cinnamon Raisin	1/8 loaf	160	1	0	170
Country White	1/8 loaf (1.6 oz)	170	3	0	170

FOOD	PORTION	CALS	FAT	CHOL	SOD
Cranberry Orange	1/8 loaf	150	2	0	150
Honey Oatmeal	1/8 loaf	160	1	0	270
Italian Herb	1/8 loaf	160	2	0	310
Sourdough	1/8 loaf	150	2	0	160
Stoneground Wheat	1/8 loaf	160	1	0	180
BREADCRUMBS					
fresh	2/3 cup	76	1	0	153
Progresso					
Garlic & Herb	1/4 cup (1 oz)	100	2	0	530
Italian Style	1/4 cup (1 oz)	110	2	0	430
Parmesan	1/4 cup (1 oz)	100	2	0	870
Plain	1/4 cup (1 oz)	110	2	0	210
BREADFRUIT					
fresh	1/4 small	99	tr	0	2
BREADSTICKS					
Bread Du Jour					
Original	1 (1.9 oz)	130	1	0	290
Sourdough	1 (1.9 oz)	130	1	0	280
New York					
Garlic Soft	1 (1.5 oz)	140	4	0	220
Pillsbury					
Soft	1 (1.4 oz)	110	2	0	290
Soft Garlic & Herb	1 (2.1 oz)	180	7	0	580
Stella D'Oro					
Garlic	1 (0.4 oz)	40	1	0	60
Grissini Style Fat Free	3 (0.5 oz)	60	0	0	130
Original	1 (9 g)	40	1	0	40
Potato 'N Onion	1 (0.4 oz)	45	1	0	210
Roasted Garlic	1 (0.4 oz)	45	1	0	210
Sesame	1 (0.4 oz)	50	3	0	45
Snack Stix Cracked Pepper	4 (0.5 oz)	70	2	0	290
Snack Stix Salted	4 (0.5 oz)	70	2	0	290
Sodium Free	1 (0.4 oz)	45	1	0	0
Wheat	1 (0.3 oz)	40	1	0	20
BREAKFAST BAR					
(*see* CEREAL BARS, ENERGY BARS)					
BREAKFAST DRINKS					
(*see also* ENERGY DRINKS, NUTRITION SUPPLEMENTS)					
Carnation					
Instant Breakfast Vanilla as prep w/ skim milk	1 serv	220	1	5	220
Instant Breakfast Vanilla as prep w/ whole milk	1 serv	280	8	35	220
BROAD BEANS					
canned	1 cup	183	1	0	1161
dried cooked	1 cup	186	1	0	8
fresh cooked	3 1/2 oz	56	tr	0	41

FOOD	PORTION	CALS	FAT	CHOL	SOD
BROCCOFLOWER					
fresh raw	1/2 cup (1.8 oz)	16	tr	0	12
BROCCOLI					
fresh					
chinese broccoli (gai lan)	1 cup (3.1 oz)	19	1	0	6
cooked					
frozen					
chopped cooked	1/2 cup	25	tr	0	22
spears cooked	1/2 cup	25	tr	0	22
spears cooked	10 oz pkg	69	tr	0	60
Amy's Organic					
Pocket Sandwich Broccoli & Cheese	1 (4.5 oz)	270	10	15	560
Birds Eye					
Baby Broccoli Blend	1 cup (3.4 oz)	70	2	0	30
Baby Florets	1 cup (3 oz)	25	0	0	20
In Cheese Sauce	1/2 cup (3.9 oz)	110	5	5	500
Green Giant					
Butter Sauce	4 oz	50	2	<5	330
Cheese Sauce	2/3 cup (3.9 oz)	70	3	<5	520
Chopped	3/4 cup (2.8 oz)	25	0	0	25
Cuts	1 cup (2.9 oz)	25	0	0	25
Harvest Fresh Cut	2/3 cup (3.2 oz)	25	0	0	150
Harvest Fresh Spears	3.5 oz	25	0	0	125
Select Florets	1 1/3 cups (2.9 oz)	25	0	0	25
Select Spears	3 oz	25	0	0	25
Health Is Wealth					
Broccoli Munchees	2 (1 oz)	60	2	0	170
Stouffer's					
Au Gratin	1 serv (4 oz)	100	4	10	450
BROWNIE					
frozen					
Greenfield					
Fat Free Homestyle	1 (1.3 oz)	110	0	0	60
Otis Spunkmeyer					
Blue Yonder w/ Walnuts	1 (2 oz)	230	10	20	170
Weight Watchers					
Brownie A La Mode	1 (3.14 oz)	190	4	30	190
Double Fudge Brownie Parfait	1 (5.3 oz)	190	3	5	170
mix					
Betty Crocker					
Caramel	1	190	9	25	120
Caramel No Cholesterol Recipe	1	170	5	0	125
Chocolate Chunk Supreme	1	180	9	20	100
Dark Chocolate Fudge	1	170	7	20	110
Dark Chocolate w/ Hershey Syrup	1	170	7	20	110

FOOD	PORTION	CALS	FAT	CHOL	SOD
Frosted Supreme	1	210	9	20	125
Fudge	1	190	7	20	125
Fudge No Cholesterol Recipe	1	140	4	0	105
German Chocolate	1	220	8	20	130
Hot Fudge Supreme	1	170	8	20	110
Original Supreme	1	160	6	20	110
Peanut Butter Candies w/ Reese's Pieces	1	180	9	20	105
Pouch Dessert Fudge	1	190	8	25	130
Stir'n Bake w/ Mini Kisses	1 serv	220	8	0	150
T-Rex Fossils	1	180	8	25	100
T-Rex Fossils No Cholesterol Recipe	1	170	8	0	100
Turtle	1	170	8	20	100
Walnut Supreme	1	160	9	20	95
Estee					
Brownie Mix as prep	2	100	4	0	0
No Pudge!					
Cappuccino Fudge	1	100	0	0	90
Fudge	1	100	0	0	90
Mint Fudge	1/2 cup	100	0	0	90
Raspberry Fudge	1	100	0	0	90
Sweet Rewards					
Reduced Fat Fudge	1	140	4	20	110
Reduced Fat Fudge No Cholesterol Recipe	1	140	3	0	110
ready-to-eat					
Dolly Madison					
Fudge	1 (3 oz)	330	11	45	190
Entenmann's					
Little Bites	3 (2.2 oz)	290	16	45	200
Ultimate Fudge	1 (1.6 oz)	220	13	50	60
Greenfield					
Blondie Fat Free Apple Spice	1 (1.3 oz)	110	0	0	60
Health Valley					
Bar w/ Fudge Filling	1 bar	110	0	0	30
Hostess					
Brownie Bites	3 (1.3 oz)	170	9	30	80
Fudge	1 (3 oz)	330	11	45	190
Light	1 (1.4 oz)	140	3	1	80
Lance					
Fudge Nut	1 (2.25 oz)	340	13	20	180
Little Debbie					
Brownie Lights	1 (2 oz)	190	3	0	200
Brownie Loaves	1 (2.1 oz)	260	15	40	160
Fudge	1 pkg (2.1 oz)	270	13	15	170

FOOD	PORTION	CALS	FAT	CHOL	SOD
Sweet Rewards					
Low Fat Homestyle	1 (1.1 oz)	120	2	0	105
Tastykake					
Fudge Walnut	1 (3 oz)	370	17	80	150
Tom's					
Fudge Nut	1 pkg (2.5 oz)	300	13	5	95
take-out					
plain	1 2 in sq (2.1 oz)	243	10	10	153
BRUSSELS SPROUTS					
fresh					
cooked	1 sprout	8	tr	0	4
frozen					
Birds Eye					
Brussels Sprouts	6 (3 oz)	35	0	0	15
Green Giant					
Butter Sauce	2/3 cup (3.6 oz)	60	2	<5	270
BUCKWHEAT					
groats roasted cooked	1 cup (5.9 oz)	647	1	0	7
BUFFALO					
water buffalo roasted	3 oz	111	2	52	48
BULGUR					
cooked	1 cup (6.3 oz)	151	tr	0	9
BURBOT (FISH)					
fresh baked	3 oz	98	1	65	106
BURDOCK ROOT					
cooked	1 cup	110	tr	0	5
BUTTER					
(*see also* BUTTER BLENDS, BUTTER SUBSTITUTES, MARGARINE)					
stick	1 pat (5 g)	36	4	11	41
whipped	1 pat (4 g)	27	3	8	31
Breakstone's					
Salted	1 tbsp (0.5 oz)	100	11	30	85
Hotel Bar					
Stick	1 tbsp (0.5 oz)	100	11	30	90
Keller's					
European	1 tbsp (0.5 oz)	100	11	30	0
Organic Valley					
Butter	1 tbsp (0.5 oz)	100	11	30	75
Unsalted	1 tbsp (0.5 oz)	110	12	30	0
BUTTER BEANS					
canned					
Green Giant					
Butter Beans	1/2 cup (4.5 oz)	90	0	0	450
Van Camp					
Butter Beans	1/2 cup (4.6 oz)	110	1	0	430

FOOD	PORTION	CALS	FAT	CHOL	SOD
frozen					
Birds Eye					
Butter Beans	1/2 cup (2.7 oz)	100	0	0	130
Speckled	1/2 cup (2.7 oz)	100	0	0	130
BUTTER BLENDS					
(*see also* BUTTER, BUTTER SUBSTITUTES, MARGARINE)					
Brummel & Brown					
Spread Made With Yogurt	1 tbsp (0.5 oz)	50	5	0	95
BUTTER SUBSTITUTES					
(*see also* BUTTER BLENDS, MARGARINE)					
Molly McButter					
Cheese	1 tsp	5	0	0	125
Light Sodium	1 tsp	5	0	0	90
Natural Butter	1 tsp	5	0	0	180
Roasted Garlic	1 tsp	5	0	0	125
Mrs. Bateman's					
Butterlike Baking Butter	1 tbsp (0.5 oz)	36	1	<5	20
Butterlike Saute Butter	1 tbsp (0.5 oz)	40	2	5	60
BUTTERBUR					
canned fuki chopped	1 cup	3	tr	0	5
BUTTERFISH					
baked	3 oz	159	9	71	97
fillet baked	1 oz	47	3	21	29
BUTTERNUTS					
dried	1 oz	174	16	0	0
BUTTERSCOTCH					
(*see also* CANDY)					
Hershey					
Chips	1 tbsp (0.5 oz)	80	4	0	10
Nestle					
Morsels	1 tbsp	80	4	0	15
CABBAGE					
(*see also* COLESLAW)					
chinese pak-choi shredded cooked	1/2 cup	10	tr	0	29
chinese pe-tsai shredded cooked	1 cup	16	tr	0	11
danish shredded cooked	1/2 cup (2.6 oz)	17	tr	0	6
green raw shredded	1/2 cup (1.2 oz)	9	tr	0	6
green shredded cooked	1/2 cup (2.6 oz)	17	tr	0	6
napa cooked	1 cup (3.8 oz)	13	tr	0	12
red raw shredded	1/2 cup	10	tr	0	4
red shredded cooked	1/2 cup	16	tr	0	6
savoy raw shredded	1/2 cup	10	tr	0	10
savoy shredded cooked	1/2 cup	18	tr	0	17

FOOD	PORTION	CALS	FAT	CHOL	SOD
CAKE					
(*see also* BROWNIE, CAKE MIX, COOKIES, DANISH PASTRY, DOUGHNUTS, PIE)					
jelly roll lemon filled	1 slice (3 oz)	210	2	35	300
sponge	1/12 cake (1.3 oz)	110	1	39	93
sponge cake dessert shell	1 (0.8 oz)	75	1	33	165
Baby Watson					
Cheesecake	1 slice (3 oz)	260	18	65	150
Carousel					
New York Cheese Cake	1 cake (3 oz)	250	19	95	180
Dolly Madison					
Angel Food	1 slice (2.1 oz)	160	2	0	190
Apple Crumb	1 (1.6 oz)	160	5	15	160
Banana Dream Flip	1 (3.5 oz)	390	16	30	240
Bear Claw	1 (2.75 oz)	270	10	25	330
Carrot	1 (4 oz)	360	8	0	500
Chocolate Snack Squares	1 (1.6 oz)	210	10	10	150
Cinnamon Buttercrumb	1 (1.6 oz)	170	6	15	170
Cinnamon Buttercrumb Low Fat	1 (1.5 oz)	140	2	0	150
Cinnamon Stix	1 (1.3 oz)	170	9	15	140
Creme Cakes	2 (1.9 oz)	210	8	25	230
Cupcakes Chocolate	1 (2 oz)	210	7	5	330
Cupcakes Spice	1 (2 oz)	230	10	20	160
Dunkin' Stix	1 (1.3 oz)	170	9	15	130
Frosty Angel	1 (3.5 oz)	330	6	0	270
Holiday Cupcakes	1 (1.9 oz)	180	3	5	190
Honey Bun	1 (3.7 oz)	440	25	15	260
Koo Koos	1 (1.8 oz)	200	9	5	90
Mini Coconut Loaf	1 (3.5 oz)	350	10	5	350
Mini Pound Cake	1 (3.2 oz)	310	11	15	390
Raspberry Square	1 (1.8 oz)	190	8	5	110
Sweet Roll Apple	1 (2.2 oz)	200	6	5	240
Sweet Roll Cherry	1 (2.2 oz)	210	6	10	180
Sweet Roll Cinnamon	1 (2.2 oz)	230	7	10	200
Texas Cinnamon Bun	1 (4.2 oz)	440	15	25	410
Zingers Devil's Food	2 (2.6 oz)	270	8	5	230
Zingers Lemon	1 (1.4 oz)	150	6	5	90
Zingers Raspberry	1 (1.4 oz)	150	6	5	90
Zingers Yellow	2 (2.5 oz)	280	8	5	160
Drake's					
Coffee Cake Low Fat	1 (1.1 oz)	110	2	10	110
Mini Coffee Cakes	4 (1.83 oz)	220	9	18	140
Yodel's	1 (1 oz)	150	9	5	65
Entenmann's					
Cupcakes Light Chocolate Creme Filled	1 (2 oz)	160	0	0	150
Hot Cross Buns	1 (2.3 oz)	230	7	20	160
Stollen Fruit	1/8 cake (2 oz)	210	7	15	125

FOOD	PORTION	CALS	FAT	CHOL	SOD
Greenfield					
Blondie Fat Free Chocolate Chip	1 (1.3 oz)	110	0	0	60
Hostess					
Angel Food	1/8 cake (2 oz)	160	2	0	180
Chocodiles	1 (1.6 oz)	240	11	20	180
Chocolicious	1 (1.6 oz)	190	7	10	210
Coffee Crumb	1 (1.1 oz)	130	5	10	110
Crumb Cake Light	1 (1 oz)	90	1	0	100
Cupcakes Chocolate	1 (1.8 oz)	180	6	5	290
Cupcakes Orange	1 (1.5 oz)	160	5	10	160
Cupcakes Light Chocolate	1 (1.6 oz)	140	2	0	190
Ding Dongs	2 (2.7 oz)	360	19	15	240
Ho Ho's	2 (2 oz)	250	12	20	150
Honey Bun Glazed	1 (2.7 oz)	320	19	15	210
Honey Bun Iced	1 (3.4 oz)	410	24	10	270
Shortcake Dessert Cups	1 (1 oz)	100	2	15	120
Sno Balls	1 (1.8 oz)	180	5	5	190
Suzy Q's	2 (2 oz)	230	9	10	270
Sweet Roll Cherry	1 (2.2 oz)	210	6	10	180
Sweet Roll Cinnamon	1 (2.2 oz)	230	7	10	200
Twinkies	1 (1.5 oz)	150	5	20	200
Twinkies Light	1 (1.5 oz)	130	2	10	190
Jell-O					
Dessert Delights Cheesecake	1 bar (1.4 oz)	160	7	5	100
Dessert Delights Chocolate Fudge Pudding	1 bar (1.4 oz)	150	6	0	80
Kellogg's					
Pop-Tarts Apple Cinnamon	1 (1.8 oz)	210	6	0	180
Pop-Tarts Blueberry	1 (1.8 oz)	210	5	0	190
Pop-Tarts Brown Sugar Cinnamon	1 (1.8 oz)	210	6	0	190
Pop-Tarts Cherry	1 (1.8 oz)	200	5	0	180
Pop-Tarts Chocolate Graham	1 (1.8 oz)	210	6	0	230
Pop-Tarts Frosted Apple Cinnamon	1 (1.8 oz)	190	3	0	230
Pop-Tarts Frosted Blueberry	1 (1.8 oz)	200	5	0	170
Pop-Tarts Frosted Brown Sugar Cinnamon	1 (1.8 oz)	210	7	0	180
Pop-Tarts Frosted Cherry	1 (1.8 oz)	200	5	0	170
Pop-Tarts Frosted Chocolate Vanilla Creme	1 (1.8 oz)	200	5	0	220
Pop-Tarts Frosted Chocolate Fudge	1 (1.8 oz)	200	5	0	220
Pop-Tarts Frosted Grape	1 (1.8 oz)	200	5	0	170
Pop-Tarts Frosted Raspberry	1 (1.8 oz)	210	5	0	170

FOOD	PORTION	CALS	FAT	CHOL	SOD
Kellogg's (cont.)					
Pop-Tarts Frosted S'mores	1 (1.8 oz)	200	6	0	200
Pop-Tarts Frosted Strawberry	1 (1.8 oz)	200	5	0	170
Pop-Tarts Frosted Wild Berry	1 (2 oz)	210	5	0	170
Pop-Tarts Frosted Wild Watermelon	1 (2 oz)	210	5	0	170
Pop-Tarts Low Fat Blueberry	1 (1.8 oz)	190	3	0	230
Pop-Tarts Low Fat Cherry	1 (1.8 oz)	190	3	0	230
Pop-Tarts Low Fat Frosted Brown Sugar Cinnamon	1 (1.8 oz)	190	3	0	230
Pop-Tarts Low Fat Frosted Chocolate Fudge	1 (1.8 oz)	190	3	0	270
Pop-Tarts Low Fat Frosted Strawberry	1 (1.8 oz)	190	3	0	210
Pop-Tarts Low Fat Strawberry	1 (1.8 oz)	190	3	0	230
Pop-Tarts Strawberry	1 (1.8 oz)	200	5	0	190
Lance					
Dunking Sticks	1 (2.75 oz)	180	10	<5	130
Fig Cake	1/2 piece (2.1 oz)	110	2	0	70
Fig Cake Fat Free	1/2 piece (2.1 oz)	100	0	0	85
Honey Bun	1 (3 oz)	330	13	0	200
Pecan Twirls	1 pkg (2 oz)	220	9	5	140
Swiss Rolls	1 (2.5 oz)	170	9	10	130
Little Debbie					
Angel Cakes Lemon	1 (1.6 oz)	130	1	0	135
Angel Cakes Raspberry	1 (1.6 oz)	130	1	0	125
Banana Nut Loaves	1 (1.9 oz)	220	10	10	220
Banana Twins	1 (2.2 oz)	250	10	10	170
Be My Valentine Chocolate	1 (2.2 oz)	280	13	0	140
Be My Valentine Vanilla	1 (2.2 oz)	290	14	0	125
Blueberry Loaves	1 (2 oz)	220	10	0	200
Chocolate Chip	1 (2.4 oz)	310	15	0	210
Christmas Tree Cake	1 pkg (1.5 oz)	190	10	0	100
Coconut Creme	1 (1.7 oz)	210	10	0	140
Coffee Cake Apple	1 (2.1 oz)	230	7	10	190
Cupcake Creme Filled Chocolate	1 (1.6 oz)	180	9	5	135
Cupcake Creme Filled Orange	1 (1.7 oz)	210	10	0	110
Cupcake Creme Filled Strawberry	1 (1.7 oz)	210	10	0	100
Devil Cremes	1 (1.6 oz)	190	8	0	170
Devil Squares	1 (2.2 oz)	270	13	0	180
Easter Basket Cake Chocolate	1 (2.4 oz)	300	14	0	160
Easter Basket Cake Vanilla	1 (2.5 oz)	320	10	0	150
Fall Party Cake Chocolate	1 (2.4 oz)	290	14	0	170
Fall Party Cake Vanilla	1 (2.5 oz)	310	15	0	170

FOOD	PORTION	CALS	FAT	CHOL	SOD
Fancy Cakes	1 (2.4 oz)	300	15	0	190
Frosted Fudge	1 (1.5 oz)	200	10	<5	105
Golden Cremes	1 (1.5 oz)	150	5	10	120
Holiday Cake Roll Cherry Creme	1 (2.1 oz)	260	12	13	170
Holiday Snack Cake Chocolate	1 (2.4 oz)	300	14	0	150
Holiday Snack Cake Vanilla	1 (2.5 oz)	320	15	0	180
Honey Bun	1 (1.8 oz)	220	13	<5	170
Pecan Spinwheels	1 (1 oz)	110	4	0	80
Snack Cake Chocolate	1 (2.5 oz)	310	15	0	180
Strawberry Shortcake Roll	1 (2.1 oz)	230	8	15	230
Swiss Rolls	1 (2.1 oz)	270	12	15	140
Zebra Cakes	1 (2.6 oz)	330	16	0	160
Natural Touch					
Toaster Square Blueberry	1 (2.8 oz)	180	2	0	65
Toaster Squares Date Walnut	1 (2.8 oz)	200	3	0	50
Nature's Choice					
Toaster Pastries Fat Free Apple Cinnamon	1 (1.9 oz)	180	0	0	180
Toaster Pastries Fat Free Blueberry	1 (1.9 oz)	180	0	0	180
Toaster Pastries Fat Free Raspberry	1 (1.9 oz)	180	0	0	190
Toaster Pastries Fat Free Strawberry	1 (1.9 oz)	180	0	0	190
Toaster Pastries Low Fat Cherry	1 (1.9 oz)	180	3	0	30
Toaster Pastries Low Fat Frosted Blueberry	1 (1.9 oz)	190	2	0	40
Toaster Pastries Low Fat Frosted Chocolate	1 (1.9 oz)	200	3	0	45
Toaster Pastries Low Fat Frosted Cinnamon	1 (1.9 oz)	190	2	0	40
Toaster Pastries Low Fat Frosted Strawberry	1 (1.9 oz)	190	2	0	40
Toaster Pastries Low Fat Peach Apricot	1 (1.9 oz)	180	3	0	30
Pepperidge Farm					
Apple Turnover	1 (3.1 oz)	330	14	0	180
Blueberry Turnovers	1 (3.1 oz)	340	16	0	200
Cherry Turnover	1 (3.1 oz)	320	13	0	190
Large Layer Chocolate Fudge	1/8 cake (2.4 oz)	260	11	30	160
Large Layer Coconut	1/8 cake (2.4 oz)	260	11	35	115
Large Layer Vanilla	1/8 cake (2.4 oz)	250	11	25	120
Mini Turnover Apple	1 (1.4 oz)	140	8	0	80
Mini Turnover Cherry	1 (1.4 oz)	140	8	0	70

FOOD	PORTION	CALS	FAT	CHOL	SOD
Pepperidge Farm (cont.)					
Mini Turnover Strawberry	1 (1.4 oz)	140	7	0	100
Peach Turnover	1 (3.1 oz)	340	15	0	180
Raspberry Turnovers	1 (3.1 oz)	330	14	0	190
Philadelphia					
Snack Bars Classic Cheesecake	1 (1.5 oz)	200	13	35	85
Pillsbury					
Apple Turnovers	1 (2 oz)	170	8	0	310
Cherry Turnovers	1 (2 oz)	180	8	0	310
Sara Lee					
Banana	1/6 cake (2.3 oz)	230	8	20	210
Banana Sundae	1/10 cake (2.8 oz)	270	14	20	140
Carrot	1/6 cake (3.2 oz)	320	17	30	340
Cheesecake Cherry	1/4 cake (4.7 oz)	350	12	35	310
Cheesecake Chocolate Chip	1/4 cake (4.2 oz)	410	21	65	300
Cheesecake Chocolate Mousse	1/5 cake	400	25	30	190
Cheesecake French	1/6 cake	350	21	20	280
Cheesecake Singles Fudge Brownie Crumble	1 slice (4 oz)	400	22	90	250
Cheesecake Singles Strawberry Drizzle	1 slice (4 oz)	380	20	85	240
Cheesecake Strawberry	1/4 pie (4.7 oz)	330	12	40	310
Cheesecake Strawberry French	1/6 cake	320	14	20	230
Cheesecake Bars Chocolate Dipped Original	1 bar (2.7 oz)	190	14	20	50
Cheesecake Bites Chocolate Praline Pecan	1 piece (0.8 oz)	100	6	15	60
Cheesecake Bites Chocolate Dipped Original	1 piece (0.8 oz)	100	7	15	60
Cheesecake Bits Toasted Almond Crunch	1 (0.8 oz)	90	6	15	65
Coffee Cake Butter Streusel	1/6 cake (1.9 oz)	220	12	35	240
Coffee Cake Cheese	1/6 cake (1.9 oz)	180	6	20	230
Coffee Cake Crumb	1/8 cake (2 oz)	220	9	15	210
Coffee Cake Pecan	1/6 cake (1.9 oz)	230	12	25	170
Coffee Cake Raspberry	1/6 cake (1.9 oz)	200	8	15	220
Harvest Pumpkin Spice	1/8 cake (2.9 oz)	270	14	25	200
Layer Cake Coconut	1/8 cake (2.8 oz)	280	14	30	170
Layer Cake Double Chocolate	1/8 cake (2.8 oz)	260	13	25	180
Layer Cake Fudge Golden	1/8 cake (2.8 oz)	270	13	15	160
Layer Cake German Chocolate	1/8 cake (2.9 oz)	280	15	30	160
Layer Cake Vanilla	1/8 cake (2.8 oz)	250	13	35	140
Original Cheesecake Reduced Fat	1/4 cake (4.2 oz)	310	13	70	310

FOOD	PORTION	CALS	FAT	CHOL	SOD
Pound Cake	1/4 cake (2.7 oz)	320	16	85	280
Pound Cake Chocolate Swirl	1 slice (1 oz)	110	5	25	115
Pound Cake Family Size	1/6 cake (2.7 oz)	310	177	75	360
Pound Cake Free & Light	1/4 cake (2.5 oz)	200	4	0	290
Pound Cake Golden	1 slice (1 oz)	120	5	41	90
Pound Cake Reduced Fat	1 slice (1 oz)	100	4	25	125
Pound Cake Strawberry	1/4 cake (2.9 oz)	290	11	60	140
Red White & Blueberry	1/10 cake (3 oz)	210	8	15	135
Slice Chocolate	1 (3 oz)	320	16	40	115
Strawberry Shortcake	1/8 cake (2.5 oz)	180	7	15	140
SnackWell's					
Streusal Squares Apple Cinnamon	1 (1.5 oz)	150	3	0	90
Streusal Squares Cherry	1 (1.5 oz)	150	3	0	110
Tastykake					
Banana Creamie	1 (1.5 oz)	170	7	5	105
Bear Claw Apple	1 (3 oz)	280	7	0	320
Bear Claw Cinnamon	1 (3 oz)	300	8	0	310
Big Texas	1 (3 oz)	300	9	0	360
Breakfast Bun Chocolate Raisin	1 (3.2 oz)	330	8	0	320
Bunny Trail Treats	1 (1.3 oz)	150	6	30	105
Chocolate Creamie	1 (1.5 oz)	180	8	15	120
Chocolate Krimpies	2 (2.2 oz)	240	10	45	250
Coffee Roll Glazed	1 (3 oz)	300	9	0	360
Coffee Roll Vanilla	1 (3.2 oz)	320	9	0	360
Cupcakes Butter Cream Cream Filled Iced	2 (2.2 oz)	240	8	10	250
Cupcakes Chocolate Cream Filled Iced	2 (2.2 oz)	230	8	10	240
Cupcakes	2 (2.1 oz)	200	5	10	240
Cupcakes Low Fat Chocolate Cream Filled	2 (2.2 oz)	200	3	0	250
Cupcakes Low Fat Vanilla Cream Filled	2 (2.2 oz)	190	2	0	210
Cupid Kake	1 (1.3 oz)	150	6	30	105
Honey Bun Glazed	1 (3.2 oz)	350	17	10	210
Honey Bun Iced	1 (3.2 oz)	350	17	10	210
Junior Chocolate	1 (3.3 oz)	330	12	80	180
Junior Coconut	1 (3.3 oz)	310	8	75	180
Junior Koffee Kake	1 (2.5 oz)	270	9	45	200
Junior Pound Kake	1 (3 oz)	320	13	100	320
Kandy Kakes Chocolate	3 (2 oz)	250	13	0	90
Kandy Kakes Coconut	2 (2.7 oz)	330	18	5	105
Kandy Kakes Peanut Butter	2 (1.3 oz)	190	9	10	85
Koffee Kake Cream Filled	2 (2 oz)	240	10	30	150
Koffee Kake Low Fat Apple	2 (2 oz)	170	2	0	170
Koffee Kake Low Fat Lemon	2 (2 oz)	180	3	10	180

FOOD	PORTION	CALS	FAT	CHOL	SOD
Tastykake (cont.)					
Koffee Kake Low Fat Raspberry	2 (2 oz)	170	2	0	180
Kreepy Kakes	2 (2.2 oz)	240	8	20	230
Kreme Krimpies	2 (2 oz)	230	9	55	200
Krimpets Butterscotch Iced	2 (2 oz)	210	5	60	220
Krimpets Jelly Fillled	2 (2 oz)	190	3	45	170
Krimpets Strawberry	2 (2 oz)	210	5	65	220
Kringle Kake	1 (1.3 oz)	150	6	30	105
Santa Snacks	2 (2.2 oz)	240	8	20	230
Sparkle Kake	1 (1.3 oz)	150	6	30	105
Tasty Tweets	2 (2.2 oz)	240	8	20	230
Tropical Delight Coconut	2 (2 oz)	190	9	30	230
Tropical Delight Guava	2 (2 oz)	190	7	15	200
Tropical Delight Papaya	2 (2 oz)	200	7	20	220
Tropical Delight Pineapple	2 (2 oz)	200	7	20	220
Vanilla Creamie	1 (1.5 oz)	190	9	35	115
Witchy Treat	1 (1.3 oz)	150	6	30	90
Tom's					
Honey Bun	1 pkg (3 oz)	360	20	10	200
Honey Bun Jelly Filled	1 pkg (4 oz)	490	29	0	490
Marble Pound	1 pkg (2.5 oz)	300	16	50	380
Texas Cinnamon Roll	1 pkg (4 oz)	360	6	0	470
Tortuga					
Cayman Island Rum Cake	1 piece (2 oz)	194	9	0	198
Weight Watchers					
Chocolate Raspberry Royale	1 (3.5 oz)	190	3	20	220
Chocolate Eclair	1 (2.1 oz)	150	4	30	170
Danish Coffee Cake Apple Cinnamon	1 piece (1.9 oz)	160	3	0	170
Danish Coffee Cake Cheese	1 piece (1.9 oz)	160	3	5	200
Danish Coffee Cake Raspberry	1 piece (1.9 oz)	160	3	0	170
Double Fudge	1 piece (2.75 oz)	190	4	25	200
French Style Cheesecake	1 piece (3.9 oz)	170	4	15	230
New York Style Cheesecake	1 piece (2.5 oz)	150	5	15	140
Strawberry Parfait Royale	1 (5.24 oz)	180	2	10	100
Triple Chocolate Eclair	1 (2.14 oz)	160	5	30	190
take-out					
angelfood	1/12 cake (1 oz)	73	tr	0	212
apple crisp	1/2 cup (5 oz)	230	5	0	257
basbousa namoura	1 piece (1 oz)	60	3	0	144
boston cream pie	1/6 cake (3.3 oz)	293	12	43	309
carrot w/ cream cheese icing	1/12 cake (3.9 oz)	484	29	60	273
cheesecake w/ cherry topping	1/12 cake (5 oz)	359	23	106	254
coffeecake crumb topped cinnamon	1/9 cake (2.2 oz)	263	15	20	221

FOOD	PORTION	CALS	FAT	CHOL	SOD
cream puff w/ custard filling	1 (4.6 oz)	336	20	174	444
french apple tart	1 (3.5 oz)	302	15	60	326
fruitcake	1/36 cake (2.9 oz)	302	10	24	121
gingerbread	1/9 cake (2.6 oz)	264	12	24	242
petit fours	2 (0.9 oz)	120	7	0	15
pineapple upside down	1/9 cake (4 oz)	367	14	25	367
pound fat free	1 oz	80	tr	0	96
pound cake	1 slice (1 oz)	120	5	32	96
sheet cake w/ white frosting	1/9 cake	445	14	70	275
tiramisu	1 piece (5.1 oz)	409	30	171	79
CAKE ICING					
Betty Crocker					
Mix Coconut Pecan as prep	2 tbsp	160	8	0	55
Mix White Fluffy as prep	6 tbsp	100	0	0	60
Ready-To-Spread Butter Cream	2 tbsp (1.3 oz)	150	6	0	70
Ready-To-Spread Cherry	2 tbsp (1.2 oz)	140	5	0	40
Ready-To-Spread Chocolate	2 tbsp (1.2 oz)	130	5	0	95
Ready-To-Spread Chocolate w/ Stars	2 tbsp (1.2 oz)	140	5	0	105
Ready-To-Spread Coconut Pecan	2 tbsp (1.2 oz)	140	8	0	50
Ready-To-Spread Cream Cheese	2 tbsp (1.2 oz)	140	5	0	65
Ready-To-Spread Dark Chocolate	2 tbsp (1.3 oz)	140	6	0	50
Ready-To-Spread French Vanilla	2 tbsp (1.2 oz)	140	5	0	20
Ready-To-Spread Lemon	2 tbsp (1.2 oz)	140	5	0	65
Ready-To-Spread Milk Chocolate	2 tbsp (1.3 oz)	150	6	0	70
Ready-To-Spread Rainbow Chip	2 tbsp (1.2 oz)	140	6	0	25
Ready-To-Spread Sour Cream Chocolate	2 tbsp (1.3 oz)	150	6	0	105
Ready-To-Spread Sour Cream White	2 tbsp (1.3 oz)	150	6	0	45
Ready-To-Spread Strawberry Cream Cheese	2 tbsp (1.3 oz)	150	6	0	70
Ready-To-Spread Vanilla	2 tbsp (1.2 oz)	140	5	0	35
Ready-To-Spread Vanilla w/ Stars	2 tbsp (1.2 oz)	140	5	0	65
Ready-To-Spread Whipped Deluxe Chocolate	2 tbsp (0.8 oz)	100	5	0	45
Ready-To-Spread Whipped Deluxe Cream Cheese	2 tbsp (0.8 oz)	100	5	0	45
Ready-To-Spread Whipped Deluxe Fluffy White	2 tbsp (0.8 oz)	100	4	0	25

FOOD	PORTION	CALS	FAT	CHOL	SOD
Betty Crocker (cont.)					
Ready-To-Spread Whipped Deluxe Lemon	2 tbsp (0.8 oz)	100	5	0	25
Ready-To-Spread Whipped Deluxe Milk Chocolate	2 tbsp (0.8 oz)	100	5	0	50
Ready-To-Spread Whipped Deluxe Strawberry	2 tbsp (0.8 oz)	100	5	0	25
Ready-To-Spread Whipped Deluxe Vanilla	2 tbsp (0.8 oz)	100	5	0	25
Ready-To-Spread White Chocolate	2 tbsp (1.2 oz)	140	5	0	70
Duncan Hines					
Chocolate Creamy Homestyle	2 tbsp	130	5	0	95
Milk Chocolate Creamy Homestyle	2 tbsp	130	5	0	95
Vanilla Creamy Homestyle	2 tbsp	140	5	0	60
Estee					
Frosting as prep	1/5 pkg	100	0	0	0
Sweet Rewards					
Ready-To-Spread Reduced Fat Chocolate	2 tbsp (1.2 oz)	120	3	0	65
Ready-To-Spread Reduced Fat Milk Chocolate	2 tbsp (1.2 oz)	120	3	0	60
Ready-To-Spread Reduced Fat Vanilla	2 tbsp (1.2 oz)	120	2	0	65
CAKE MIX					
(*see also* CAKE)					
Betty Crocker					
Angel Food Confetti	1/12 cake	150	0	0	300
Angel Food One-Step White	1/12 cake	140	0	0	320
Angel Food Swirl	1/12 cake	150	0	0	300
Angel Food Traditional	1/12 cake	130	0	0	160
Butter Chocolate	1/12 cake	270	13	75	380
Butter Pecan	1/12 cake	250	11	55	300
Butter Pecan No Cholesterol Recipe	1/12 cake	210	7	0	300
Butter Yellow	1/12 cake	260	11	75	330
Carrot	1/10 cake	320	15	65	350
Carrot No Cholesterol Recipe	1/10 cake	260	9	0	350
Cherry Chip	1/10 cake	290	12	65	360
Chocolate Chip	1/12 cake	280	14	55	290
Chocolate Chip No Cholesterol Recipe	1/12 cake	210	7	0	290
Chocolate Fudge	1/12 cake	270	12	55	340
Coffee Cake Cinnamon Streusel	1/12 cake	170	7	20	180

FOOD	PORTION	CALS	FAT	CHOL	SOD
Devils Food	1/12 cake	240	11	55	360
Devils Food No Cholesterol Recipe	1/12 cake	200	6	0	360
Double Chocolate Swirl	1/12 cake	250	11	55	390
Double Chocolate Swirl No Cholesterol Recipe	1/12 cake	230	9	0	390
Easy Angel Food	1/4 cake	170	0	0	330
Fat Free Apple Cinnamon	1/8 cake	170	0	0	270
Fat Free Banana	1/8 cake	170	0	0	290
Fat Free Chocolate	1/8 cake	170	0	0	330
Fat Free Lemon	1/8 cake	170	0	0	290
French Vanilla	1/12 cake	250	10	55	280
French Vanilla No Cholesterol Recipe	1/12 cake	210	7	0	280
Fudge Marble	1/12 cake	250	11	55	270
Fudge Marble No Cholesterol Recipe	1/12 cake	220	7	0	270
German Chocolate	1/12 cake	250	11	55	410
German Chocolate No Cholesterol Recipe	1/12 cake	220	7	0	410
Gingerbread	1/8 cake	230	6	25	350
Gingerbread No Cholesterol Recipe	1/8 cake	220	6	0	350
Golden Vanilla	1/12 cake	280	14	55	260
Golden Vanilla No Cholesterol Recipe	1/12 cake	220	7	0	260
Lemon	1/12 cake	280	14	55	260
Lemon No Cholesterol Recipe	1/12 cake	230	8	0	260
Milk Chocolate	1/12 cake	240	10	55	300
Milk Chocolate No Cholesterol Recipe	1/12 cake	230	9	0	300
Party Swirl	1/12 cake	250	11	55	280
Party Swirl No Cholesterol Recipe	1/12 cake	220	7	0	280
Peanut Butter Chocolate Swirl	1/12 cake	240	10	55	320
Peanut Butter Chocolate Swirl No Cholesterol Recipe	1/12 cake	210	6	0	320
Pineapple Upside Down	1/6 cake	400	15	35	350
Pineapple Upside Down No Cholesterol Recipe	1/6 cake	390	14	0	350
Pound Cake	1/8 cake	260	8	55	210
Pound Cake No Cholesterol Recipe	1/8 cake	250	7	0	220
Rainbow Chip	1/12 cake	250	11	55	310
Reduced Fat White	1/12 cake	190	4	0	310

FOOD	PORTION	CALS	FAT	CHOL	SOD
Betty Crocker (cont.)					
Sour Cream White	1/10 cake	280	12	0	380
Spice	1/12 cake	250	11	55	310
Spice No Cholesterol Recipe	1/12 cake	220	7	0	310
Stir'n Bake Carrot Cake w/ Cream Cheese	1 serv	250	7	0	290
Stir'n Bake Cinnamon Streusel Coffee Cake	1 serv	200	6	10	220
Stir'n Bake Devils Food w/ Chocolate	1 serv	240	7	0	260
Strawberry Swirl	1/10 cake	290	12	65	330
Strawberry Swirl No Cholesterol Recipe	1/10 cake	250	7	0	330
White No Cholesterol Recipe	1/12 cake	230	10	0	320
White Richer Recipe	1/12 cake	250	11	55	320
White Chocolate Swirl	1/12 cake	250	11	55	290
White Chocolate Swirl No Cholesterol Recipe	1/12 cake	210	7	0	290
White Olympic Party Cake	1/12 cake	240	11	0	280
White Olympic Party Cake Richer Recipe	1/12 cake	250	11	35	280
Yellow	1/12 cake	250	10	55	300
Yellow No Cholesterol Recipe	1/12 cake	230	9	0	300
Bisquick					
Reduced Fat	1/3 cup (1.4 oz)	150	3	0	460
Dromedary					
Date Bread	1/11 cake (2 oz)	190	7	0	288
Duncan Hines					
Angel Food as prep	1/12 pkg (1.3 oz)	140	0	0	310
Butter Recipe Golden as prep	1/12 cake	320	16	80	190
Cupcake Yellow as prep	1	180	0	6	140
Dark Chocolate Fudge as prep	1/12 cake	290	15	55	360
Devil's Food Moist Deluxe as prep	1/12 cake (1.5 oz)	290	15	55	360
French Vanilla	1/12 cake (1.5 oz)	250	11	55	290
Fudge Marble Moist Deluxe as prep	1/12 cake (1.5 oz)	250	17	45	290
Lemon Supreme Moist Deluxe	1/12 cake (1.5 oz)	250	17	55	290
White Moist Deluxe as prep	1/12 cake	190	6	0	300
Yellow Moist Deluxe as prep	1.5 oz	250	17	55	270
Yellow Moist Deluxe as prep	1/12 cake	250	11	55	290
Estee					
Chocolate as prep	1/5 cake	190	4	0	240
White as prep	1/5 cake	200	4	0	170
Jell-O					
No Bake Cherry Cheesecake as prep	1/8 cake (4.8 oz)	340	12	5	400

FOOD	PORTION	CALS	FAT	CHOL	SOD
No Bake Double Layer Chocolate as prep	1/8 cake (4.4 oz)	260	12	<5	410
No Bake Double Layer Cookies And Creme as prep	1/8 cake (4.5 oz)	390	19	<5	480
No Bake Double Layer Lemon as prep	1/8 cake (4.4 oz)	260	12	<5	370
No Bake Homestyle Cheesecake as prep	1/6 cake (4.6 oz)	360	15	10	550
No Bake Peanut Butter Cup as prep	1/8 cake (3.8 oz)	380	23	<5	380
No Bake Reduced Fat Strawberry Swirl Cheesecake as prep	1/8 cake (4 oz)	250	6	5	430
No Bake Strawberry Cheesecake as prep	1/8 cake (4.8 oz)	340	12	5	400
Real Cheesecake as prep	1/8 cake (4.6 oz)	360	16	5	510
Sweet Rewards					
Reduced Fat Devils Food	1/12 cake	200	5	55	380
Reduced Fat Devils Food No Cholesterol Recipe	1/12 cake	190	4	0	380
Reduced Fat White Whole Egg Recipe	1/12 cake	200	5	35	310
Reduced Fat Yellow	1/12 cake	200	5	55	300
Reduced Fat Yellow No Cholesterol Recipe	1/12 cake	190	4	0	300
CALZONE					
take-out					
cheese	1 (12 oz)	1020	54	100	1760
CANADIAN BACON					
Boar's Head					
Canadian Bacon	2 oz	70	3	30	560
Hormel					
Sandwich Style	3 slices (2 oz)	70	3	30	640
Oscar Mayer					
Canandian Bacon	2 slices (1.6 oz)	50	2	25	620
Yorkshire Farms					
Uncured	3 oz	100	4	44	350
CANADIAN BACON SUBSTITUTES					
Yves					
Canadian Veggie Bacon	1 serv (2 oz)	80	1	0	480
CANDY					
(*see also* CHEWING GUM, MARSHMALLOW)					
butterscotch	1 piece (6 g)	24	tr	1	3
candy corn	1 oz	105	0	0	57
caramels	1 piece (8 g)	31	1	1	20
dark chocolate	1 oz	150	10	0	5
gumdrops	10 sm (0.4 oz)	135	0	0	15

FOOD	PORTION	CALS	FAT	CHOL	SOD
jelly beans	10 sm (0.4 oz)	40	tr	0	3
lollipop	1 (6 g)	22	0	0	2
marzipan	1 oz	128	7	0	5
3 Musketeers					
Bar	2 fun size (1.2 oz)	140	4	5	60
Bar	1 (2.1 oz)	260	8	5	110
5th Avenue					
Snack Size	1 bar (0.58)	80	4	0	25
100 Grand					
Bar	1 bar (1.5 oz)	200	8	10	75
Almond Joy					
Snack Size	1 (0.68 oz)	90	5	0	30
Andes					
Chocolate Covered Mint Patties	1 (0.5 oz)	60	1	0	2
Baby Ruth					
Bar	1 bar (2.1 oz)	270	13	0	130
Fun Size	1 bar (1 oz)	130	6	0	60
Barricini					
Dark Chocolate Raspberry Creme Shells	1 piece (0.3 oz)	47	3	0	4
Bittyfinger					
Bars	2	170	7	0	85
Butterfinger					
BB's	1 pkg (1.7 oz)	230	9	0	95
Bar	1 (2.1 oz)	270	11	0	130
Fun Size	1 bar	100	4	0	45
Cape Cod Provisions					
Cranberry Bog Frogs	3 pieces (1.9 oz)	250	12	7	65
Carmello					
Snack Size	1 (0.66 oz)	90	4	<5	20
Charms					
Blow Pop	1 (0.6 oz)	70	0	0	0
Lollipop Sour	1 (0.6 oz)	70	0	0	0
Lollipop Sweet	1 (0.6 oz)	70	0	0	0
Chunky					
Bar	1 (1.4 oz)	210	11	5	20
Crunch					
Fun Size	4 bars	210	11	10	60
Del Monte					
Radical Raizins Cinnamon	1 pkg (0.7 oz)	70	0	0	0
Radical Raizins Rainbow	1 pkg (0.7 oz)	70	0	0	0
Dove					
Dark Chocolate	1/4 bar (1.5 oz)	230	14	5	0
Dark Chocolate	1 bar (1.3 oz)	200	12	5	0
Dark Chocolate Minatures	7 (1.5 oz)	220	14	5	0
Milk Chocolate	1/4 bar (1.5 oz)	230	13	10	30

FOOD	PORTION	CALS	FAT	CHOL	SOD
Milk Chocolate	1 bar (1.3 oz)	200	12	5	25
Milk Chocolate Minatures	7 (1.5 oz)	230	13	10	30
Estee					
Caramels Vanilla & Chocolate	5	115	5	0	65
Dark Chocolate	1/2 bar (1.4 oz)	200	14	10	10
Milk Chocolate	1/2 bar (1.4 oz)	230	17	20	65
Milk Chocolate w/ Almonds	1/2 bar (1.4 oz)	230	17	20	65
Milk Chocolate w/ Crisp Rice	1/2 bar (1.2 oz)	370	26	30	110
Milk Chocolate w/ Fruit & Nuts	1/2 bar (1.4 oz)	220	16	20	65
Mint Chocolate	1/2 bar (1.4 oz)	200	14	10	10
Peanut Brittle	1/3 box (1.3 oz)	160	9	10	115
Peanut Butter Cups	5	200	12	<5	70
Sugar Free Assorted Fruit	5	30	0	0	0
Sugar Free Assorted Mint	5	30	0	0	0
Sugar Free Butterscotch	2	25	0	0	50
Sugar Free Fruit Gum Drops	23	80	0	0	0
Sugar Free Gourmet Jelly Beans	26	70	0	0	30
Sugar Free Gummy Apple Rings	5	70	0	0	5
Sugar Free Gummy Bears Assorted Fruit	17	100	0	0	5
Sugar Free Licorice Gum Drops	11	90	0	0	65
Sugar Free Peppermint Swirl	3	30	0	0	0
Sugar Free Sour Citrus Slices	9	60	0	0	50
Sugar Free Toffee	5	30	0	0	0
Sugar Free Tropical Fruit	5	30	0	0	0
Godiva					
Chocolatier Dark Chocolate w/ Raspberry	1 bar (1.5 oz)	220	11	3	10
Chocolatier Milk Chocolate	1 bar (1.5 oz)	230	13	10	30
Mochaccino Mousse	2 pieces (1.25 oz)	210	15	4	10
Truffles Assorted	2 pieces (1.5 oz)	220	13	10	15
Goetze's					
Cow Tales	1 pkg (1 oz)	110	3	tr	40
Goo Goo Supreme					
With Pecans	1 pkg (1.5 oz)	188	5	0	51
Goobers					
Peanuts	1 pkg (1.38 oz)	210	13	5	15
Haviland					
Chocolate Covered Thin Mints	6 (1.5 oz)	170	5	0	5
Hershey					
Amazin'Fruit Gummy Candy	1 snack pkg (0.7 oz)	60	0	0	25
Bar	1 (0.6 oz)	100	6	0	5

FOOD	PORTION	CALS	FAT	CHOL	SOD
Hershey (cont.)					
Candy-Coated Milk Chocolate Eggs	4 pieces	90	5	<5	10
Cookies 'n' Mint	1 bar (0.6 oz)	90	5	<5	30
Hugs	1 piece	25	2	0	0
Hugs w/ Almonds	1 piece	25	2	0	0
Kisses	1	25	2	0	0
Kisses w/ Almond	1	25	2	0	0
Milk Chocolate	1 bar (0.6 oz)	90	5	<5	15
Milk Chocolate w/ Almonds	1 bar (0.6 oz)	100	6	<5	15
Miniature Milk Chocolate	1 (0.3 oz)	45	3	0	5
Nuggets Cookies 'n' Creme	1 (0.35 oz)	50	3	0	20
Nuggets Cookies 'n' Mint	1 (0.35 oz)	50	3	0	15
Nuggets Milk Chocolate	1 (0.35 oz)	50	3	0	10
Nuggets Milk Chocolate w/ Almonds	1 (0.35 oz)	50	3	0	10
Pot Of Gold Solitaires	5 pieces	90	6	<5	10
ReeseSticks Snack Size	2 pieces (1.2 oz)	190	11	0	85
Special Dark Miniature	1 (0.3 oz)	45	2	0	0
Sweet Escapes Chocolate Toffee Crisp	1 bar (0.66 oz)	80	4	<5	40
Sweet Escapes Peanut Butter Crispy	1 bar (0.7 oz)	70	3	0	75
Sweet Escapes Triple Chocolate Wafer	1 bar (0.7 oz)	80	3	0	30
Tastetations Butterscotch	3 pieces (0.6 oz)	60	2	<5	85
Tastetations Caramel	3 pieces (0.6 oz)	60	2	<5	85
Tastetations Chocolate	3 pieces (0.6 oz)	60	1	<5	30
Tastetations Chocolate Mint	3 pieces (0.6 oz)	60	2	<5	30
Tastetations Peppermint	3 pieces (0.6 oz)	60	0	0	15
Jolly Rancher					
Lollipops All Flavors	1 (0.6 oz)	60	0	0	10
Junior Mints					
Snack Size	1 pkg (0.7 oz)	75	1	0	5
Just Born					
Hot Tamales	1 pkg (2.1 oz)	220	0	0	25
Mike and Ike Berry Fruits	1 pkg (2.1 oz)	220	0	0	85
Mike and Ike Cherry & Bubble Gum	1 pkg (2.1 oz)	220	0	0	25
Mike and Ike Chewy Grape	1 pkg (2.1 oz)	220	0	0	25
Mike and Ike Lemon Watermelon	1 pkg (2.1 oz)	220	0	0	25
Mike and Ike Original	1 pkg (1.2 oz)	220	0	0	25
Mike and Ike Strawberry & Banana	1 pkg (2.1 oz)	220	0	0	25
Mike and Ike Tropical Fruits	1 pkg (2.1 oz)	220	0	0	25
Super Hot Tamales	1 pkg (2.1 oz)	220	0	0	25

FOOD	PORTION	CALS	FAT	CHOL	SOD
Teenee Beanee Assorted Fruits	36 pieces (1.4 oz)	150	0	0	15
Teenee Beanee Berry Berry	36 pieces (1.4 oz)	150	0	0	15
Teenee Beanee Tropical Mix	36 pieces (1.4 oz)	150	0	0	15
Kit Kat					
Bar	1 (0.56 oz)	80	4	0	10
Krackel					
Bar	1 (0.6 oz)	90	5	<5	25
Miniature	1 (0.3 oz)	45	3	0	10
Lance					
Chocolaty Peanut Bar	1 (2 oz)	290	15	0	90
Cinnamon Chews	1 pkg (1.06 oz)	120	1	0	0
Fruit Chews	1 pkg (1.06 oz)	120	1	0	0
Gum Ball Pops	1 (0.45 oz)	45	0	0	0
K-Nuts	4 pieces (1.5 oz)	240	15	5	130
Mint Chews	1 pkg (1.06 oz)	120	1	0	0
Peanut Bar	1 (1.75 oz)	270	15	0	80
Pop-A-Lance	1 piece (0.42 oz)	45	0	0	0
Popcorn'n'Carmel	1 bar (0.75 oz)	90	0	0	120
Starlight Mints	3 pieces (1 oz)	60	0	0	0
Strawberry Chews	1 pkg (1.06 oz)	120	1	0	0
Suckers	3 pieces (0.5 oz)	50	0	0	6
Whistle Pop	1 (0.67 oz)	70	0	0	0
Lifesavers					
Roll Five Flavor	2 pieces (5 g)	20	0	0	0
Lindt					
Truffles Milk Chocolate	3 pieces (1.3 oz)	210	17	5	20
M&M's					
Peanut	1/2 bag king size	240	12	5	25
Peanut	1 pkg (1.7 oz)	250	13	5	25
Peanut	1.5 oz	220	11	5	20
Peanut	1 fun size (0.7 oz)	110	5	5	10
Peanut Butter	1 fun size (0.7 oz)	110	6	0	45
Peanut Butter	1 pkg (1.6 oz)	240	13	5	100
Peanut Butter	1.5 oz	220	12	5	90
Plain	1 pkg fun size	100	4	5	15
Plain	1.5 oz	200	9	5	30
Plain	1/2 pkg king size	220	9	5	30
Plain	1 pkg (1.7 oz)	230	10	6	35
Mars					
Almond Bar	2 fun size (1.3 oz)	190	10	5	55
Almond Bar	1 bar (1.8 oz)	240	13	5	70
Milk Duds					
Snack Size	4 boxes (1.3 oz)	160	6	0	70
Milky Way					
Bar	2 fun size (1.4 oz)	180	7	5	60
Bar	1/3 king size	160	6	5	50
Bar	1 (2.1 oz)	280	11	5	90

FOOD	PORTION	CALS	FAT	CHOL	SOD
Milky Way (cont.)					
Dark	1 fun size (0.7 oz)	90	3	0	35
Dark	1 bar (1.8 oz)	220	8	5	85
Miniature	5 (1.5 oz)	190	7	5	65
Mounds					
Bar	1 (0.68 oz)	90	5	0	30
Mr. Goodbar					
Miniature	1 (0.3 oz)	45	3	0	0
Necco					
Bridge Mix	1/4 cup (1.5 oz)	180	9	5	35
Chocolate Covered Raisins	30 pieces (1.5 oz)	170	7	0	35
Malted Milk Balls	11 pieces (1.5 oz)	180	6	0	35
SkyBar	1 bar (1.5 oz)	190	9	5	45
Nestle					
Buncha Crunch	1 pkg (1.4 oz)	90	10	10	60
Crunch	1 bar (1.55 oz)	230	12	10	65
Crunch Disk	1 (1.2 oz)	180	9	5	50
Crunchkins	5 pieces	190	10	5	45
Milk Chocolate	1 bar (1.45 oz)	220	13	10	25
Treasures Butterfinger	3 pieces	180	9	5	40
Treasures Crunch	4 pieces (1.4 oz)	210	11	10	60
Treasures Peanut Butter	4 pieces	250	17	5	90
Turtles	2 pieces (1.2 oz)	160	9	<5	40
Turtles Bite Size	1 piece (0.4 oz)	50	2	1	11
White Crunch	1 bar (1.4 oz)	220	13	10	70
Newman's Own					
Organic Peanut Butter Cups Dark Chocolate	3 pieces (1.2 oz)	180	12	0	55
Organic Peanut Butter Cups Milk Chocolate	3 pieces (1.2 oz)	180	12	0	70
Organic Peppermint Cups	3 pieces (1.2 oz)	180	12	0	15
Nibs					
Cherry	1 pkg (0.49 oz)	45	0	0	30
Licorice	1 pkg (0.49 oz)	40	0	0	75
Nips					
Butter Rum	2 pieces	60	2	0	40
Caramel	2 pieces	60	2	0	40
Chocolate	2 pieces	60	2	0	40
Chocolate Parfait	2 pieces	60	2	0	30
Coffee	2 pieces	50	2	0	40
Vanilla Almond Cafe	2 pieces	50	1	0	40
Oh Henry!					
Bar	1 (1.8 oz)	120	5	<5	60
Palmer					
Milk Chocolate Lollipop	1 (0.9 oz)	130	7	4	35
Pearson's					
Irish Cream Parfait	2 pieces	60	2	0	30
Mint Patties	5 (1.3 oz)	150	3	0	70

FOOD	PORTION	CALS	FAT	CHOL	SOD
Pez					
Sugar Free	1 roll (0.3 oz)	30	0	0	0
Planters					
Original Peanut Bar	1 pkg (1.6 oz)	230	14	0	70
Raisinets					
Candy	1 pkg (1.58 oz)	200	8	<5	15
Fun Size	3 pkg (1.7 oz)	200	8	5	15
Reese's					
Nutrageous	1 (0.6 oz)	90	5	0	25
Peanut Butter Cups	1 (0.28 oz)	40	3	0	25
Pieces	25 (0.7 oz)	100	4	0	30
ResseSticks Peanut Butter	2 pieces (1.2 oz)	190	11	0	85
Rokeach					
Cotton Candy	2 cups (1 oz)	110	0	0	0
Rolo					
Caramels In Milk Chocolate	3 pieces (0.64 oz)	90	4	<5	40
Russell Stover					
Assorted Creams	3 pieces (1.4 oz)	180	7	<5	50
Looney Tunes Peanut Butter Nougat w/ Peanuts in Milk Chocolate	1 snack size (0.7 oz)	90	5	<5	60
Peanut Butter & Grape Jelly	1 piece (0.8 oz)	100	6	<5	30
Peanut Butter & Red Raspberry Cups	2 (1.2 oz)	140	9	<5	40
Pecan Delights	1 pkg (1.8 oz)	250	17	10	60
Pecan Roll	1 (1.75 oz)	260	18	<5	80
S'mores	3 (1.4 oz)	210	12	<5	80
Simply Lite					
Sugar Free Lil'l Bits Chocolately	36 pieces (1.4 oz)	130	5	0	55
Sugar Free Lil'l Bits Peanut Buttery	36 pieces (1.4 oz)	140	5	0	50
Sugar Free Patteez	5 pieces (1.3 oz)	110	3	0	10
Skittles					
Original	1.5 oz	170	2	0	5
Tropical	1.5 oz	170	2	0	5
Smucker's					
Fruit Fillers Strawberry	1 pkg (0.9 oz)	80	0	0	25
Jelly Beans	1 pkg (0.7 oz)	70	0	0	10
Snickers					
Bar	1 bar (2.1 oz)	280	14	10	150
Bar	2 bars fun size	190	9	5	100
Sno Caps					
Candies	1 pkg (2.3 oz)	300	13	0	0
Starburst					
Original Fruits	1 stick (2.1 oz)	240	5	0	35
Steel's					
Salt Water Taffy Assorted	3 pieces (1 oz)	90	1	0	50

FOOD	PORTION	CALS	FAT	CHOL	SOD
Swedish Fish					
Original	19 pieces (1.4 oz)	160	0	0	25
Sweet'N Low					
Sugar Free Butter Toffee	4 pieces (0.5 oz)	30	1	<5	80
Sugar Free Butterscotch	1 piece	7	0	0	0
Sugar Free Cinnamon	1 piece	7	0	0	0
Sugar Free Fancy Fruit	1 piece	7	0	0	0
Sugar Free Fruit Flavors	1 piece	7	0	0	0
Sugar Free Hard Candy Coffee	4 pieces (0.5 oz)	30	0	0	20
Sugar Free Peppermint	1 piece	7	0	0	0
Sugar Free Watermelon	1 piece	7	0	0	0
Sugar Free Wild Cherry	1 piece	7	0	0	0
Symphony					
Bar	1 (0.6 oz)	100	6	<5	15
W/ Almonds & Chocolate Chips	1 bar (0.6 oz)	90	6	<5	25
Terry's					
Orange Milk Chocolate	5 pieces (1.5 oz)	240	14	10	40
Tom's					
Cherry Sours	1 pkg (2.25 oz)	210	0	0	30
Jelly Beans	1 pkg (2.25 oz)	230	0	0	30
Twix					
Caramel	1 (1 oz)	140	7	0	60
Caramel	1 fun size (0.5 oz)	80	4	0	30
Caramel	1 pkg (2 oz)	280	14	5	115
Caramel	1 king size (0.8 oz)	120	6	0	45
Peanut Butter	1 (0.9 oz)	130	8	0	70
Twizzlers					
Cherry	1 pieces	35	0	0	35
Chocolate	1 piece	30	0	0	35
Licorice	1 piece	35	0	0	60
Pull'n'Peel Cherry	1 piece (1 oz)	90	0	0	70
Strawberry	1 piece	35	0	0	30
Very Special					
Chocolate Bottles Liquor Filled	3 pieces (1 oz)	150	6	0	10
Whatchamacallit					
Bar	1 (0.58 oz)	80	4	0	35
Whitman's					
Snoopy Treats Caramel Peanuts Milk Chocolate	1 snack size (1.4 oz)	80	5	5	90
York					
Chocolate Covered Peppermint Bites	15 pieces (1 oz)	150	3	0	20
Peppermint Patty	1 (0.49 oz)	50	1	0	0

FOOD	PORTION	CALS	FAT	CHOL	SOD
CANTALOUPE					
dried	3.5 pieces (1.4 oz)	140	0	0	110
fresh cubed	1 cup	57	tr	0	14
fresh half	1/2	94	1	0	23
CARAWAY					
seed	1 tsp	7	tr	0	tr
CARDAMOM					
ground	1 tsp	6	tr	0	tr
CARDOON					
fresh cooked	3 1/2 oz	22	tr	0	176
raw shredded	1/2 cup	36	tr	0	151
CARIBOU					
roasted	3 oz	142	4	93	51
CARISSA					
fresh	1	12	tr	0	1
CAROB					
carob mix	3 tsp	45	0	0	12
carob mix as prep w/ whole milk	9 oz	195	8	33	132
flour	1 tbsp	14	tr	0	3
flour	1 cup	185	1	0	36
CARP					
fresh cooked	3 oz	138	6	72	54
CARROT JUICE					
canned	6 oz	73	tr	0	54
CARROTS					
canned					
Green Giant					
Sliced	1/2 cup (4.2 oz)	25	0	0	380
LeSueur					
Baby Whole	1/2 cup (4.2 oz)	35	0	0	410
fresh					
baby raw	1 (1/2 oz)	6	tr	0	5
raw	1 (2.5 oz)	31	tr	0	25
raw shredded	1/2 cup	24	tr	0	19
slices cooked	1/2 cup	35	tr	0	52
Dole					
Shredded	1 cups (3 oz)	40	0	0	45
frozen					
Birds Eye					
Baby Whole	2/3 cup (3 oz)	35	0	0	45
Green Giant					
Harvest Fresh Baby	2/3 cup (3 oz)	20	0	0	70
Select Baby Cut	3/4 cup (2.8 oz)	30	0	0	40
CASABA					
cubed	1 cup	45	tr	0	20
fresh	1/10 melon	43	tr	0	20

FOOD	PORTION	CALS	FAT	CHOL	SOD
CASHEWS					
cashew butter w/o salt	1 tbsp	94	8	0	2
dry roasted w/ salt	18 nuts (1 oz)	160	13	0	180
Frito Lay					
Salted	1 oz	180	15	0	190
Lance					
Cashews	1 pkg (1 1/8 oz)	200	16	0	90
CASSAVA					
raw	3 1/2 oz	120	tr	0	8
CATFISH					
channel breaded & fried	3 oz	194	11	69	238
CATSUP					
(*see* KETCHUP)					
CAULIFLOWER					
fresh					
cooked	1/2 cup (2.2 oz)	14	tr	0	9
flowerets raw	3 (2 oz)	14	tr	0	17
green cooked	1 1/2 cup (3.2 oz)	29	tr	0	21
frozen					
Birds Eye					
In Cheese Sauce	1/2 cup (4.1 oz)	80	5	5	630
Green Giant					
Cheese Sauce	1/2 cup (3.5 oz)	60	3	<5	510
Florets	1 cup (2.8 oz)	25	0	0	25
CAVIAR					
black	1 tbsp	40	3	94	240
red	1 tbsp	40	3	94	240
CELERIAC					
fresh cooked	3 1/2 oz	25	tr	0	61
CELERY					
diced cooked	1/2 cup	13	tr	0	68
fresh	1 stalk (1.3 oz)	6	tr	0	35
raw diced	1/2 cup	10	tr	0	52
seed	1 tsp	8	tr	0	3
CELTUCE					
raw	3 1/2 oz	22	tr	0	11
CEREAL					
Albers					
Hominy Quick Grits uncooked	1/4 cup	140	1	0	0
Barbara's					
Apple Cinnamon Toasted O's	3/4 cup	110	1	0	90
Bite Size Shredded Oats	1 1/4 cups (2 oz)	220	3	0	260
Breakfast O's	1 cup (1 oz)	120	2	0	115
Brown Rice Crisps	1 cup (1 oz)	120	1	0	125
Cocoa Crunch Stars	1 cup (1 oz)	110	1	0	140
Corn Flakes	1 cup (1 oz)	110	0	0	130
Frosted Corn Flakes	1 cup (1 oz)	110	0	0	100

FOOD	PORTION	CALS	FAT	CHOL	SOD
Honey Crunch Stars	1 cup (1 oz)	110	0	0	50
Honey Nut Toasted O's	3/4 cup	120	2	0	90
Organic Ultra Minis Frosted	3/4 cup (1.9 oz)	190	1	0	200
Organic Ultra Minis Original	3/4 cup (1.9 oz)	190	1	0	240
Organic Fruity Punch	1 cup (1 oz)	110	1	0	120
Puffins	3/4 cup (0.9 oz)	90	1	0	150
Shredded Spoonfuls	3/4 cup (1.1 oz)	120	2	0	200
Shredded Wheat	2 biscuits (1.4 oz)	140	1	0	0
Barbara's Bakery					
Apple Cinnamon O's	3/4 cup	110	1	0	90
Bite Size Shredded Oats	1 1/4 cups (2 oz)	220	3	0	260
Cinnamon Puffins	1 1/4 cup (2 oz)	100	1	0	150
Cocoa Crunch Stars	1 cup (1 oz)	110	1	0	140
Frosted Corn Flakes	1 cup (1 oz)	110	1	0	100
Fruit Juice Sweetened Breakfast O's	1 cup (1 oz)	120	2	0	115
Fruit Juice Sweetened Brown Rice Crisps	1 cup (1 oz)	120	1	0	125
Fruit Juice Sweetened Corn Flakes	1 cup (1 oz)	110	0	0	130
GrainShop	2/3 cup (1 oz)	90	1	0	110
Honey Crunch Stars	1 cup (1 oz)	110	0	0	50
Honey Nut Toasted O's	3/4 cup	120	2	0	90
Organic Fruity Punch	1 cup (1 oz)	110	1	0	120
Organic Soy Essence	3/4 cup (1 oz)	100	1	0	110
Puffins	3/4 cup (0.9 oz)	90	1	0	190
Shredded Spoonfuls	3/4 cup (1.1 oz)	110	2	0	200
Shredded Wheat	2 biscuits (1.4 oz)	140	1	0	0
Betty Crocker					
Dutch Apple	1 cup (1.9 oz)	220	2	0	330
Streusel	3/4 cup (1 oz)	120	2	0	170
General Mills					
Apple Cinnamon Cheerios	3/4 cup (1 oz)	120	2	0	160
Basic 4	1 cup (1.9 oz)	200	2	0	320
Berry Berry Kix	3/4 cup (1 oz)	120	2	0	180
Body Buddies Natural Fruit	1 cup (1 oz)	120	2	0	290
Boo Berry	1 cup (1 oz)	120	1	0	220
Cheerios	1 cup (1 oz)	110	2	0	280
Chex Multi-Bran	1 cup (2 oz)	200	2	0	390
Cinnamon Grahams	3/4 cup (1 oz)	120	1	0	240
Cinnamon Toast Crunch	3/4 cup (1 oz)	130	4	0	210
Cocoa Puffs	1 cup (1 oz)	120	1	0	190
Cookie Crisp	1 cup (1 oz)	120	2	0	115
Corn Chex	1 cup (1 oz)	110	0	0	300
Count Chocula	1 cup (1 oz)	120	1	0	180
Country Corn Flakes	1 cup (1 oz)	120	1	0	290
Crispy Wheaties 'n Raisins	1 cup (1.9 oz)	190	1	0	270
Fiber One	1/2 cup (1 oz)	60	1	0	135

FOOD	PORTION	CALS	FAT	CHOL	SOD
General Mills (cont.)					
Frankenberry	1 cup (1 oz)	120	1	0	210
French Toast Crunch	3/4 cup (1 oz)	120	2	0	170
Frosted Cheerios	1 cup (1 oz)	120	1	0	210
Golden Grahams	3/4 cup (1 oz)	120	1	0	280
Grand Slams Major League	1 cup (1 oz)	120	1	0	160
Honey Frosted Wheaties	3/4 cup (1 oz)	110	1	0	200
Honey Nut Cheerios	1 cup (1 oz)	120	2	0	270
Honey Nut Clusters	1 cup (1.9 oz)	210	3	0	270
Honey Nut Chex	3/4 cup (1 oz)	120	1	0	220
Jurassic Park Crunch	1 cup (1 oz)	120	1	0	200
Kaboom	1 1/4 cup (1 oz)	120	2	0	280
Kix	1 1/3 cup (1 oz)	120	1	0	270
Lucky Charms	1 cup (1 oz)	120	1	0	210
Multi-Bran Chex	1 cup (2 oz)	200	2	0	360
Multi-Grain Cheerios Plus	1 cup (1 oz)	110	1	0	210
Oatmeal Crisp Almond	1 cup (1.9 oz)	220	5	0	250
Oatmeal Crisp Apple Cinnamon	1 cup (1.9 oz)	210	2	0	280
Oatmeal Crisp Raisin	1 cup (1.9 oz)	210	3	0	210
Raisin Nut Bran	3/4 cup (1.9 oz)	200	4	0	250
Reese's Peanut Butter Puffs	3/4 cup (1 oz)	130	3	0	210
Rice Chex	1 1/4 cup (1.1 oz)	120	0	0	280
Sunrise Organic	3/4 cup (1 oz)	110	1	0	190
Team Cheerios	1 cup (1 oz)	120	1	0	220
Total Corn Flakes	1 1/3 cup (1 oz)	110	1	0	210
Total Raisin Bran	1 cup (1.9 oz)	180	1	0	240
Total Whole Grain	3/4 cup (1 oz)	110	1	0	200
Trix	1 cup (1 oz)	120	2	0	200
USA Olympic Crunch	1 cup (1 oz)	120	1	0	200
Wheat Chex	1 cup (1.9 oz)	180	1	0	420
Wheat Hearts	1/4 cup (1.3 oz)	130	1	0	0
Wheaties	1 cup (1 oz)	110	1	0	220
Health Valley					
10 Bran O's Apple Cinnamon	3/4 cup	100	0	0	90
Bran w/ Apples & Cinnamon	3/4 cup	160	0	0	10
Golden Flax	1/2 cup	190	3	0	30
Granola 98% Fat Free Date Almond	2/3 cup	180	1	0	90
Healthy Crunches & Flakes Almond	3/4 cup	130	0	0	35
Healthy Crunches & Flakes Apple Cinnamon	3/4 cup	130	0	0	35
Healthy Crunches & Flakes Honey Crunch	3/4 cup	130	0	0	35
Hot Cereal Cups Amazing Apple!	1 pkg	220	2	0	230

FOOD	PORTION	CALS	FAT	CHOL	SOD
Hot Cereal Cups Banana Gone Nuts	1 pkg	240	3	0	240
Hot Cereal Cups Maple Madness!	1 pkg	240	2	0	290
Hot Cereal Cups Terrific 10 Grain!	1 pkg	220	3	0	210
Oat Bran O'S	3/4 cup	100	0	0	90
Organic Amaranth Flakes	3/4 cup	100	0	0	35
Organic Blue Corn Bran Flakes	3/4 cup	100	0	0	10
Organic Bran w/ Raisin	3/4 cup	160	0	0	10
Organic Fiber 7 Flakes	3/4 cup	100	0	0	15
Organic Healthy Fiber Flakes	3/4 cup	100	0	0	10
Organic Oat Bran Flakes	3/4 cup	100	0	0	15
Organic Oat Bran Flakes w/ Raisins	3/4 cup	110	0	0	15
Puffed Honey Sweetened Corn	1 cup	110	0	0	0
Puffed Honey Sweetened Crisp Brown Rice	1 cup	110	0	0	0
Raisin Bran Flakes	1 1/4 cup	190	0	0	90
Real Oat Bran	1/2 cup	200	3	0	90
Healthy Choice					
Almond Crunch w/ Raisins	1 cup (2 oz)	210	3	0	230
Golden Multi-Grain Flakes	3/4 cup (1.1 oz)	110	0	0	180
Toasted Brown Sugar Squares	1 cup (2 oz)	190	1	0	5
Kashi					
Breakfast Pilaf as prep	1/2 cup (4.9 oz)	170	3	0	15
Go Apple Spice	1/2 cup (4.9 oz)	270	3	0	0
Go Banana Almond	1/2 cup (4.9 oz)	280	4	0	5
Go Berry Tart	1/2 cup (4.9 oz)	260	3	0	5
Go Blueberry Bliss	1/2 cup (4.9 oz)	260	3	0	5
Go Cherry Vanilla	1/2 cup (4.9 oz)	260	3	0	15
Go Just Peachy	1/2 cup (4.9 oz)	260	3	0	0
GoLean	3/4 cup (1.4 oz)	120	1	0	35
Good Friends	3/4 cup (1 oz)	90	1	0	70
Honey Puffed	1 cup (1 oz)	120	1	0	6
Medley	1/2 cup (1 oz)	100	1	0	50
Pillows Apple	3/4 cup (1.9 oz)	200	1	0	30
Pillows Chocolate	3/4 cup (1.9 oz)	200	1	0	50
Pillows Strawberry Crisp	3/4 cup (1.9 oz)	200	1	0	25
Puffed	1 cup (0.9 oz)	70	tr	0	0
Kellogg's					
All-Bran	1/2 cup (1.1 oz)	80	1	0	65
All-Bran Bran Buds	1/3 cup (1 oz)	80	1	0	210
All-Bran Extra Fiber	1/2 cup (0.9 oz)	50	1	0	120
Apple Jacks	1 cup (1.2 oz)	120	0	0	150

FOOD	PORTION	CALS	FAT	CHOL	SOD
Kellogg's (cont.)					
Cocoa Frosted Flakes	3/4 cup (1.1 oz)	120	0	0	210
Cocoa Krispies	3/4 cup (1.1 oz)	120	1	0	220
Complete Oat Bran Flakes	3/4 cup (1 oz)	110	1	0	270
Complete Wheat Bran Flakes	3/4 cup (1 oz)	90	1	0	220
Corn Flakes	1 cup (1 oz)	100	0	0	300
Corn Pops K-Sentials	1 oz	100	0	0	110
Cracklin' Oat Bran	3/4 cup (1.7 oz)	190	7	0	170
Crispix	1 cup (1 oz)	110	0	0	210
Froot Loops K-Sentials	1 oz	100	1	0	130
Frosted Flakes	3/4 cup (1.1 oz)	120	0	0	200
Granola Low Fat	1/2 cup (1.7 oz)	190	3	0	120
Honey Crunch Corn Flakes	3/4 cup (1.1 oz)	120	1	0	210
Just Right Crunchy Nuggets	1 cup (2 oz)	210	2	0	320
Just Right Fruit & Nut	1 cup (2.1 oz)	220	2	0	280
Low Fat w/ Raisins	2/3 cup (2.1 oz)	220	3	0	150
Mini-Wheats Apple Cinnamon Squares	3/4 cup (1.9 oz)	180	1	0	20
Mini-Wheats Blueberry Squares	3/4 cup (1.9 oz)	180	1	0	20
Mini-Wheats Frosted	1 cup (1.8 oz)	180	1	0	5
Mini-Wheats Frosted Bite Size	24 pieces (2.1 oz)	200	1	0	5
Mini-Wheats Raisin Squares	3/4 cup (1.9 oz)	180	1	0	5
Mini-Wheats Strawberry Squares	3/4 cup (1.8 oz)	170	1	0	15
Mueslix Apple & Almond Crunch	3/4 cups (1.9 oz)	200	5	0	260
Mueslix Raisin & Almond	2/3 cup (1.9 oz)	200	3	0	160
Nutri-Grain Almond Raisin	1 1/4 cup (1.7 oz)	180	3	0	170
Nutri-Grain Golden Wheat	3/4 cup (1 oz)	100	1	0	210
Product 19	1 cup (1 oz)	100	0	0	210
Raisin Bran	1 cup (2.1 oz)	200	2	0	370
Rice Krispies	1 1/4 cup (1.2 oz)	120	0	0	350
Rice Krispies Razzle Dazzle	3/4 cup (1 oz)	110	0	0	170
Rice Krispies Treats	3/4 cup (1 oz)	120	2	0	190
Smacks	3/4 cup (1 oz)	100	1	0	50
Smart Start	1 cup (1.8 oz)	180	1	0	310
Special K	1 cup (1.1 oz)	110	0	0	220
Kolln					
Crispy Oats	1 cup (1.8 oz)	190	3	0	210
Oat Bran Crunch	2/3 cup (2.1 oz)	220	5	0	0
Oat Muesli Fruit	3/4 cup (2 oz)	200	5	0	15
Lundberg					
Purely Organic Hot'n Creamy Rice	1/3 cup	190	2	0	0
McCann's					
Irish Oatmeal	1 oz	110	2	0	0

FOOD	PORTION	CALS	FAT	CHOL	SOD
Morning Traditions					
Banana Nut Crunch	1 cup (2 oz)	250	6	0	240
Blueberry Morning	1 1/4 cup (1.9 oz)	220	3	0	250
Cranberry Almond Crunch	1 cup (1.9 oz)	220	3	0	200
Great Grains Crunchy Pecan	2/3 cup (1.9 oz)	220	6	0	190
Great Grains Raisins Dates & Pecans	2/3 cup (1.9 oz)	210	5	0	160
Nabisco					
100% Bran	1/3 cup (1 oz)	80	1	0	120
Frosted Shredded Wheat Bite Size	1 cup (1.8 oz)	190	1	0	10
Honey Nut Shredded Wheat Bite Size	1 cup (1.8 oz)	200	2	0	40
Original Shredded Wheat	2 biscuits (1.6 oz)	160	1	0	0
Original Shredded Wheat 'N Bran	1 1/4 cup (2.1 oz)	200	1	0	0
Original Shredded Wheat Spoon Size	1 cup (1.7 oz)	170	1	0	0
Nature Valley					
Granola Low Fat Fruit	2/3 cup (1.9 oz)	210	3	0	210
Post					
Alpha-Bits	1 cup (1 oz)	130	2	0	210
Alpha-Bits Marshmallow	1 cup (1 oz)	120	1	0	160
Bran Flakes	3/4 cup (1 oz)	100	1	0	220
Cocoa Pebbles	3/4 cup (1 oz)	120	1	0	160
Fruit & Fibre Dates Raisins & Walnuts	1 cup (1.9 oz)	210	3	0	250
Fruit & Fibre Peaches Raisins & Almonds	1 cup (1.9 oz)	210	3	0	260
Fruity Pebbles	3/4 cup (1 oz)	110	1	0	160
Golden Crisp	3/4 cup (1 oz)	110	0	0	40
Grape-Nuts	3/4 cup (1 oz)	100	1	0	140
Grape-Nuts Flakes	3/4 cup (1 oz)	100	1	0	140
Honey Bunches Of Oats	3/4 cup (1 oz)	120	2	0	190
Honey Bunches Of Oats With Almonds	3/4 cup (1.1 oz)	130	3	0	180
Honeycomb	1 1/3 cups (1 oz)	110	1	0	220
Post Toasties	1 cup (1 oz)	100	0	0	270
Raisin Bran	1 cup (2 oz)	190	1	0	300
Selects Blueberry Morning	3/4 cup (1.3 oz)	140	2	0	150
Waffle Crisp	1 cup (1 oz)	130	3	0	120
Quaker					
Instant Grits Original	1 pkg (1 oz)	100	0	0	300
Multigrain	1/2 cup (1.4 oz)	130	2	0	10
Oatmeal Instant	1 pkg (1 oz)	100	2	0	80
Oatmeal Instant Apples & Cinnamon	1 pkg (1.2 oz)	130	2	0	170

FOOD	PORTION	CALS	FAT	CHOL	SOD
Quaker (cont.)					
Oatmeal Instant Bananas & Cream	1 pkg (1.2 oz)	130	3	0	170
Oatmeal Instant Blueberries & Cream	1 pkg (1.2 oz)	130	3	0	160
Oatmeal Instant Cinnamon & Spice	1 pkg (1.6 oz)	170	2	0	240
Oatmeal Instant Kid's Choice Chocolate Chip Cookie	1 pkg (1.5 oz)	160	3	0	200
Oatmeal Instant Kid's Choice Cookie'n Cream	1 pkg (1.5 oz)	160	3	0	200
Oatmeal Instant Kid's Choice Fruity Marshmallow	1 pkg (1.4 oz)	150	2	0	190
Oatmeal Instant Kid's Choice Oatmeal Raisin Cookie	1 pkg (1.5 oz)	160	2	0	220
Oatmeal Instant Kid's Choice Radical Raspberry	1 pkg (1.4 oz)	150	3	0	180
Oatmeal Instant Kid's Choice S'mores	1 pkg (1.5 oz)	160	3	0	220
Oatmeal Instant Kid's Choice Strawberries'n Stuff	1 pkg (1.4 oz)	150	2	0	180
Oatmeal Instant Kid's Choice Twisted Strawberry Banana	1 pkg (1.4 oz)	150	2	0	180
Oatmeal Instant Maple & Brown Sugar	1 pkg (1.5 oz)	160	2	0	240
Oatmeal Instant Peaches & Cream	1 pkg (1.2 oz)	140	3	0	170
Oatmeal Instant Raisin & Spice	1 pkg (1.5 oz)	150	2	0	250
Oatmeal Instant Raisin Date & Walnut	1 pkg (1.3 oz)	140	3	0	240
Oatmeal Instant Strawberries & Cream	1 pkg (1.2 oz)	140	3	0	170
Oatmeal Nutrition for Women Golden Brown Sugar	1 pkg (1.6 oz)	170	2	0	310
Oatmeal Quick'n Hearty Microwave	1 pkg (1 oz)	110	2	0	150
Oatmeal Quick'n Hearty Microwave Apple Spice	1 pkg (1.6 oz)	170	2	0	280
Oatmeal Quick'n Hearty Microwave Brown Sugar Cinnamon	1 pkg (1.5 oz)	150	2	0	260
Oatmeal Quick'n Hearty Microwave Cinnamon Double Raisin	1 pkg (1.6 oz)	170	2	0	280

FOOD	PORTION	CALS	FAT	CHOL	SOD
Oatmeal Quick'n Hearty Microwave Honey Bran	1 pkg (1.4 oz)	150	2	0	250
Oats Old Fashion	1/2 cup (1.4 oz)	150	3	0	0
Oats Quick	1/2 cup (1.4 oz)	150	3	0	0
Oats Steel Cut	1/2 cup (1.4 oz)	150	3	0	0
Whole Wheat Hot Natural	1/2 cup (1.4 oz)	130	1	0	0
Sunbelt					
Berry Basic	1/2 cup (1.9 oz)	220	6	0	200
Granola Banana Nut	1/2 cup (1.9 oz)	250	9	0	60
Granola Cinnamon Raisins	1/2 cup (1.9 oz)	200	3	0	80
Granola Fruit & Nut	1/2 cup (1.9 oz)	240	7	0	70
Muesli 5 Whole Grains	1/2 cup (1.9 oz)	210	2	0	70
Wheatena					
Cereal	1/3 cup (1.4 oz)	150	1	0	0

CEREAL BARS

(*see also* ENERGY BARS, NUTRITION SUPPLEMENTS)

FOOD	PORTION	CALS	FAT	CHOL	SOD
Barbara's Bakery					
Nature's Choice Apple Cinnamon	1 bar (1.3 oz)	120	2	0	75
Nature's Choice Blueberry	1 bar (1/3 oz)	120	2	0	75
Nature's Choice Cherry	1 bar (1.3 oz)	120	2	0	75
Nature's Choice Granola Carob Chip	1 bar (0.7 oz)	80	2	0	5
Nature's Choice Granola Cinnamon & Raisin	1 bar (0.7 oz)	80	2	0	5
Nature's Choice Granola Oats 'N Honey	1 bar (0.7 oz)	80	2	0	5
Nature's Choice Granola Peanut Butter	1 bar (0.7 oz)	80	3	0	5
Nature's Choice Raspberry	1 bar (1.3 oz)	120	2	0	75
Nature's Choice Strawberry	1 bar (1.3 oz)	120	2	0	75
Nature's Choice Triple Berry	1 bar (1.3 oz)	120	2	0	75
Cap'n Crunch					
Bar	1 (0.8 oz)	90	2	0	105
Berries Bar	1 (0.8 oz)	90	2	0	110
Dolly Madison					
Apple	1 (1.3 oz)	120	2	0	90
Blueberry	1 (1.3 oz)	120	2	0	90
Raspberry	1 (1.3 oz)	120	2	0	100
Strawberry	1 (1.3 oz)	120	2	0	100
Entenmann's					
Apple Cinnamon	1 (1.3 oz)	140	3	0	85
Blueberry	1 (1.3 oz)	140	3	0	90
Oatmeal Apple Cinnamon	1 (1.3 oz)	140	3	0	110
Oatmeal Apple Raisin	1 (1.3 oz)	140	3	0	110
Raspberry	1 (1.3 oz)	140	3	0	110
Strawberry	1 (1.3 oz)	140	3	0	90

FOOD	PORTION	CALS	FAT	CHOL	SOD
Estee					
Rice Crunchie Chocolate	1 (0.7 oz)	50	0	0	40
Rice Crunchie Chocolate Chip	1 (0.7 oz)	50	0	0	40
Rice Crunchie Peanut Butter	1 (0.7 oz)	60	1	0	35
Rice Crunchie Vanilla	1 (0.7 oz)	60	0	0	35
General Mills					
Golden Grahams Treats	1 (0.8 oz)	90	2	0	110
Golden Grahams Treats Marshmallow Graham	1 (0.8 oz)	90	3	0	110
Golden Grahams Treats S'mores Chocolate Chunk	1 (0.8 oz)	90	3	0	100
Milk 'N Cereal Bars Chex	1 bar (1.6 oz)	160	4	0	150
Milk 'N Cereal Bars Cinnamon Toast Crunch	1 bar (1.6 oz)	180	4	0	160
Milk 'N Cereal Bars Honey Nut Cherrios	1 bar (1.6 oz)	160	4	0	150
Glenny's					
Chocolate Crunch Creamy Low Fat	1 bar (1.75 oz)	190	3	0	113
Chocolate Crunch Roasted Peanut	1 bar (1.75 oz)	200	4	0	100
Chocolate Crunch Toasted Almond	1 bar (1.75 oz)	200	4	0	100
Health Valley					
98% Fat Free Raisin Cinnamon	2/3 cup	180	1	0	90
98% Fat Free Tropical	2/3 cup	180	1	0	90
Blueberry	1 bar	140	0	0	5
Breakfast Bakes Apple Cinnamon	1 bar	110	0	0	25
Breakfast Bakes California Strawberry	1 bar	110	0	0	25
Breakfast Bakes Mountain Blueberry	1 bar	110	0	0	25
Breakfast Bakes Red Raspberry	1 bar	110	0	0	25
Chocolate Chip	1 bar	140	0	0	5
Crisp Rice Bars Apple Cinnamon	1 bar	110	0	0	5
Crisp Rice Bars Orange Date	1 bar	110	0	0	5
Crisp Rice Bars Tropical Fruit	1 bar	110	0	0	5
Date Almond	1 bar	140	0	0	5
Fiber 7 Flakes w/ Strawberry	1 bar	110	0	0	25
O's Almond	3/4 cup	120	0	0	90
O's Apple Cinnamon	3/4 cup	120	0	0	90
O's Honey Crunch	3/4 cup	120	0	0	90
Oat Bran Flakes w/ Blueberry	1 bar	110	0	0	25
Raisin	1 bar	140	0	0	5

FOOD	PORTION	CALS	FAT	CHOL	SOD
Raisin Bran Flakes w/ Apple Raisin	1 bar	110	0	0	25
Raspberry	1 bar	140	0	0	5
Strawberry	1 bar	140	0	0	5
Hershey's					
Crispy Rice Snacks Peanut Butter	1 bar (0.5 oz)	60	2	0	57
Hostess					
Apple	1 (1.3 oz)	120	2	0	90
Banana Nut	1 (1.3 oz)	120	2	0	80
Blueberry	1 (1.3 oz)	120	2	0	90
Raspberry	1 (1.3 oz)	120	2	0	100
Strawberry	1 (1.3 oz)	120	2	0	100
Kellogg's					
Nutri-Grain Apple Cinnamon	1 (1.3 oz)	140	3	0	110
Nutri-Grain Blueberry	1 (1.3 oz)	140	3	0	110
Nutri-Grain Cherry	1 (1.3 oz)	140	3	0	110
Nutri-Grain Mixed Berry	1 (1.3 oz)	140	3	0	110
Nutri-Grain Peach	1 (1.3 oz)	140	3	0	110
Nutri-Grain Raspberry	1 (1.3 oz)	140	3	0	110
Nutri-Grain Strawberry	1 (1.3 oz)	140	3	0	110
Nutri-Grain Twists Low Fat Apple Cinnamon	1 (1.3 oz)	140	3	0	105
Nutri-Grain Twists Low Fat Banana Strawberry	1 (1.3 oz)	140	3	0	100
Nutri-Grain Twists Low Fat Strawberry Blueberry	1 (1.3 oz)	140	3	0	110
Rice Krispies Treats	1 (0.8 oz)	90	2	0	100
Rice Krispies Treats Cocoa	1 (0.8 oz)	100	4	0	105
Rice Krispies Treats Peanut Butter Chocolate	1 (0.8 oz)	110	4	0	100
Kudos					
Chocolate Coated Chocolate Chip	1	120	5	0	75
Chocolate Coated Peanut Butter	1	90	3	0	105
Snickers	1	100	4	0	105
With M&M's	1	90	3	0	105
Little Debbie					
Raspberry	1 (1.3 oz)	130	3	0	75
S'mores Granola Treats	1 (1 oz)	130	5	0	45
Strawberry	1 (1.3 oz)	130	3	0	75
Nabisco					
Nutter Butter Granola Bar	1 (1 oz)	120	8	0	45
Oreo Granola Bar	1 (1 oz)	120	4	0	65
Nature Valley					
Crunchy Cinnamon	2 bars (1.6 oz)	200	6	0	170
Crunchy Oats'n Honey	2 bars (1.6 oz)	200	6	0	170

FOOD	PORTION	CALS	FAT	CHOL	SOD
Nature Valley (cont.)					
Crunchy Peanut Butter	2 bars (1.6 oz)	200	6	0	170
Low Fat Chewy Apple Brown Sugar	1 bar (1 oz)	110	2	0	80
Low Fat Chewy Chocolate Chip	1 bar (1 oz)	110	2	0	90
Low Fat Chewy Honey Nut	1 bar (1 oz)	110	2	0	80
Low Fat Chewy Oatmeal Raisin	1 bar (1 oz)	110	2	0	70
Low Fat Chewy Orchard Blend	1 bar (1 oz)	110	2	0	65
Low Fat Chewy Triple Berry	1 bar (1 oz)	110	2	0	60
Nature's Choice					
Carob Chip	1 bar (0.7 oz)	80	3	0	5
Cinnamon & Raisin	1 bar (0.7 oz)	80	2	0	5
Fat Free Apple	1 bar (1.3 oz)	110	0	0	90
Fat Free Blueberry	1 bar (1.3 oz)	110	0	0	90
Fat Free Cranberry	1 bar (1.3 oz)	110	0	0	110
Fat Free Peach	1 bar (1.3 oz)	110	0	0	90
Fat Free Raspberry	1 bar (1.3 oz)	110	0	0	110
Fat Free Strawberry	1 bar (1.3 oz)	110	0	0	110
Low Fat Triple Berry	1 bar (1.3 oz)	130	2	0	190
Low Fat Very Cherry	1 bar (1.3 oz)	130	2	0	190
Oats 'n Honey	1 bar (0.7 oz)	80	2	0	5
Peanut Butter	1 bar (0.7 oz)	80	3	0	5
Nutri-Grain					
Fruit-full Squares Apple	1 (1.7 oz)	180	4	0	95
Fruit-full Squares Banana	1 (1.7 oz)	190	5	0	95
Fruit-full Squares Cinnamon Raisin	1 (1.7 oz)	180	4	0	95
Quaker					
Chewy Chocolate Chip	1 (1 oz)	120	4	0	70
Chewy Cookies 'n Cream	1 (1 oz)	110	3	0	80
Chewy Peanut Butter Chocolate Chunk	1 (1 oz)	120	3	0	105
Chewy Graham Slam Chocolate Chip	1 (1 oz)	110	2	0	75
Chewy Graham Slam Peanut Butter	1 (1 oz)	110	2	0	80
Chewy Low Fat Chocolate Chunk	1 (1 oz)	110	2	0	80
Chewy Low Fat Oatmeal Raisin	1 (1 oz)	110	2	0	70
Chewy Low Fat S'mores	1 (1 oz)	110	2	0	80
Fruit & Oatmeal Apple Cinnamon	1 (1.3 oz)	130	3	0	95
Fruit & Oatmeal Low Fat Cherry Cobbler	1 (1.3 oz)	140	3	0	95

FOOD	PORTION	CALS	FAT	CHOL	SOD
Fruit & Oatmeal Low Fat Strawberry	1 (1.3 oz)	140	3	0	125
Fruit & Oatmeal Low Fat Strawberry Banana	1 (1.3 oz)	130	3	0	100
Fruit & Oatmeal Low Fat Strawberry Cheesecake	1 (1.3 oz)	130	3	0	125
SnackWell's					
Country Fruit Medley	1 (1.3 oz)	130	3	0	75
Fat Free Apple Cinnamon	1 (1.3 oz)	120	0	0	115
Fat Free Blueberry	1 (1.3 oz)	120	0	0	85
Fat Free Strawberry	1 (1.3 oz)	120	0	0	115
Hearty Fruit'n Grain Crisp Autumn Apple	1 (1.3 oz)	130	3	0	95
Hearty Fruit'n Grain Mixed Berry	1 (1.3 oz)	120	3	0	95
Hearty Fruit'n Grain Orchard Cherry	1 (1.3 oz)	130	5	0	90
Sunbelt					
Apple	1 (1.3 oz)	130	3	0	75
Blueberry	1 (1.3 oz)	130	3	0	75
Chewy Granola Almond	1 (1 oz)	130	7	0	65
Chewy Granola Apple Cinnamon	1 (1.2 oz)	140	3	0	105
Chewy Granola Chocolate Chip	1 (1.2 oz)	160	7	0	70
Chewy Granola Oatmeal Raisin	1 (1.2 oz)	130	3	0	100
Chewy Granola Oats & Honey	1 (1 oz)	120	5	0	65
Granola Fudge Dipped Chocolate Chip	1 (1.5 oz)	200	10	0	70
Granola Fudge Dipped Macaroon	1 (1.4 oz)	190	10	0	65
Weight Watchers					
Apple Cinnamon	1 (1 oz)	100	2	0	95
Blueberry	1 (1 oz)	100	2	0	90
Raspberry	1 (1 oz)	100	2	0	90
CHAYOTE					
fresh cooked	1 cup	38	1	0	1
raw	1 (7 oz)	49	1	0	8
raw cut up	1 cup	32	tr	0	198
CHEESE					
(*see also* CHEESE DISHES, CHEESE SUBSTITUTES, COTTAGE CHEESE, CREAM CHEESE, NEUFCHATEL)					
cacio di roma sheep's milk cheese	1 oz	130	10	30	170
camembert	1 oz	85	7	20	239

FOOD	PORTION	CALS	FAT	CHOL	SOD
cantal	1 oz	105	9	26	269
chabichou	1 oz	95	8	23	189
chaource	1 oz	83	7	20	230
cheshire	1 oz	110	9	29	198
comte	1 oz	114	9	34	105
coulommiers	1 oz	88	7	23	195
crottin	1 oz	105	9	23	133
emmentaler	3 1/2 oz	403	30	92	450
feta	1 oz	75	6	25	316
goat fresh	1 oz	23	2	5	18
goat hard	1 oz	128	10	30	98
goat semisoft	1 oz	103	8	22	146
goat soft	1 oz	76	6	13	104
gouda	1 oz	101	8	32	232
gruyere	1 oz	117	9	31	95
limburger	1 oz	93	8	26	227
maroilles	1 oz	97	8	26	300
morbier	1 oz	99	8	23	283
pont l'eveque	1 oz	86	7	20	191
port du salut	1 oz	100	8	35	151
pyrenees	1 oz	101	8	26	235
quark 20% fat	3 1/2 oz	116	5	17	35
quark 40% fat	3 1/2 oz	167	11	37	34
quark made w/ skim milk	3 1/2 oz	78	tr	1	40
queso anego	1 oz	106	9	30	321
queso asadero	1 oz	101	8	30	186
queso chichuahua	1 oz	106	8	30	175
raclette	1 oz	102	8	26	217
reblochon	1 oz	88	7	23	240
rouy	1 oz	95	8	23	138
saint marcellin	1 oz	94	8	23	171
saint nectaire	1 oz	97	8	23	169
saint paulin	1 oz	85	6	20	174
sainte maure	1 oz	99	8	23	411
selles sur cher	1 oz	93	8	20	181
tilsit	1 oz	96	7	29	213
tome	1 oz	92	7	23	231
triple creme	1 oz	113	11	34	86
vacherin	1 oz	92	8	23	129
yogurt cheese	1 oz	80	7	15	60
Alpine Lace					
American Jalapeno Peppers	1 slice (1 oz)	80	6	20	260
American Less Fat Less Sodium White	1 slice (1 oz)	50	6	20	200
American Less Fat Less Sodium Yellow	1 slice (1 oz)	80	6	20	200
Cheddar Reduced Fat	1 slice (1 oz)	70	5	15	170
Colby Reduced Fat	1 slice (1 oz)	80	5	15	115

FOOD	PORTION	CALS	FAT	CHOL	SOD
Fat Free Parmesan	2 tsp (5 g)	10	0	0	65
Feta Reduced Fat	1 oz	50	3	10	370
Feta Reduced Fat Sun Dried Tomato & Basil	1 oz	50	3	10	370
Goat Reduced Fat	1 oz	40	3	5	130
Mozzarella Reduced Fat	1 oz	70	3	10	200
Muenster Reduced Sodium	1 slice (1 oz)	100	9	25	85
Provolone Smoked Reduced Fat	1 slice (1 oz)	70	5	15	120
Swiss Reduced Fat	1 slice (1 oz)	90	6	20	35
Boar's Head					
American	1 oz	100	9	25	380
Baby Swiss	1 oz	110	9	25	135
Canadian Cheddar	1 oz	110	10	35	170
Double Glouster Yellow	1 oz	110	10	35	200
Havarti	1 oz	110	10	35	210
Havarti w/ Dill	1 oz	110	10	35	210
Havarti w/ Jalapeno	1 oz	110	10	35	210
Lacey Swiss	1 oz	90	6	15	35
Longhorn Colby	1 oz	110	9	30	170
Monerey Jack	1 oz	100	9	25	170
Monerey Jack w/ Jalapeno	1 oz	100	9	25	170
Mozzarella	1 oz	90	7	25	140
Muenster	1 oz	100	8	25	180
Muenster Low Sodium	1 oz	100	8	20	75
Provolone Picante Sharp	1 oz	100	8	25	250
Swiss	1 oz	110	8	20	65
Swiss No Salt Added	1 oz	110	8	25	10
Breakstone's					
Ricotta	1/4 cup (2.2 oz)	110	8	25	90
Cabot					
Cheddar	1 oz	110	9	30	180
Cheddar Five Peppercorn	1 oz	110	9	30	180
Cheddar Mediterranean	1 oz	110	9	30	180
Cheddar Sundried Tomato Basil	1 oz	110	9	30	180
Cheddar Toasted Onion & Chive	1 oz	110	9	30	180
Cheddar Light 50% Reduced Fat	1 oz	70	5	15	170
Cheddar Light 50% Reduced Fat Jalapeno	1 oz	70	5	15	170
Cheddar Light 50% Reduced Fat Tomato Basil	1 oz	70	5	15	170
Cheddar Light 75% Reduced Fat	1 oz	60	3	10	200
Dehyrdated Cheddar Powder	2 tsp (5 g)	25	2	5	210
Monterey Jack	1 oz	110	9	30	170

FOOD	PORTION	CALS	FAT	CHOL	SOD
Cedar Grove					
Marble Colby	1 oz	110	9	30	185
Organic Tomato Basil Cheddar	1 oz	110	9	30	185
Cheez Whiz					
Light	2 tbsp (1.2 oz)	80	3	15	540
Cracker Barrel					
Baby Swiss	1 oz	110	9	25	110
Cheddar Extra Sharp	1 oz	120	10	30	180
Cheddar Marbled Sharp	1 oz	110	9	30	180
Cheddar New York Aged	1 oz	120	10	30	180
Cheddar Sharp	1 oz	120	10	30	180
Cheddar Vermont Sharp	1 oz	110	9	30	180
Reduced Fat Cheddar Extra Sharp	1 oz	90	6	20	240
Reduced Fat Cheddar Sharp	1 oz	90	6	20	240
Reduced Fat Cheddar Vermont Sharp	1 oz	90	6	20	240
Whipped Spreadable Cream Cheese & Extra Sharp Cheddar	2 tbsp (0.9 oz)	80	8	20	180
Whipped Spreadable Cream Cheese & Sharp Cheddar	2 tbsp (0.9 oz)	80	8	20	180
Whipped Spreadable Cream Cheese & Sharp Cheddar w/ Herbs	2 tbsp (0.9 oz)	80	8	20	180
Di Giorno					
Parmesan Grated	2 tsp (5 g)	25	2	5	85
Parmesan Shredded	2 tsp (5 g)	20	2	5	75
Romano Grated	2 tsp (5 g)	25	2	5	90
Romano Shredded	2 tsp (5 g)	20	2	5	70
Friendship					
Farmer	2 tbsp (1 oz)	50	3	10	120
Handi-Snacks					
Cheez'n Breadsticks	1 pkg (1.1 oz)	120	6	15	320
Cheez'n Crackers	1 pkg (1.1 oz)	110	7	15	300
Cheez'n Pretzels	1 pkg (1 oz)	100	5	15	410
Mozzarella String Cheese	1 piece (1 oz)	80	6	20	240
Nacho Stix'n Cheez	1 pkg (1.1 oz)	110	6	15	320
Hollow Road Farms					
Sheep's Milk	1 oz	45	3	15	65
Kraft					
Cheddar Extra Sharp	1 oz	120	10	30	180
Cheddar Medium	1 oz	110	9	30	180
Cheddar Mild	1 oz	110	9	30	180
Cheddar Sharp	1 oz	120	10	30	180

FOOD	PORTION	CALS	FAT	CHOL	SOD
Cheddary Melts Medium Cheddar	1 oz	110	9	30	390
Cheddary Melts Mild Cheddar	1 oz	110	9	30	390
Cheddary Melts Shreds Medium Cheddar	1/4 cup (1.1 oz)	120	9	30	420
Cheddary Melts Shreds Mild Cheddar	1/4 cup (1.1 oz)	120	9	30	420
Cheese Food w/ Garlic	1 oz	90	7	20	370
Cheese Food w/ Jalapeno Peppers	1 oz	90	7	20	370
Colby	1 oz	110	9	30	180
Colby Monterey Jack	1 oz	110	9	30	180
Deluxe American	1 oz	100	9	25	430
Deluxe American White	1 oz	100	9	25	430
Deluxe Singles American	1 (0.7 oz)	70	6	15	310
Deluxe Singles American	1 (1 oz)	110	9	30	460
Deluxe Singles Pimento	1 (1 oz)	100	8	25	430
Deluxe Singles Swiss	1 slice (0.7 oz)	70	5	20	310
Deluxe Singles Swiss	1 (1 oz)	90	7	25	410
Free Grated	2 tsp (5 g)	15	0	0	75
Free Shredded Cheddar	1/4 cup (0.9 oz)	40	0	<5	270
Free Shredded Mozzarella	1/4 cup (1 oz)	45	0	<5	340
Grated Parm Plus! Garlic Herb	2 tsp (5 g)	15	0	0	110
Grated Parm Plus! Zesty Red Pepper	2 tsp (5 g)	15	0	0	110
Grated Parmesan	2 tsp (5 g)	20	2	5	85
Grated Romano	2 tsp (5 g)	20	2	<5	70
Marbled Cheddar Mild	1 oz	110	9	30	180
Marbled Cheddar & Monterey Jack	1 oz	110	9	30	190
Marbled Cheddar & Whole Milk Mozzarella	1 oz	100	8	25	190
Marbled Colby Monterey Jack	1 oz	110	9	30	180
Monterey Jack	1 oz	110	9	30	190
Monterey Jack w/ Jalapeno Peppers	1 oz	110	9	30	190
Mozzarella Part Skim Low Moisture	1 oz	80	5	15	200
Mozzarella String Cheese Low Moisture Part Skim	1 piece (1 oz)	80	6	20	240
Pizza Shredded Four Cheese	1/4 cup (0.9 oz)	90	7	20	220
Pizza Shredded Mozzarella & Cheddar	1/3 cup (1.1 oz)	120	9	20	220
Pizza Shredded Mozzarella & Provolone w/ Smoke Flavor	1/4 cup (0.9 oz)	90	7	20	200
Reduced Fat Cheddar Mild	1 oz	90	6	20	240
Reduced Fat Cheddar Sharp	1 oz	90	6	20	240

FOOD	PORTION	CALS	FAT	CHOL	SOD
Kraft (cont.)					
Reduced Fat Colby	1 oz	80	6	20	220
Reduced Fat Monterey Jack	1 oz	80	6	20	240
Shredded Cheddar Medium	1/4 cup (0.9 oz)	100	8	30	170
Shredded Cheddar Mild	1/4 cup (0.9 oz)	100	8	30	170
Shredded Cheddar Sharp	1 oz (0.9 oz)	110	9	25	170
Shredded Cheddar & Monterey Jack	1/4 cup (0.9 oz)	100	8	25	170
Shredded Colby & Monterey Jack	1/4 cup (0.9 oz)	100	8	25	170
Shredded Hearty Italian	1/3 cup (1.1 oz)	100	8	25	230
Shredded Italian Style Classic Garlic	1/3 cup (1.1 oz)	100	8	25	240
Shredded Italian Style Mozzarella & Parmesan	1/3 cup (1.1 oz)	100	8	25	240
Shredded Lower Fat Cheddar Mild	1/4 cup (0.9 oz)	80	6	20	220
Shredded Lower Fat Cheddar Sharp	1/4 cup (0.9 oz)	80	6	20	220
Shredded Lower Fat Colby & Monterey Jack	1/4 cup (0.9 oz)	80	5	15	210
Shredded Lower Fat Mozzarella	1/3 cup (1.1 oz)	80	5	15	210
Shredded Lower Fat Pizza Cheese	1/3 cup (1.1 oz)	90	6	20	240
Shredded Mexican Style Cheddar & Monterey Jack	1/3 cup (1.1 oz)	120	10	30	200
Shredded Mexican Style Cheddar & Monterey Jack w/ Jalapeno Peppers	1/3 cup (1.1 oz)	120	10	30	200
Shredded Mexican Style Four Cheese	1/3 cup (1.1 oz)	120	10	30	210
Shredded Mexican Style Taco Cheese	1/3 cup (1.1 oz)	120	10	30	240
Shredded Monterey Jack	1/4 cup (0.9 oz)	100	8	25	170
Shredded Parmesan	2 tsp (5 g)	20	2	2	75
Shredded Part Skim Mozzarella	1/4 cup (1.1 oz)	90	6	20	220
Shredded Swiss	1/4 cup (0.9 oz)	100	8	25	25
Shredded Whole Milk Mozzarella	1/4 cup (1.1 oz)	100	8	25	220
Shredded Finely Cheddar Mild	1/4 cup (1.1 oz)	120	10	30	190
Shredded Finely Cheddar Sharp	1/4 cup (1.1 oz)	120	10	30	190
Shredded Finely Colby & Monterey Jack	1/4 cup (1 oz)	110	9	30	190
Shredded Finely Lower Fat Cheddar Mild	1/3 cup (1.1 oz)	100	7	20	260

FOOD	PORTION	CALS	FAT	CHOL	SOD
Shredded Finely Lower Fat Cheddar Sharp	1/3 cup (1.1 oz)	100	7	20	260
Shredded Finely Part Skim Mozzarella	1/4 cup (1.1 oz)	90	6	20	220
Shredded Finely Swiss	1/4 cup (0.9 oz)	110	8	25	45
Singles American	1 (1.2 oz)	110	8	25	460
Singles American	1 (0.7 oz)	60	5	15	260
Singles Mild Mexican	1 (0.7 oz)	70	5	15	280
Singles Monterey	1 slice (0.7 oz)	70	5	15	290
Singles Pimento	1 (0.7 oz)	60	5	15	260
Singles Reduced Fat American	1 (0.7 oz)	50	3	10	320
Singles Reduced Fat American White	1 (0.7 oz)	50	3	10	320
Singles Sharp	1 slice (0.7 oz)	70	6	20	300
Singles Swiss	1 slice (0.7 oz)	70	5	15	320
Singles Nonfat American	1 (0.7 oz)	30	0	<5	270
Singles Nonfat American White	1 (0.7 oz)	30	0	<5	270
Singles Nonfat Sharp Cheddar	1 (0.7 oz)	35	0	<5	300
Singles Nonfat Swiss	1 slice (0.7 oz)	30	0	<5	270
Slices Cheddar Mild	1 (1 oz)	110	9	30	180
Slices Colby	1 (1.6 oz)	180	14	45	290
Slices Part Skim Mozzarella	1 (1.6 oz)	130	8	25	320
Slices Part Skim Mozzarella	1 (1.5 oz)	120	8	25	310
Slices Provolone Smoke Flavor	1 (1.5 oz)	150	11	35	370
Slices Swiss	1 (1.5 oz)	170	13	45	45
Slices Swiss	1 (1.3 oz)	150	12	40	65
Slices Swiss	1 (0.8 oz)	90	7	25	40
Slices Swiss	1 (1.6 oz)	180	14	45	45
Slices Swiss Aged	1 (1.5 oz)	170	13	45	75
Slices Deli-Thin Part Skim Mozzarella	1 (1 oz)	80	5	15	200
Slices Deli-Thin Swiss	1 (0.8 oz)	90	7	25	40
Slices Deli-Thin Swiss Aged	1 (0.8 oz)	90	7	25	40
Slices Reduced Fat Swiss	1 (1.3 oz)	130	9	25	90
Spread Bacon	2 tbsp (1.1 oz)	90	8	25	570
Spread Olive & Pimento	2 tbsp (1.1 oz)	70	6	20	220
Spread Pimento	2 tbsp (1.1 oz)	80	6	20	170
Spread Pineapple	2 tbsp (1.1 oz)	70	5	15	115
Spread Roka Brand Blue	2 tbsp (1.1 oz)	90	8	25	520
Swiss	1 oz	110	9	30	50
Land O'Lakes					
American	1 slice (0.7 oz)	80	6	20	320
American Jalapeno	1 slice (0.6 oz)	70	6	15	320
American Light	1 oz	70	5	20	400

FOOD	PORTION	CALS	FAT	CHOL	SOD
Land O'Lakes (cont.)					
American Reduced Salt	1 oz	110	9	30	270
American Sharp	2 slices (1 oz)	100	9	30	420
American & Swiss	1 slice (0.6 oz)	70	5	15	310
Baby Swiss	1 oz	110	9	25	125
Chedarella	1 oz	100	8	25	200
Cheddar	1 oz	100	9	30	180
Cheddar Extra Sharp	1 oz	110	8	30	360
Cheddar Sharp	1 oz	110	9	30	180
Cheese Spread Golden Velvet	1 oz	80	6	20	370
Colby	1 oz	110	9	30	180
Jalapeno Light	1 oz	70	4	15	400
Monterey Jack	1 oz	110	8	30	170
Monterey Jack Hot Pepper	1 oz	110	8	30	140
Mozzarella	1 oz	80	6	15	190
Muenster	1 oz	100	8	25	220
Parmesan Grated	1 tbsp	35	4	10	95
Provolone	1 oz	100	8	20	240
Swiss	1 oz	110	8	25	75
Swiss Light	1 oz	80	4	15	60
Lifetime					
Cheddar Fat Free	1 oz	40	0	<5	220
Cheddar Fat Free Lactose Free	1 oz	40	0	<5	220
Garden Vegetable Fat Free	1 oz	40	0	<5	220
Jalapeno Jack Fat Free	1 oz	40	0	<5	220
Jalapeno Jack Fat Free Lactose Free	1 oz	40	0	<5	220
Mild Mexican Fat Free	1 oz	40	0	<5	220
Monterey Jack Fat Free	1 oz	40	0	<5	220
Mozzarella Fat Free	1 oz	40	0	<5	220
Mozzarella Fat Free Lactose Free	1 oz	40	0	<5	220
Onions & Chives Fat Free	1 oz	40	0	<5	220
Sharp Cheddar Fat Free	1 oz	40	0	<5	220
Smoked Cheddar Fat Free	1 oz	40	0	<5	220
Swiss Fat Free	1 oz	40	0	<5	220
Light N'Lively					
Singles American	1 (0.7 oz)	45	3	10	280
Old English					
American Sharp	1 slice (1 oz)	100	9	30	460
Organic Valley					
Aged Swiss Unpasteurized	1 oz	100	8	25	60
Cheddar Reduced Fat Low Sodium	1 oz	90	6	15	135
Cheddar Sharp & Mild	1 oz	110	9	25	190
Cheddar Sharp & Mild Unpasteurized	1 oz	110	9	25	190

FOOD	PORTION	CALS	FAT	CHOL	SOD
Colby	1 oz	110	9	28	175
Colby Unpasteurized	1 oz	110	9	28	175
Farmer Reduced Fat	1 oz	90	6	15	110
Feta	1 oz	90	7	20	180
Monterey Jack	1 oz	100	8	20	170
Monterey Jack Reduced Fat	1 oz	80	5	15	170
Mozzarella Part Skim	1 oz	80	5	16	170
Muenster	1 oz	100	8	25	165
Pepper Jack	1 oz	110	9	20	160
Provolone	1 oz	100	8	20	245
String Part Skim	1 oz	80	5	16	170
Wisconsin Raw Milk Cheese	1 oz	100	8	20	170
Polly-O					
String Lite	1 piece (1 oz)	60	3	10	230
President					
Feta Fat Free	1 oz	30	0	0	450
Sargento					
Blue Crumbled	1/4 cup (1 oz)	100	8	20	380
Cheddar	1 slice (1 oz)	110	9	30	160
Cheddar Shredded	1/4 cup (1 oz)	110	9	30	160
Cheese For Nachos & Tacos Shredded	1/4 cup (1 oz)	110	9	25	240
Cheese For Pizza Shredded	1/4 cup (1 oz)	90	6	20	210
Cheese For Tacos Shredded	1/4 cup (1 oz)	110	9	25	220
Colby	1 slice (1 oz)	110	9	30	190
Colby-Jack Shredded	1/4 cup (1 oz)	110	9	25	190
Jarlsberg	1 slice (1.2 oz)	120	9	20	160
Monterey Jack	1 slice (1 oz)	100	9	30	190
Monterey Jack Shredded	1/4 cup (1 oz)	100	9	30	190
MooTown Snackers Cheddar	1 piece (0.8 oz)	100	8	25	130
MooTown Snackers Cheddar Mild Light	1 piece (0.8 oz)	60	4	10	170
MooTown Snackers Cheese & Pretzels	1 pkg (0.9 oz)	90	3	10	320
MooTown Snackers Colby-Jack	1 piece (0.8 oz)	90	8	20	160
MooTown Snackers Pizza Cheese & Sticks	1 pkg (1 oz)	100	4	10	260
MooTown Snackers String	1 piece (0.8 oz)	70	5	15	170
MooTown Snackers String Light	1 piece (0.8 oz)	60	3	10	200
Mozzarella	1 slice (1.5 oz)	130	9	25	230
Mozzarella Shredded	1/4 cup (1 oz)	80	6	15	150
Muenster	1 slice (1 oz)	100	9	25	200
Parmesan Grated	1 tbsp (5 g)	25	2	<5	75
Parmesan Shredded	1/4 cup (1 oz)	110	7	25	300
Parmesan & Romano Shredded	1/4 cup (1 oz)	110	7	25	340

FOOD	PORTION	CALS	FAT	CHOL	SOD
Sargento (cont.)					
Parmesan & Romano Grated	1 tbsp (5 g)	25	2	<5	70
Pizza Double Cheese Shredded	1/4 cup (1 oz)	90	6	20	150
Preferred Light Cheddar Mild Shredded	1/4 cup (1 oz)	70	5	10	200
Preferred Light Cheese For Tacos Shredded	1/4 cup (1 oz)	70	5	15	240
Preferred Light Mozzarella	1 slice (1.5 oz)	90	5	15	230
Preferred Light Mozzarella Shredded	1/4 cup (1 oz)	70	3	10	140
Preferred Light Swiss	1 slice (1 oz)	80	4	15	50
Provolone	1 slice (1 oz)	100	8	25	190
Recipe Blend 4 Cheese Mexican Shredded	1/4 cup (1 oz)	110	9	25	200
Recipe Blend 6 Cheese Italian Shredded	1/4 cup (1 oz)	90	7	20	180
Ricotta Light	1/4 cup (2.2 oz)	60	3	15	55
Ricotta Old Fashioned	1/4 cup (2.2 oz)	90	6	25	75
Ricotta Part-Skim	1/4 cup (2.2 oz)	80	5	20	75
Swiss	1 slice (0.7 oz)	80	6	20	30
Swiss Shredded	1/4 cup (1 oz)	110	8	30	40
Swiss Wafer Thin	2 slices (1 oz)	110	9	25	40
Smart Beat					
American Fat Free	1 slice (0.6 oz)	25	0	0	180
Lactose Free Fat Free	1 slice (0.6 oz)	25	0	0	180
Mellow Cheddar Fat Free	1 slice (0.6 oz)	25	0	0	180
Sharp Cheddar Fat Free	1 slice (0.6 oz)	25	0	0	220
Sorrento					
Mozzarella Part Skim Jalapeno	1 oz	80	5	15	180
Velveeta					
Light	1 oz	60	3	10	440
Shredded	1/4 cup (1.3 oz)	130	9	30	500
Shredded Mild Mexican w/ Jalapeno Pepper	1/4 cup (1.3 oz)	120	9	30	520
Spread	1 oz	90	6	25	420
Spread Hot Mexican	1 oz	90	6	20	420
Spread Mild Mexican	1 oz	90	6	25	420
Weight Watchers					
Cheddar Mild Yellow	1 oz	80	5	15	180
Cheddar Sharp Yellow	1 oz	80	5	15	180
Fat Free Grated Italian Topping	1 tbsp	20	0	0	60
Fat Free Reduced Sodium Yellow	2 slices (0.75 oz)	30	0	0	160
Fat Free Sharp Cheddar	2 slices (0.75 oz)	30	0	0	320
Fat Free Swiss	2 slices (0.75 oz)	30	0	0	320

FOOD	PORTION	CALS	FAT	CHOL	SOD
Fat Free White	2 slices (0.75 oz)	30	0	0	320
Fat Free Yellow	2 slices (0.75 oz)	30	0	0	320
Wholesome Valley					
Organic American Reduced Fat	1 slice (0.7 oz)	50	3	10	290
CHEESE DISHES					
frozen					
Health Is Wealth					
Mozzarella Sticks	2 (1.3 oz)	120	5	15	250
Stouffer's					
Welsh Rarebit	1/2 cup (2.5 oz)	120	9	20	280
take-out					
fondue	1/2 cup (3.8 oz)	247	15	49	142
souffle	1 serv (7 oz)	504	38	370	848
CHEESE SUBSTITUTES					
Sargento					
Cheddar Shredded	1/4 cup (1 oz)	90	7	0	420
Mozzarella Shredded	1/4 cup (1 oz)	80	6	0	320
Yves					
Good Slice American	1 slice (0.7 oz)	35	2	0	290
Good Slice Cheddar	1 slice (0.7 oz)	35	2	0	280
Good Slice Jalapeno Jack	1 slice (0.7 oz)	35	2	0	250
Good Slice Mozzarella	1 slice (0.7 oz)	30	2	0	270
Good Slice Swiss	1 slice (0.7 oz)	35	2	0	260
CHERRIES					
canned					
sour in heavy syrup	1/2 cup	232	tr	0	18
sour in light syrup	1/2 cup	189	tr	0	18
sour water packed	1 cup	87	tr	0	17
sweet in heavy syrup	1/2 cup	107	tr	0	3
sweet in light syrup	1/2 cup	85	tr	0	3
sweet juice pack	1/2 cup	68	tr	0	3
sweet water pack	1/2 cup	57	tr	0	2
dried					
Sonoma					
Pitted	1/4 cup (1.4 oz)	140	0	0	0
fresh					
sour	1 cup	51	tr	0	3
sweet	10	49	1	0	0
frozen					
sour unsweetened	1 cup	72	1	0	1
sweet sweetened	1 cup	232	tr	0	3
CHERRY JUICE					
Capri Sun					
Wild Cherry Drink	1 pkg (7 oz)	100	0	0	20
Juicy Juice					
Drink	1 box (8.5 oz)	140	0	0	15
Drink	1 box (4.23 oz)	70	0	0	10

FOOD	PORTION	CALS	FAT	CHOL	SOD
Kool-Aid					
Black Cherry Drink as prep w/ sugar	1 serv (8 oz)	100	0	0	15
Bursts Cherry Drink	1 (7 oz)	100	0	0	30
Splash Drink	1 serv (8 oz)	110	0	0	35
Sugar Free Drink Mix as prep	1 serv (8 oz)	5	0	0	5
Mott's					
Cherry	1 box (8 oz)	120	0	0	15
Ocean Spray					
Black Cherry Blast	8 oz	140	0	0	35
Veryfine					
Juice-Ups	8 oz	130	0	0	15
CHERVIL					
seed	1 tsp	1	tr	0	tr
CHESTNUTS					
chinese cooked	1 oz	44	tr	0	1
chinese dried	1 oz	103	tr	0	2
chinese roasted	1 oz	68	tr	0	1
cooked	1 oz	37	tr	0	8
creme de marrons	1 oz	73	tr	0	1
dried peeled	1 oz	105	1	0	11
japanese cooked	1 oz	16	tr	0	1
japanese dried	1 oz	102	tr	0	10
roasted	2 to 3 (1 oz)	70	1	0	1
CHEWING GUM					
bubble gum	1 block (8 g)	27	0	0	0
stick	1 (3 g)	10	0	0	0
Arm & Hammer					
Dental Care Spearmint or Peppermint	2 pieces (2.5 g)	5	0	0	30
Beech-Nut					
Peppermint	1 stick (3 g)	10	0	0	0
Spearmint	1 stick (3 g)	10	0	0	0
Big Red					
Stick	1	10	tr	0	0
Bubble Yum					
Regular	1 piece (0.3 oz)	25	0	0	0
*Care*Free*					
Sugarless Wild Cherry	1 stick (3 g)	10	0	0	0
Doublemint					
Chewing Gum	1 piece	10	tr	0	0
Extra Sugar Free					
Cinnamon	1 piece	8	tr	0	0
Spearmint & Peppermint	1 stick	8	tr	0	0
Winter Fresh	1 piece	8	tr	0	0
Freedent					
Spearmint Peppermint & Cinnamon	1 stick	10	tr	0	0

FOOD	PORTION	CALS	FAT	CHOL	SOD
Fruit Stripe					
Bubble Gum Jumbo Pack	1 stick (3 g)	10	0	0	0
Hubba Bubba					
Bubble Gum Cola	1 piece	23	tr	0	0
Bubble Gum Sugarfree Grape	1 piece	13	tr	0	0
Bubble Gum Sugarfree Original	1 piece	14	tr	0	0
Original	1 piece	23	tr	0	0
Strawberry Grape Raspberry	1 piece	23	tr	0	0
Juicy Fruit					
Stick	1	10	tr	0	0
Lance					
Big Red Cinnamon	1 piece (3 g)	10	0	0	0
Double Bubble	1 piece (7 g)	25	0	0	0
Double Mint	1 piece (3 g)	10	0	0	0
Winterfresh					
Stick	1 stick (3 g)	10	0	0	0
Wrigley's					
Spearmint	1 stick	10	tr	0	0

CHICKEN

(*see also* CHICKEN DISHES, CHICKEN SUBSTITUTES, DINNER, HOT DOG)

FOOD	PORTION	CALS	FAT	CHOL	SOD
fresh					
broiler/fryer back w/ skin batter dipped & fried	1/2 back (2.5 oz)	238	16	63	228
broiler/fryer back w/ skin floured & fried	1.5 oz	146	9	39	40
broiler/fryer back w/ skin roasted	1 oz	96	7	28	28
broiler/fryer back w/ skin stewed	1/2 back (2.1 oz)	158	11	48	39
broiler/fryer breast w/ skin batter dipped & fried	1/2 breast (4.9 oz)	364	18	119	385
broiler/fryer breast w/ skin roasted	1/2 breast (3.4 oz)	193	8	83	69
broiler/fryer breast w/ skin stewed	1/2 breast (3.9 oz)	202	8	83	68
broiler/fryer breast w/o skin fried	1/2 breast (3 oz)	161	4	78	68
broiler/fryer breast w/o skin roasted	1/2 breast (3 oz)	142	3	73	63
broiler/fryer drumstick w/ skin batter dipped & fried	1 (2.6 oz)	193	11	62	194
broiler/fryer drumstick w/ skin floured & fried	1 (1.7 oz)	120	7	44	44
broiler/fryer drumstick w/ skin roasted	1 (1.8 oz)	112	6	48	47
broiler/fryer drumstick w/ skin stewed	1 (2 oz)	116	6	48	43

FOOD	PORTION	CALS	FAT	CHOL	SOD
broiler/fryer drumstick w/o skin fried	1 (1.5 oz)	82	3	40	40
broiler/fryer drumstick w/o skin roasted	1 (1.5 oz)	76	2	41	42
broiler/fryer drumstick w/o skin stewed	1 (1.6 oz)	78	3	40	37
broiler/fryer leg w/ skin batter dipped & fried	1 (5.5 oz)	431	26	142	442
broiler/fryer leg w/ skin floured & fried	1 (3.9 oz)	285	16	105	99
broiler/fryer leg w/ skin roasted	1 (4 oz)	265	15	105	99
broiler/fryer leg w/ skin stewed	1 (4.4 oz)	275	16	105	92
broiler/fryer leg w/o skin fried	1 (3.3 oz)	195	9	93	90
broiler/fryer leg w/o skin roasted	1 (3.3 oz)	182	8	89	87
broiler/fryer leg w/o skin stewed	1 (3.5 oz)	187	8	90	78
broiler/fryer neck w/ skin stewed	1 (1.3 oz)	94	7	27	20
broiler/fryer skin batter dipped & fried	from 1/2 chicken (6.7 oz)	748	55	140	1105
broiler/fryer skin floured & fried	from 1/2 chicken (2 oz)	281	24	41	30
broiler/fryer skin roasted	from 1/2 chicken (2 oz)	254	23	46	36
broiler/fryer skin stewed	from 1/2 chicken (2.5 oz)	261	24	45	40
broiler/fryer thigh w/ skin batter dipped & fried	1 (3 oz)	238	14	80	248
broiler/fryer thigh w/ skin floured & fried	1 (2.2 oz)	162	9	60	55
broiler/fryer thigh w/ skin roasted	1 (2.2 oz)	153	10	58	52
broiler/fryer thigh w/ skin stewed	1 (2.4 oz)	158	10	57	49
broiler/fryer thigh w/o skin fried	1 (1.8 oz)	113	5	53	49
broiler/fryer thigh w/o skin roasted	1 (1.8 oz)	109	6	49	46
broiler/fryer thigh w/o skin stewed	1 (1.9 oz)	107	5	49	41
broiler/fryer w/o skin roasted	1 cup (5 oz)	266	10	125	120
broiler/fryer w/o skin stewed	1 cup (5 oz)	248	9	116	98
broiler/fryer w/o skin stewed	1 oz	54	3	22	18
broiler/fryer wing w/ skin	1 (1.7 oz)	159	11	39	157

FOOD	PORTION	CALS	FAT	CHOL	SOD
batter dipped &fried					
broiler/fryer wing w/ skin	1 (1.1 oz)	103	7	26	25
floured & fried					
broiler/fryer wing w/ skin	1 (1.2 oz)	99	7	29	28
roasted					
broiler/fryer wing w/ skin	1 (1.4 oz)	100	7	28	27
stewed					
capon w/ skin neck & giblets	1 chicken (3.1 lbs)	3211	165	1458	704
roasted					
cornish hen w/ skin roasted	1 hen (8 oz)	595	42	299	146
cornish hen w/ skin roasted	1/2 hen (4 oz)	296	21	149	73
Tyson					
Broth Marinated Breast Filet	1 (4.7 oz)	140	4	70	330
Broth Marinated Drums	2 (4 oz)	140	7	90	290
Broth Marinated Thighs	1 (4.9 oz)	380	34	110	350
Broth Marinated Wings	4 pieces (4.2 oz)	240	18	95	340
Chicken Broccoli & Cheese	1 piece (5.9 oz)	320	16	50	670
Chicken Stuffed w/ Wild	1 piece (5.9 oz)	300	12	50	860
Rice & Mushroom					
Cordon Bleu	1 piece (5.9 oz)	350	17	55	640
Cornish Hen	1 serv (4 oz)	180	12	130	65
Kiev	1 piece (5.9 oz)	460	32	115	570
Wampler					
Breast Tenders	4 oz	130	2	70	55
frozen					
Health Is Wealth					
Nuggets	4 (3 oz)	150	6	40	180
Patties	1 (3 oz)	150	6	40	180
Tenders	3 (3 oz)	130	3	35	230
Weaver					
Breast Strips	3 pieces (3.3 oz)	210	11	35	430
Breast Tenders	5 pieces (3 oz)	220	15	35	290
Croquettes	1 serv (3.5 oz)	290	18	45	540
Dutch Frye Nuggets	5 pieces (3.3 oz)	280	20	45	410
Honey Battered Tenders	5 pieces (2.9 oz)	230	15	35	380
Hot Wings Buffalo Style	3 pieces (2.7 oz)	190	13	95	370
Mini Drums Crispy	5 pieces (3.3 oz)	250	16	40	410
Nuggets	4 pieces (2.7 oz)	210	15	35	360
Patties	1 (2.6 oz)	180	11	30	430
Rondelet	1 (2.6 oz)	170	10	20	410
Rondelet Dutch Frye	1 (2.6 oz)	230	16	35	360
Rondelet Italian	1 (2.6 oz)	210	14	20	470
ready-to-eat					
chicken roll light meat	1 pkg (6 oz)	271	13	85	992
chicken roll light meat	2 oz	90	4	28	331
poultry salad sandwich spread	1 tbsp (13 g)	109	2	4	49
poultry salad sandwich	1 oz	238	4	9	107
spread					

FOOD	PORTION	CALS	FAT	CHOL	SOD
Banquet					
Breast Tenders Fat Free	3 (3.2 oz)	130	0	30	480
Boar's Head					
Breast Hickory Smoked	2 oz	60	1	30	440
Breast Oven Roasted	2 oz	50	1	30	420
Breast Bar B Q Sauce Basted	2 oz	60	1	30	490
Carl Buddig					
Chicken Sliced	1 pkg (2.5 oz)	110	7	40	680
Lean Slices Honey Smoked Breast	1 pkg (2.5 oz)	70	1	30	630
Lean Slices Roasted Breast	1 pkg (2.5 oz)	60	1	30	630
Chicken By George					
Cajun	1 breast (4 oz)	130	4	60	700
Caribbean Grill	1 breast (4 oz)	150	4	60	550
Garlic & Herb	1 breast (4 oz)	120	3	60	600
Italian Bleu Cheese	1 breast (4 oz)	130	5	60	790
Lemon Herb	1 breast (4 oz)	120	3	60	800
Lemon Oregano	1 breast (4 oz)	130	4	50	600
Mesquite Barbecue	1 breast (4 oz)	130	3	60	700
Mustard Dill	1 breast (4 oz)	140	5	60	650
Roasted	1 breast (4 oz)	110	3	55	500
Teriyaki	1 breast (4 oz)	130	3	55	530
Tomato Herb With Basil	1 breast (4 oz)	140	5	60	630
Louis Rich					
Carving Board Classic Baked	2 slices (1.6 oz)	45	1	25	510
Carving Board Grilled	2 slices (1.6 oz)	45	1	25	510
Deli-Thin Oven Roasted Breast	4 slices (1.8 oz)	50	1	25	620
Oven Roasted Deluxe Breast	1 slice (1 oz)	30	1	15	330
Oscar Mayer					
Free Oven Roasted Breast	4 slices (1.8 oz)	45	0	25	650
Perdue					
Cafe Meal Kit Stir Fry	1 serv (8.2 oz)	360	2	25	1180
Seasoned Whole Chicken Dark Meat	3 oz	190	14	100	330
Seasoned Whole Chicken White Meat	3 oz	160	9	75	320
Short Cuts Italian	3 oz	110	2	55	540
Short Cuts Lemon Pepper	1/2 cup (2.5 oz)	90	2	50	530
Short Cuts Oven Roasted	1/2 cup (2.5 oz)	100	3	60	580
Short Cuts Southwestern Seasoned	1/2 cup (2.5 oz)	100	2	45	310
Shady Brook					
Slow Roasted Breast	2 oz	60	1	30	400
Tyson					
Breaded Breast Chunks	6 pieces (2.9 oz)	230	16	20	440
Breaded Breast Fillet	2 pieces (2.8 oz)	180	8	25	440

FOOD	PORTION	CALS	FAT	CHOL	SOD
Breaded Breast Pattie	1 (2.6 oz)	190	12	25	320
Breaded Breast Tenders	5 pieces (3 oz)	220	15	35	290
Breaded Chicken Chunks	6 pieces (3 oz)	220	14	40	480
Chick'n Quick Chick'n Cheddar	1 patty (2.6 oz)	220	14	40	270
Chicken Bits Southern Fried	6 pieces (2.9 oz)	260	19	40	540
Chicken Strips	1 serv (3 oz)	90	1	45	240
Chicken Strips Southwestern	1 serv (3 oz)	110	3	40	400
Country Fried Chicken Fritter	5 pieces (2.9 oz)	260	18	40	470
Drumsticks Hot BBQ Style	2 (3.5 oz)	160	7	100	620
Glazed Grilled Breast Pattie	1 (2.7 oz)	120	7	40	440
Grilled Chicken Pattie	1 (2.9 oz)	170	12	55	340
Nuggets Breaded White Meat	6 pieces (2.9 oz)	250	18	35	450
Patties Southern Fried	1 (2.9 oz)	260	19	40	540
Roasted Drumsticks	3 (5.6 oz)	320	15	230	1200
Roasted Drumsticks w/o Skin	2 (3.3 oz)	140	5	120	730
Roasted Half Chicken	1 serv (3 oz)	160	11	75	490
Roasted Whole Chicken	1 serv (3 oz)	160	11	75	490
Roasted Breast Boneless w/o Skin	1 (3.7 oz)	130	3	70	580
Roasted Breast Half w/o Skin	1 (4.3 oz)	150	3	80	660
Roasted Half Breast w/ Skin	1 (5.1 oz)	260	13	110	670
Roasted Half Chicken w/o Skin	1 serv (3 oz)	120	6	75	510
Roasted Tabasco Wings	3 (3 oz)	190	13	100	520
Roasted Thigh w/ Skin	1 (3.6 oz)	270	21	120	650
Roasted Thigh w/o Skin	1 (2.9 oz)	150	8	95	560
Roll White Meat	2 oz	90	6	25	440
Southern Fried Breaded Breast Pattie	1 (2.6 oz)	180	12	30	360
Southern Fried Breast Fillets	2 pieces (3.4 oz)	210	11	30	480
Southern Fried Chunks	6 pieces (2.9 oz)	260	19	40	540
Tenders Breaded Honey Battered	5 pieces (2.9 oz)	230	15	35	380
Tenders Breaded Pattie	3 pieces (3.2 oz)	100	0	0	540
Thick'n Crispy Pattie	1 (2.6 oz)	200	14	40	320
Wings BBQ	3 pieces (3.2 oz)	200	13	110	330
Wings Hot N'Spicy	4 (3.2 oz)	210	14	100	1020
Wings Teriyaki	4 pieces (3.4 oz)	190	12	120	210
Wings Of Fire	4 pieces (3.4 oz)	220	15	110	560

CHICKEN DISHES

(*see also* CHICKEN SUBSTITUTES, DINNER)

canned

Dinty Moore

Noodles & Chicken	1 can (7.5 oz)	180	8	30	1010
Stew	1 cup (8.5 oz)	220	11	40	980

FOOD	PORTION	CALS	FAT	CHOL	SOD
mix					
Chicken Skillet Helper					
Stir-Fried Chicken as prep	1 cup	270	9	105	760
Hamburger Helper					
Reduced Sodium Cheddar Spirals Chicken Recipe as prep	1 cup	240	6	40	630
Reduced Sodium Italian Herb Chicken Recipe as prep	1 cup	200	2	35	630
Reduced Sodium Southwestern Recipe as prep	1 cup	220	3	35	600
Tyson					
Mandarin Wrap Kit	1 1/2 wraps (14.6 oz)	630	15	50	1840
ready-to-eat					
Shady Brook					
Chicken Breast w/ Rice Pilaf	1 serv (12 oz)	350	13	120	270
Teriyaki Breast	1 serv (12 oz)	490	3	15	1600
Wampler					
Cacciatore	1 cup	260	9	90	600
Fajitas	1 cup	210	7	70	1360
Salad	1/3 cup	200	14	30	420
Salad Lite	1/3 cup	130	7	25	370
Salad Low Fat	1/3 cup	90	2	20	440
Smokey Barbecue Chicken	1 cup	430	15	140	1020
Sweet-n-Sour	1 cup	250	4	55	510
shelf-stable					
Dinty Moore					
Microwave Cup Chicken & Dumpling	1 pkg (7.5 oz)	200	6	35	890
Microwave Cup Stew	1 pkg (7.5 oz)	180	8	30	920
Lunch Bucket					
Chicken Fiesta	1 pkg (7.5 oz)	160	2	5	530
Dumplings'n Chicken	1 pkg (7.5 oz)	140	5	10	780
take-out					
boneless breaded & fried w/ barbecue sauce	6 pieces (4.6 oz)	330	18	61	830
boneless breaded & fried w/ honey	6 pieces (4 oz)	339	18	61	537
boneless breaded & fried w/ mustard sauce	6 pieces (4.6 oz)	323	17	62	791
boneless breaded & fried w/ sweet & sour sauce	6 pieces (4.6 oz)	346	18	61	791

FOOD	PORTION	CALS	FAT	CHOL	SOD
breast & wing breaded & fried	2 pieces (5.7 oz)	494	30	149	975
chicken & dumplings	3/4 cup	256	12	109	1283
chicken & noodles	1 cup	365	18	103	600
chicken a la king	1 cup	470	34	221	760
chicken cacciatore	3/4 cup	394	24	99	671
drumstick breaded & fried	2 pieces (5.2 oz)	430	27	165	756
groundnut stew hkatenkwan	1 serv (15.7 oz)	576	40	116	1009
jamaican jerk wings	4 wings (9.9 oz)	709	51	172	1045
thigh breaded & fried	2 pieces (5.2 oz)	430	27	165	756
CHICKEN SUBSTITUTES					
Health Is Wealth					
Buffalo Wings	3 pieces (2.2 oz)	100	2	0	490
Chicken-Free Nuggets	3 pieces (2.25 oz)	90	1	0	330
Chicken-Free Patties	1 (3 oz)	120	2	0	440
Loma Linda					
Chicken Supreme Mix not prep	1/3 cup (0.9 oz)	90	1	0	720
Chik Nuggets	5 pieces (3 oz)	240	16	0	710
Fried Chik'n w/ Gravy	2 pieces (2.8 oz)	160	10	0	440
Morningstar Farms					
Chik Nuggets	4 pieces (3 oz)	160	4	0	670
Chik Patties	1 (2.5 oz)	150	6	0	570
Meatless Buffalo Wings	5 pieces (3 oz)	200	9	0	730
Soy Is Us					
Chicken Not!	1/2 cup (1.75 oz)	140	2	0	5
Worthington					
Chic-Ketts	2 slices (1.9 oz)	120	7	0	390
Chicken Sliced or Roll	2 slices (2 oz)	80	5	0	370
Chicken Sliced	2 slices (2 oz)	80	5	0	270
ChikStiks	1 (1.6 oz)	110	7	0	360
CrispyChik Patties	1 (2.5 oz)	150	6	0	600
Cutlets	1 slice (2.1 oz)	70	1	0	340
Diced Chik	1/4 cup (1.9 oz)	40	0	0	270
FriChik	2 pieces (3.2 oz)	120	8	0	430
FriChik Low Fat	2 pieces (3 oz)	80	3	0	430
Golden Croquettes	4 pieces (3 oz)	210	10	0	600
Yves					
Veggie Chicken Burgers	1 (3 oz)	120	3	0	390
CHICKPEAS					
canned					
Green Giant					
Garbanzo	1/2 cup (4.4 oz)	110	2	0	380
Progresso					
Chick Peas	1/2 cup (4.6 oz)	120	3	0	280
Garbanzo	1/2 cup (4.4 oz)	110	2	0	380
dried					
cooked	1 cup	269	4	0	11

FOOD	PORTION	CALS	FAT	CHOL	SOD
CHICORY					
greens raw chopped	1/2 cup	21	tr	0	41
root raw	1 (2.1 oz)	44	tr	0	30
roots raw cut up	1/2 cup (1.6 oz)	33	tr	0	23
witloof head raw	1 (1.9 oz)	9	tr	0	1
witloof raw	1/2 cup (1.6 oz)	8	tr	0	1
CHILI					
powder	1 tsp	8	tr	0	26
Amy's Organic					
Whole Meals Chili & Cornbread	1 pkg (10.5 oz)	320	6	10	780
Armour					
Chili No Beans	1 cup (8.7 oz)	390	29	70	1200
Chili w/ Beans Western Style	1 cup (8.8 oz)	370	22	60	1130
Chili w/ Beans	1 cup (8.9 oz)	370	21	50	1220
Chili w/ Beans Hot	1 cup (8.9 oz)	370	21	50	1220
Vienna Sausage & Chili	1 cup (8.7 oz)	410	27	80	1270
Eden					
Organic Chili Beans w/ Jalapeno & Red Peppers	1/2 cup (4.6 oz)	130	0	0	250
Gebhardt					
Chili Powder	1/4 tsp (0.3 g)	1	tr	0	tr
Chili Quik Seasoning	1 tbsp (0.3 oz)	43	1	0	985
Plain	1 cup (9.4 oz)	232	19	0	737
With Beans	1 cup (9.4 oz)	322	15	29	673
Health Valley					
Burrito	1 cup	160	1	0	360
Enchilada	1 cup	160	1	0	320
Fajita	1 cup	80	0	0	160
In A Cup Black Bean Mild	3/4 cup	120	1	0	290
In A Cup Texas Style Spicy	3/4 cup	120	1	0	290
Vegetarian Lentil Mild	1 cup	160	1	0	200
Vegetarian Lentil No Salt	1 cup	80	0	0	50
Vegetarian Mild	1 cup	160	1	0	200
Vegetarian Mild No Salt	1 cup	160	1	0	65
Vegetarian Spicy	1 cup	160	1	0	200
Vegetarian Spicy No Salt	1 cup	160	1	0	65
Vegetarian w/ 3 Beans Mild	1 cup	160	1	0	320
Vegetarian w/ Black Beans Mild	1 cup	160	1	0	320
Vegetarian w/ Black Beans Spicy	1 cup	160	1	0	320
Hormel					
Chunky w/ Beans	1 cup (8.7 oz)	270	7	35	1240
Hot No Beans	1 cup (8.3 oz)	210	9	35	910
Hot With Beans	1 cup (8.7 oz)	270	7	35	1240
Microcup Meals Chili Mac	1 cup (7.5 oz)	200	9	25	980

FOOD	PORTION	CALS	FAT	CHOL	SOD
Microcup Meals Hot With Beans	1 cup (7.3 oz)	220	6	30	1050
Microcup Meals No Beans	1 cup (7.3 oz)	190	8	30	800
Microcup Meals With Beans	1 cup (7.3 oz)	220	6	30	1050
No Beans	1 cup (8.3 oz)	210	9	35	910
Turkey No Beans	1 cup (8.3 oz)	190	3	75	1250
Turkey w/ Beans	1 cup (8.7 oz)	210	3	35	1180
Vegetarian	1 cup (8.7 oz)	200	1	0	780
With Beans	1 cup (8.7 oz)	270	7	35	1240
Hunt's					
Chili Beans	1/2 cup (4.5 oz)	87	1	0	597
Chili Sauce	2 tbsp (1.2 oz)	35	tr	0	393
Hurst					
HamBeens Chili Beans	1 serv	130	1	0	170
Just Rite					
With Beans	1 cup (9 oz)	379	27	35	51
Lean Cuisine					
Everyday Favorites Three Bean Chili w/ Rice	1 pkg (10 oz)	250	6	10	590
Lunch Bucket					
Chili With Beans	1 pkg (7.5 oz)	260	12	25	1040
Manwich					
Homestyle Fixins	1/2 cup (4.6 oz)	84	1	0	858
McCormick					
Original Chili Seasoning	1 1/3 tbsp (9 g)	30	1	0	310
Natural Choice					
Organic Vegan Three Bean	1/2 cup (4.6 oz)	140	1	0	510
Natural Touch					
Vegetarian	1 cup (8.1 oz)	170	1	0	870
Open Range					
Plain	1 cup (8.8 oz)	353	26	48	1216
With Beans	1 cup (9 oz)	281	16	26	1291
Stouffer's					
With Beans	1 pkg (8.75 oz)	270	10	35	1130
Ultimate					
No Beans Hot	1 cup (8.7 oz)	420	30	85	1420
Turkey w/ Beans	1 cup (8.7 oz)	260	9	50	930
W/ Beans	1 cup (8.7 oz)	320	16	50	920
W/ Beans Hot	1 cup (8.7 oz)	320	16	50	920
Van Camp					
Beanee Weenee Chilee	1 cup (7.7 oz)	240	12	35	1090
Chili With Beans	1 cup (8.9 oz)	350	21	45	1020
Mexican Style Chili Beans	1/2 cup (4.6 oz)	110	2	0	430
Wampler					
Turkey	1 cup	250	7	75	1840
Worthington					
Chili	1 cup (8.1 oz)	290	15	0	1130
Low Fat	1 cup (8.1 oz)	170	1	0	870

FOOD	PORTION	CALS	FAT	CHOL	SOD
Yves					
Veggie Chili	1 pkg (10.5 oz)	230	1	0	850
take-out					
con carne w/ bean	8.9 oz	254	8	133	1008
CHILI PEPPERS					
(*see* PEPPERS)					
CHINESE CABBAGE					
(*see* CABBAGE)					
CHINESE FOOD					
(*see* ASIAN FOOD)					
CHINESE PRESERVING MELON					
cooked	1/2 cup	11	tr	0	93
CHIPS					
(*see also* POPCORN, PRETZELS, SNACKS)					
Barbara's					
No Salt Added	1 1/4 cups (1 oz)	150	10	0	20
Pinta Chips	13 (1 oz)	130	6	0	70
Pinta Chips Salsa	12 (1 oz)	130	6	0	210
Potato	1 1/4 cups (1 oz)	150	10	0	180
Ripple	1 1/4 cups (1 oz)	150	10	0	180
Tortilla Blue Corn	15 (1 oz)	140	7	0	40
Yogurt & Green Onion	1 1/4 cups (1 oz)	150	9	0	240
Barbara's Bakery					
Potato	1 1/4 cup (1 oz)	150	10	0	180
Potato No Salt Added	1 1/4 cups (1 oz)	150	10	0	20
Potato Ripple	1 1/4 cup (1 oz)	150	10	0	180
Potato Yogurt & Green Onion	1 1/4 cup (1 oz)	150	9	0	240
Tortilla Blue Corn	15 chips (1 oz)	140	7	0	40
Tortilla Blue Corn No Salt	15 chips (1 oz)	140	7	0	0
Tortilla Pinta Salsa	15 chips (1 oz)	130	6	0	210
Bruno & Luigi's					
Pasta Chips Garlic & Herb	1 oz	117	1	0	25
Cape Cod					
Potato Golden Russet	1 pkg (0.5 oz)	70	4	0	75
Chester's					
Flamin'Hot	1 oz	140	8	0	250
Salsa	1 oz	140	7	0	290
Doritos					
3D's Cooler Ranch	27 (1 oz)	140	6	<5	350
3D's Nacho Cheesier	27 (1 oz)	140	7	<5	360
Cooler Ranch	12 (1 oz)	140	7	0	170
Flamin' Hot	11 (1 oz)	140	7	0	210
Nacho Cheesier	11 (1 oz)	140	7	0	200
Salsa Verde	12 (1 oz)	150	7	0	210
Smokey Red	12 (1 oz)	150	7	0	210
Spicy Nacho	12 (1 oz)	140	6	0	210
Toasted Corn	13 (1 oz)	140	7	0	120
Wow Nacho Cheesier	1 pkg (0.75 oz)	70	1	0	180

FOOD	PORTION	CALS	FAT	CHOL	SOD
Durangos					
Tortilla	15 (1 oz)	150	7	0	105
Fritos					
Chili Cheese	31 (1 oz)	160	10	0	240
Corn Chips BBQ	29 (1 oz)	150	9	0	290
Corn Chips King Size	12 (1 oz)	150	10	0	150
Corn Chips Sabrositas Flamin' Hot	30 (1 oz)	150	9	0	180
Corn Chips Sabrositas Lime'N Chile	28 (1 oz)	150	9	0	240
Corn Chips Wild N'Mild Ranch	28 (1 oz)	160	10	0	160
Original	32 (1 oz)	160	10	0	170
Scoops	11 (1 oz)	160	10	0	105
Texas Grill Honey BBQ	15 (1 oz)	150	9	0	200
Guiltless Gourmet					
Tortilla Baked Chili Lime	18 (1 oz)	110	2	0	200
Tortilla Baked Mucho Nacho	18 (1 oz)	110	2	0	200
Tortilla Baked Organic Blue Corn	18 (1 oz)	110	2	0	140
Tortilla Baked Picante Ranch	18 (1 oz)	110	2	0	200
Tortilla Baked Red Corn	18 (1 oz)	110	2	0	200
Tortilla Baked Spicy Black Bean	18 (1 oz)	110	2	0	200
Tortilla Baked Sweet White Corn	18 (1 oz)	110	2	0	140
Tortilla Baked Yellow Corn	18 (1 oz)	110	2	0	160
Tortilla Baked Yellow Corn Unsalted	18 (1 oz)	110	1	0	26
Herr's					
Potato	1 oz	140	8	0	180
Tortilla Restaurant Style White Corn	10 chips (1 oz)	140	6	0	90
Lance					
BBQ	22 (1 oz)	160	10	0	170
Cajun	15 (1 oz)	150	10	0	290
Corn Chips	39 (1.25 oz)	200	11	0	140
Corn Chips Hot BBQ	35 (1.25 oz)	210	13	0	210
Hot Fries	1 pkg (0.9 oz)	140	10	0	190
Mesquite BBQ	22 (1 oz)	150	10	0	280
Potato	23 (1 oz)	160	10	0	130
Ripple	15 (1 oz)	160	11	0	150
Salt & Vinegar	22 (1 oz)	160	10	0	340
Sour Cream & Onion	22 (1 oz)	160	10	0	170
Tortilla Fiesta Salsa Triangles	16 (1 oz)	140	7	0	200
Tortilla Nacho Mini Round	46 (1/25 oz)	180	9	0	240
Tortilla Nacho Triangles	15 (1 oz)	140	14	0	200

FOOD	PORTION	CALS	FAT	CHOL	SOD
Lay's					
Adobadas	16 (1 oz)	170	10	0	240
Baked KC Masterpiece BBQ	11 (1 oz)	120	3	0	210
Baked Original	11 (1 oz)	110	2	0	150
Baked Roasted Herb	12 (1 oz)	130	3	0	190
Baked Sour Cream & Onion	12 (1 oz)	120	2	0	210
Classic	20 (1 oz)	150	10	0	180
Deli Style Hot N'Tangy BBQ	18 (1 oz)	150	10	0	220
Deli Style Jalapeno	17 (1 oz)	150	10	0	230
Deli Style Original	17 (1 oz)	140	10	0	180
Deli Style Salt & Vinegar	16 (1 oz)	90	10	0	380
Flamin' Hot	17 pieces (1 oz)	150	10	0	180
KC Masterpiece BBQ	15 (1 oz)	150	10	0	200
Onion & Garlic	19 (1 oz)	150	9	0	200
Salt & Vinegar	17 pieces (1 oz)	150	10	0	300
Sour Cream & Onion	17 pieces (1 oz)	160	11	<5	200
Toasted Onion & Cheese	17 pieces (1 oz)	160	10	0	240
Wavy Au Gratin	13 (1 oz)	150	10	<5	200
Wavy Original	11 pieces (1 oz)	160	10	0	210
Wavy Ranch	11 (1 oz)	160	11	0	150
Wow Mesquite BBQ	20 (1 oz)	75	0	0	250
Wow Mesquite BBQ	20 (1 oz)	75	0	0	250
Wow Original	1 pkg (0.75 oz)	55	0	0	130
Wow Original	20 (1 oz)	75	0	0	200
Wow Sour Cream & Chive	19 (1 oz)	80	0	0	230
Wow Sour Cream & Chive	19 (1 oz)	80	0	0	230
Old Dutch Foods					
Potato	12-15 chips (1 oz)	150	8	0	130
Potato BBQ	12-15 chips (1 oz)	150	9	0	300
Potato BBQ Ripple	12-15 chips (1 oz)	150	9	0	180
Potato Cajun Ripple	12-15 chips (1 oz)	150	10	0	160
Potato Cheddar & Sour Cream Ripples	12-15 chips (1 oz)	150	9	0	190
Potato Dill	12-15 chips (1 oz)	140	8	0	310
Potato Dutch Crunch	15-20 chips (1 oz)	130	6	0	140
Potato French Onion Ripple	12-15 chips (1 oz)	150	10	0	180
Potato Jalapeno & Cheddar Dutch Crunch	15-20 chips (1 oz)	130	6	0	190
Potato Jalapeno Cheese	12-15 chips (1 oz)	150	9	0	170
Potato Mesquite BBQ Dutch Crunch	15-20 chips (1 oz)	130	6	0	230
Potato Onion & Garlic	12-15 chips (1 oz)	140	8	0	210
Potato Outback Spicy BBQ	12-15 chips (1 oz)	150	10	0	170
Potato Ripples	12-15 chips (1 oz)	150	9	0	115
Potato Salt & Vinegar Dutch Crunch	15-20 chips (1 oz)	130	6	0	360
Potato Sour Cream & Onion	12-15 chips (1 oz)	150	9	0	230
Tortilla Bite Size White Corn	20 chips (1 oz)	150	8	0	105

FOOD	PORTION	CALS	FAT	CHOL	SOD
Tortilla Nacho Cheese	15 chips (1 oz)	150	7	0	150
Tortilla Restaurant Style White	9 chips (1 oz)	140	7	0	95
Tostados White Corn	11 chips (1 oz)	140	7	0	115
Tostados Yellow	11 chips (1 oz)	140	6	0	90
Pringles					
Fat Free	15 chips (1 oz)	75	0	0	170
Original	14 chips (1 oz)	160	11	0	170
Robert's American Gourmet					
Spirulina Spirals	1 oz	120	2	0	110
Ruffles					
Baked	10 (1 oz)	110	2	0	180
Baked Cheddar & Sour Cream	9 (1 oz)	120	3	0	270
Buffalo Style	11 chips (1 oz)	160	10	0	230
Cheddar & Sour Cream	11 chips (1 oz)	160	10	0	190
French Onion	11 (1 oz)	150	10	0	190
MC Masterpiece Mesquite BBQ	11 (1 oz)	150	10	0	190
Original	12 chips (1 oz)	150	10	0	180
Ranch	13 (1 oz)	150	9	0	280
Reduced Fat	16 (1 oz)	130	7	0	130
The Works	12 (1 oz)	160	11	0	210
Wow Cheddar & Sour Cream	15 (1 oz)	75	0	0	230
Wow Original	6 (1 oz)	90	1	0	105
Wow Original	17 (1 oz)	75	0	0	200
Santitas					
100% White Corn	6 (1 oz)	130	6	0	110
Restaurant Style Chips	7 (1 oz)	130	6	0	110
Restaurant Style Strips	10 (1 oz)	130	6	0	110
Snyder's Of Hanover					
BBQ Rib	1 oz	140	7	0	290
Barbeque Corn	1.5 oz	230	14	0	350
Cheddar Bacon	1 oz	150	6	0	270
Corn Chips	1.5 oz	230	15	0	220
Grilled Steak & Onion	1 oz	140	6	0	140
Hot Buffalo	1 oz	150	7	0	330
Kosher Dill	1 oz	140	6	0	360
No Salt	1 oz	140	6	0	0
Potato	1 oz	140	6	0	90
Ripple	1 oz	140	6	0	100
Salt & Vinegar	1 oz	140	6	0	150
Sausage Pizza	1 oz	150	6	0	250
Sour Cream & Onion	1 oz	150	7	0	150
Tasty Veggie Potato Chips	1 oz	150	6	0	260
Tortilla Nacho	1 oz	140	7	0	130
Tortilla No Salt Yellow Corn	1 oz	140	6	0	0
Tortilla White Corn	1 oz	140	6	0	130

FOOD	PORTION	CALS	FAT	CHOL	SOD
Snyder's Of Hanover (cont.)					
Tortilla Yellow Corn	1 oz	140	6	0	130
Tortilla Yellow Corn Mini	1 oz	160	8	0	130
Soya King					
Soy Mongolian BBQ	23 chips (1 oz)	140	7	0	115
Soy Original	23 chips (1 oz)	140	7	0	115
Soy Sour Cream & Onion	23 chips (1 oz)	140	7	0	115
Soy Taco	23 chips (1 oz)	140	7	0	115
Sunchips					
French Onion	13 (1 oz)	140	7	0	115
Harvest Cheddar	13 (1 oz)	140	6	0	115
Original	14 (1 oz)	140	6	0	115
Tostitos					
Baked Bite Size	20 (1 oz)	110	1	0	200
Baked Bite Size Salsa & Cream Cheese	16 (1 oz)	120	3	0	190
Baked Original	13 (1 oz)	110	1	3	200
Bite Size	15 (1 oz)	140	8	0	110
Crispy Rounds	13 (1 oz)	150	8	0	85
Nacho Style	6 (1 oz)	140	6	0	100
Restaurant Style	7 (1 oz)	140	6	0	110
Restaurant Style Hint Of Lime	6 (1 oz)	140	6	0	160
Santa Fe Gold	7 (1 oz)	140	6	0	80
Tyson					
Tortilla Salted	13 (1 oz)	150	7	0	65
Tortilla Yellow Corn Salted	13 (1 oz)	150	7	0	65
Utz					
Baked Crisps	12 (1 oz)	110	2	0	180
Carolina Barbeque	20 (1 oz)	150	9	0	270
Cheddar & Sour Cream	20 (1 oz)	160	10	0	200
Corn Chips	24 (1 oz)	160	10	0	160
Corn Chips Barbecue	24 (1 oz)	160	10	0	180
Grandma	20 (1 oz)	140	8	5	120
Grandma BBQ	20 (1 oz)	140	8	5	240
Home Style Kettle	20 (1 oz)	140	8	0	120
Home Style Kettle BBQ	20 (1 oz)	140	8	0	240
Kettle Classics Crunchy	20 (1 oz)	150	9	0	95
Kettle Classics Crunchy Mesquite BBQ	20 (1 oz)	150	9	0	200
No Salt Added	20 (1 oz)	150	9	0	5
Onion & Garlic	20 (1 oz)	150	9	0	180
Potato	20 (1 oz)	150	9	0	95
Reduced Fat BBQ	22 (1 oz)	140	6	0	190
Reduced Fat Ripple	24 (1 oz)	140	7	0	120
Ripple	20 (1 oz)	150	10	0	95
Ripple Sour Cream & Onion	20 (1 oz)	160	10	0	140
Ripple Barbeque	20 (1 oz)	150	10	0	200
Salt'N Vinegar	20 (1 oz)	150	9	0	270

FOOD	PORTION	CALS	FAT	CHOL	SOD
The Crab Chip	20 (1 oz)	150	9	0	300
Tortilla Black Bean & Salsa	13 (1 oz)	150	7	0	230
Tortilla Low Fat Baked	10 (1 oz)	120	2	0	200
Tortilla Nacho	13 (1 oz)	150	8	0	200
Tortilla Restaurant Style	6 (1 oz)	140	7	0	120
Tortilla Spicy Nacho	13 (1 oz)	150	8	0	220
Tortilla White Corn	12 (1 oz)	140	7	0	120
Wavy	20 chips (1 oz)	150	9	0	95
Yes! Fat Free	20 (1 oz)	75	0	0	180
Yes! Fat Free Barbeque	20 (1 oz)	75	0	0	210
Yes! Fat Free Ripple	20 (1 oz)	75	0	0	180
Wise					
Dipsy Doodles	1 pkg (1.5 oz)	240	15	0	270
Wow					
Tortilla Nacho Cheese	11 (1 oz)	90	1	0	240
CHITTERLINGS					
pork cooked	3 oz	258	24	122	33
CHIVES					
fresh chopped	1 tbsp	1	tr	0	0
fresh chopped	1 tsp	0	tr	0	0
CHOCOLATE					

(*see also* CANDY, CAROB, COCOA, ICE CREAM, TOPPINGS, MILK DRINKS)

baking

FOOD	PORTION	CALS	FAT	CHOL	SOD
Baker's					
Bittersweet	1/2 square (0.5 oz)	70	6	0	0
German's Sweet	2 squares (0.5 oz)	60	4	0	0
Semi-Sweet	1/2 square (0.5 oz)	70	5	0	0
Unsweetened	1/2 square (0.5 oz)	70	7	0	0
White	1/2 square (0.5 oz)	80	5	<5	15
Nestle					
Choco Bake	1/2 oz	80	8	0	0
Premier White Bar	1/2 oz	80	5	<5	15
Premier White Morsels	1 tbsp	80	4	0	20
Semi-Sweet Bar	1/2 oz	70	4	0	0
Unsweetened Bar	1/2 oz	80	7	0	0
chips					
Baker's					
Real Milk Chocolate	1/2 oz	70	4	0	10
Real Semi-Sweet	1/2 oz	60	4	0	0
Semi-Sweet	1/2 oz	70	4	0	15
Hershey					
Almond Joy Bits	1 tbsp (0.5 oz)	60	4	0	0
Chocolate & Peanut Butter Chips	1 tbsp (0.5 oz)	70	3	0	40
Holiday Baking Bits	1 tbsp (0.5 oz)	70	3	0	0
Milk Chocolate	1 tbsp (0.5 oz)	80	5	<5	10
Mini Kisses For Baking Mint	11 pieces (0.5 oz)	80	5	<5	15
Chocolate	1 tbsp (0.5 oz)	80	4	0	0

FOOD	PORTION	CALS	FAT	CHOL	SOD
Hershey (cont.)					
Premier White Milk Chips	1 tbsp (0.5 oz)	80	4	0	30
Raspberry Chips	1 tbsp (0.5 oz)	80	4	0	0
Semi-Sweet	1 tbsp (0.5 oz)	80	4	0	0
Semi-Sweet Mini	1 tbsp (0.5 oz)	80	4	0	0
Skor English Toffee Baking Bits	1 tbsp (0.5 oz)	70	5	10	60
M&M's					
Baking Bits Milk Chocolate	0.5 oz	70	3	5	0
Baking Bits Semi-Sweet	0.5 oz	70	4	0	0
Nestle					
Crunch Baking Pieces	1 1/2 tbsp	80	4	0	25
Milk Chocolate Morsels	1 tbsp	70	4	<5	0
Mint Chocolate Morsels	1 tbsp	70	4	0	0
Morsels Semi-Sweet	1 tbsp	70	4	0	0
Semi-Sweet Mega Morsels	1 tbsp	70	4	0	0
Semi-Sweet Mini Morsels	1 tbsp	70	4	0	0
Toll House					
Mint-Chocolate	2 tbsp (1.5 oz)	130	3	0	30
Semi-Sweet	2 tbsp (1.5 oz)	130	4	0	30
mix					
powder as prep w/ whole milk	9 oz	226	9	33	165
Quik					
Chocolate Powder	2 tbsp (0.8 oz)	90	1	0	30
Chocolate Powder No Sugar	2 tbsp (0.4 oz)	40	1	0	45
CHOCOLATE MILK					
(*see* CHOCOLATE, COCOA, MILK DRINKS, MILKSHAKE)					
CHOCOLATE SYRUP					
syrup as prep w/ whole milk	9 oz	232	9	33	156
Estee					
Chocolate	2 tbsp	15	0	0	40
Hershey					
Chocolate Fudge (canned)	1 tbsp (0.7 oz)	70	3	<5	25
Chocolate Malt	2 tbsp (1.4 oz)	100	0	0	55
Lite	2 tbsp (1.2 oz)	50	0	0	35
Syrup	2 tbsp (1.4 oz)	100	0	0	25
Quik					
Chocolate	2 tbsp (1.3 oz)	100	1	0	30
Toll House					
Mint Chocolate	2 tbsp (1.5 oz)	130	3	0	30
Semi-Sweet	2 tbsp (1.5 oz)	130	4	0	30
CHUTNEY					
coconut	1/4 cup	74	7	0	5
CILANTRO					
fresh	1 tsp (2 g)	tr	tr	0	1
fresh	1 cup (1.6 oz)	11	tr	0	25
CINNAMON					
ground	1 tsp	6	tr	0	1

FOOD	PORTION	CALS	FAT	CHOL	SOD
CISCO					
smoked	3 oz	151	10	27	409
CLAMS					
canned					
Progresso					
Creamy Clam Sauce	1/2 cup (4.2 oz)	110	6	10	440
Minced	1/4 cup (2.1 oz)	25	0	10	250
Red Clam Sauce	1/2 cup (4.4 oz)	60	1	10	350
White Clam Sauce	1/2 cup (4.4 oz)	150	10	20	710
fresh					
cooked	20 sm	133	2	60	100
raw	20 sm	133	2	60	100
take-out					
breaded & fried	20 sm	379	21	115	684
CLOVES					
ground	1 tsp	7	tr	0	5
COCOA					
(*see* also CHOCOLATE)					
hot cocoa	1 cup	218	9	33	123
Carnation					
Hot Cocoa 70 Calorie	1 pkg (0.7 oz)	70	0	0	140
Hot Cocoa Double Chocolate Meltdown	1 pkg (1.2 oz)	150	4	0	170
Hot Cocoa Fat Free Raspberry	1 pkg (0.3 oz)	30	0	0	150
Hot Cocoa Fat Free w/ Marshmallows	1 pkg (0.4 oz)	45	0	0	100
Hot Cocoa Lactose Free	1 pkg (1 oz)	120	2	0	115
Hot Cocoa Marshmallow Blizzard	1 pkg (1.5 oz)	180	2	<5	140
Hot Cocoa Milk Chocolate	3 tbsp (1 oz)	110	1	<5	95
Hot Cocoa Rich Chocolate	3 tbsp (1 oz)	110	1	<5	100
Hot Cocoa Rich Chocolate Fat Free	1 pkg (0.3 oz)	25	0	0	135
Hot Cocoa Rich Chocolate No Sugar Added	3 tbsp (0.5 oz)	50	0	<5	140
Hot Cocoa Rich Chocolate w/ Marshmallows	3 tbsp (1 oz)	110	1	<5	95
Hershey					
Cocoa	1 tbsp (5 g)	20	1	0	0
European Cocoa	1 tbsp (5 g)	20	1	0	0
Nestle					
Cocoa	1 tbsp	15	1	0	0
Hot Cocoa Rich Chocolate	1 pkg (1 oz)	110	1	0	60
Hot Cocoa Rich w/ Marshmallows	1 pkg (1 oz)	110	1	0	60
Swiss Miss					
Hot Cocoa And Cream	1 serv	153	5	6	159

FOOD	PORTION	CALS	FAT	CHOL	SOD
Swiss Miss (cont.)					
Hot Cocoa Chocolate Sensation	1 serv	148	4	tr	171
Hot Cocoa Diet	1 serv	22	tr	tr	185
Hot Cocoa Fat Free	1 serv	52	tr	0	185
Hot Cocoa Fat Free Marshmallow Lovers	1 serv	65	tr	0	155
Hot Cocoa Lite	1 serv	76	1	0	177
Hot Cocoa Marshmallow Lovers	1 serv	142	3	2	152
Hot Cocoa Milk Chocolate	1 serv	118	3	1	118
Hot Cocoa Milk Chocolate No Sugar Added	1 serv	55	1	1	164
Hot Cocoa Milk Chocolate w/ Marshmallows	1 serv	118	3	tr	123
Hot Cocoa Rich Chocolate	1 serv	110	2	1	140
Hot Cocoa White Chocolate	1 serv	109	1	1	128
Hot Cocoa w/ Marshmallows No Sugar Added	1 serv	56	1	1	146
Premiere Hot Cocoa Almond Mocha	1 serv	144	3	1	207
Premiere Hot Cocoa English Toffee	1 serv	142	2	1	223
Premiere Hot Cocoa Raspberry Truffle	1 serv	144	3	1	220
Premiere Hot Cocoa Suisse Truffle	1 serv	142	2	1	225
Rich Hot Cocoa No Sugar Added	1 serv	54	1	1	165
Sidewalk Cafe Cappuccino	1 serv	119	4	1	35
Sidewalk Cafe Cinnamon	1 serv	126	4	1	46
Sidewalk Cafe French Vanilla	1 serv	121	4	1	32
Sidewalk Cafe Mocha	1 serv	120	4	1	43
Weight Watchers					
Hot Cocoa Mix as prep	1 pkg	70	0	0	160
COCONUT					
coconut water	1 tbsp	3	tr	0	16
coconut water	1 cup	46	tr	0	252
cream canned	1 cup	568	52	0	149
cream canned	1 tbsp	36	3	0	10
fresh	1 piece (1.5 oz)	159	15	0	9
fresh shredded	1 cup	283	27	0	16
milk canned	1 tbsp	30	3	0	2
milk canned	1 cup	445	48	0	29
Baker's					
Angel Flake	1 tbsp (0.5 oz)	70	5	0	45
Angel Flake (canned)	2 tbsp (0.5 oz)	70	6	0	0
Premium Shred	2 tbsp (0.5 oz)	70	5	0	45

FOOD	PORTION	CALS	FAT	CHOL	SOD
COD					
canned					
atlantic	3 oz	89	1	47	185
dried					
atlantic	3 oz	246	2	129	5973
fresh					
atlantic cooked	3 oz	89	1	47	66
pacific baked	3 oz	95	1	43	82
COFFEE					
(see also COFFEE BEVERAGES, COFFEE SUBSTITUTES)					
instant					
decaffeinated	1 rounded tsp (1.8 g)	4	0	0	0
decaffeinated as prep	6 oz	4	0	0	6
regular	1 rounded tsp	4	0	0	1
regular as prep	6 oz	4	0	0	6
regular w/ chicory	1 rounded tsp	6	0	0	5
regular w/ chicory as prep	6 oz	6	0	0	10
Nescafe					
Decafe	1 tsp (2 g)	0	0	0	0
Decafe w/ Chicory	1 tsp (2 g)	0	0	0	0
French Vanilla	1 tsp (2 g)	5	0	0	0
French Vanilla Decaf	1 tsp (2 g)	5	0	0	0
Hazelnut	1 tsp (2 g)	5	0	0	0
Irish Creme	1 tsp (2 g)	5	0	0	0
Regular	1 tsp (2 g)	0	0	0	0
With Chicory	1 tsp (2 g)	5	0	0	0
regular					
brewed	6 oz	4	0	0	4
Folgers					
Colombian Supreme	1 tbsp	16	tr	0	tr
Custom Roast	1 tbsp	16	tr	0	tr
Decaffeinated	1 tbsp	17	tr	0	tr
French Roast	1 tbsp	16	tr	0	tr
Gourmet Supreme	1 tbsp	16	tr	0	tr
Instant	1 tsp	8	tr	0	1
Instant Decaffeinated	1 tsp	8	tr	0	2
Singles	1 bag	21	tr	0	1
Singles Decaffeinated	1 bag	21	tr	0	2
Special Roast	1 tbsp	16	tr	0	tr
Vacuum Pack	1 tbsp	16	tr	0	tr
Nescafe					
Cafe Mocha	1 can (10 oz)	140	3	10	115
Caffe Latte	1 can (10 oz)	130	3	15	130
Caffe Latte Decaffeinated	1 can (10 oz)	130	3	15	100
Espresso	1 tsp (2 g)	0	0	0	0
Espresso Cafe Latte	1 pkg (0.6 oz)	70	2	10	50
Espresso Cafe Mocha	1 pkg (1 oz)	110	3	10	35
Espresso Cappuccino	1 pkg (0.6 oz)	80	3	10	40

FOOD	PORTION	CALS	FAT	CHOL	SOD
Nescafe (cont.)					
Espresso Roast	1 can (10 oz)	90	1	<5	75
French Vanilla	1 can (10 oz)	150	4	15	140
Hazelnut	1 can (10 oz)	130	3	15	100
Roasted Ground Decaffeinated as prep	1 cup (6 oz)	0	0	0	0
Roasted Ground as prep	1 cup (6 oz)	0	0	0	0
take-out					
cafe au lait	1 cup (8 fl oz)	77	4	17	62
cafe brulot	1 cup (4.8 fl oz)	48	0	0	2
cappuccino	1 cup (8 fl oz)	77	4	17	62
coffee con leche	1 cup (8 fl oz)	77	4	17	62
espresso	1 cup (3 fl oz)	2	0	0	2
irish coffee	1 serv (9 fl oz)	107	3	12	25
latte w/ skim milk	13 oz	88	tr	4	128
latte w/ whole milk	13 oz	152	8	33	122
mocha	1 mug (9.6 fl oz)	202	15	40	28
COFFEE BEVERAGES					
(*see also* COFFEE SUBSTITUTES)					
Arizona					
Iced Latte Supreme	8 oz	110	2	6	95
Iced Mocha Latte	8 oz	110	2	5	98
Coffee House USA					
All Flavors	1 bottle (9.5 oz)	100	4	15	160
Gehl's					
Iced Cappuccino	1 can (11 oz)	190	2	13	330
General Foods					
Cappuccino Coolers French Vanilla as prep w/ 2% milk	1 serv	180	5	21	120
International Coffees Sugar Free Cafe Vienna as prep	1 serv (8 oz)	30	2	0	75
International Coffees Sugar Free Fat Free Suisse Mocha as prep	1 serv (8 oz)	25	0	0	35
International Coffees Cafe Francais as prep	1 serv (8 oz)	60	4	0	95
International Coffees Cafe Vienna as prep	1 serv (8 oz)	70	3	0	110
International Coffees Decaffeinated French Vanilla Cafe as prep	1 serv (8 oz)	60	3	0	55
International Coffees Decaffeinated Suisse Mocha as prep	1 serv (8 oz)	60	2	0	35
International Coffees French Vanilla Cafe as prep	1 serv (8 oz)	60	3	0	55
International Coffees Hazelnut Belgian Cafe as prep	1 serv (8 oz)	70	2	0	60

FOOD	PORTION	CALS	FAT	CHOL	SOD
International Coffees Irish Creme Cafe as prep	1 serv (8 oz)	60	2	0	45
International Coffees Italian Cappuccino as prep	1 serv (8 oz)	60	2	0	50
International Coffees Kahlua Cafe as prep	1 serv (8 oz)	60	2	0	55
International Coffees Orange Cappuccino as prep	1 serv (8 oz)	70	2	0	100
International Coffees Suisse Mocha as prep	1 serv (8 oz)	60	2	0	35
International Coffees Viennese Chocolate Cafe as prep	1 serv (8 oz)	50	2	0	30
International Coffees Sugar Free Fat Free Decaffeinated French Vanilla	1 serv (8 oz)	25	0	0	65
International Coffees Sugar Free Fat Free Decaffeinated Suisse Mocha	1 serv (8 oz)	25	0	0	35
International Coffees Sugar Free Fat Free French Vanilla Cafe as prep	1 serv (8 oz)	25	0	0	65
Maxwell House					
Cafe Cappuccino Amaretto as prep	1 serv (8 oz)	90	1	0	65
Cafe Cappuccino Decaffeinated Mocha as prep	1 serv (8 oz)	100	3	0	70
Cafe Cappuccino Decaffeinated Vanilla as prep	1 serv (8 oz)	90	1	0	65
Cafe Cappuccino Irish Cream as prep	1 serv (8 oz)	90	1	0	65
Cafe Cappuccino Mocha as prep	1 serv (8 oz)	100	3	0	65
Cafe Cappuccino Sugar Free Mocha as prep	1 serv (8 oz)	60	3	0	80
Cafe Cappuccino Sugar Free Vanilla as prep	1 serv (8 oz)	60	3	0	85
Cafe Cappuccino Vanilla as prep	1 serv (8 oz)	90	1	0	65
Iced Cappuccino as prep w/ 2% milk	1 serv (8 oz)	180	5	20	125
Starbucks					
Frappuccino	1 bottle (9.5 fl oz)	190	3	12	110

FOOD	PORTION	CALS	FAT	CHOL	SOD
COFFEE SUBSTITUTES					
Natural Touch					
Kaffree Roma	1 tsp (2 g)	10	0	0	0
Roma Cappuccino	3 tbsp (0.4 oz)	50	3	0	15
Pero					
Instant Grain Beverage	1 tsp (1.5 g)	5	0	0	0
Postum					
Instant Coffee Flavor as prep	1 serv (8 oz)	10	0	0	0
Instant as prep	1 serv (8 oz)	10	0	0	0
COFFEE WHITENERS					
(*see also* MILK SUBSTITUTES)					
liquid nondairy frozen	1 tbsp (0.5 oz)	20	2	0	12
powder nondairy	1 tsp	11	tr	0	4
N-Rich					
Coffee Creamer	1 tsp (2 g)	10	1	0	4
COLESLAW					
take-out					
coleslaw w/ dressing	1/2 cup	42	2	5	14
vinegar & oil coleslaw	3.5 oz	150	9	0	480
COLLARDS					
fresh cooked	1/2 cup	17	tr	0	10
frozen chopped cooked	1/2 cup	31	tr	0	42
COOKIES					
(*see also* BROWNIE, CAKE, DOUGHNUTS, PIE)					
mix					
Betty Crocker					
Chocolate Peanut Butter	1 bar	200	9	20	190
Easy Layer Dessert Bar	1 bar	140	6	0	105
Hershey Bars	1 bar	150	6	15	120
Pouch Dessert Chocolate Chip	2	160	8	10	105
Pouch Dessert Double Chocolate Chunk	2	150	6	10	105
Pouch Dessert Oatmeal Chocolate Chip	2	160	7	10	125
Pouch Dessert Peanut Butter	2	160	8	10	135
Pouch Dessert Sugar	2	170	8	10	130
Sunkist Lemon	1 bar	140	5	40	90
GoldnBrown					
Fat Free	1 (1.1 oz)	120	0	0	135
ready-to-eat					
australian anzac biscuit	1	98	3	0	59
graham chocolate covered	1 (0.49 oz)	68	3	0	41
hermits	1 (1 oz)	117	5	23	54
jumbles coconut	1 (1 oz)	121	7	26	19

FOOD	PORTION	CALS	FAT	CHOL	SOD
ladyfingers	1 (0.38 oz)	40	1	40	16
macaroons	1 (0.8 oz)	97	3	0	59
madeleines	1 (0.8 oz)	86	5	46	34
meringue	1 (0.3 oz)	20	0	0	20
neapolitan tri-color cookie	1 (0.6 oz)	79	5	17	10
pinenut cookies	1 (1.1 oz)	134	9	0	11
reginette queen'a biscuit	1 (0.8 oz)	86	3	tr	83
toll house original	1 (0.8 oz)	105	6	15	57
zeppole	1 (0.8 oz)	78	6	24	14
Alternative Baking					
Vegan Chocolate Chip	1 serv (2.5 oz)	280	10	0	150
Vegan Expresso Chocolate Chip	1 serv (2 oz)	230	9	0	125
Vegan Lemon	1 serv (2.25 oz)	250	7	0	170
Vegan Oatmeal	1 serv (2.25 oz)	250	10	0	105
Vegan Peanut Butter	1 serv (2.25 oz)	270	10	0	115
Vegan Pumpkin	1 serv (2 oz)	200	6	0	120
Vegan Wheat Free Choco Cherry Chunk	1 serv (1.75 oz)	190	6	0	30
Vegan Wheat Free Hula Nut	1 serv (1.75 oz)	190	6	0	65
Vegan Wheat Free P-nut Fudge Fusion	1 serv (1.75 oz)	190	7	0	75
Vegan Wheat Free Snickerdoodle	1 serv (1.75 oz)	170	3	0	70
Amay's					
Chinese Style Almond	1 (0.5 oz)	80	4	4	13
Archway					
Alpine Fudge	1 (1.3 oz)	160	6	<5	80
Carrot Cake	1 (1 oz)	130	5	5	200
Chocolate Chip	1 (0.9 oz)	120	6	5	85
Chocolate Chip Sugar Free	1 (0.8 oz)	110	5	0	65
Coconut Macaroon	2 (1.4 oz)	180	11	0	500
Devils Food Chocolate Drop Fat Free	1 (0.7 oz)	60	0	0	70
Dutch Cocoa	1 (0.9 oz)	100	4	0	65
Frosty Lemon	1 (0.9 oz)	100	4	0	100
Fruit & Honey Bar	1 (0.9 oz)	110	3	5	100
Fruit Bar Fat Free	1 (0.9 oz)	90	0	0	90
Ginger Snaps	5 (1 oz)	120	5	0	150
Homestyle Chocolate Chip	3 (1 oz)	130	7	5	60
Iced Spice	1 (1 oz)	120	5	0	140
Oatmeal	1 (0.9 oz)	100	4	5	100
Oatmeal Apple Filled	1 (0.9 oz)	90	3	<5	70
Oatmeal Pecan	1 (0.9 oz)	110	4	5	120
Oatmeal Raisin Bran	1 (0.9 oz)	100	3	0	65
Oatmeal Raspberry Fat Free	1 (1.1 oz)	100	0	0	170
Oatmeal Sugar Free	1 (0.8 oz)	110	5	0	75

FOOD	PORTION	CALS	FAT	CHOL	SOD
Archway (cont.)					
Oatmeal Raisin	1 (0.9 oz)	100	4	0	65
Oatmeal Raisin Fat Free	1 (1.1 oz)	100	0	0	60
Old Dutch Apple	1 (0.9 oz)	110	4	5	115
Peanut Butter	1 (1 oz)	150	9	5	110
Peanut Butter Fudge	1 (1.3 oz)	220	13	<5	135
Peanut Butter Sugar Free	1 (0.8 oz)	110	6	0	85
Pecan Crunch	3 (1.2 oz)	180	10	5	140
Raspberry Filled	1 (0.8 oz)	90	4	5	80
Rocky Road	1 (0.8 oz)	110	5	10	70
Rocky Road Sugar Free	1 (0.8 oz)	100	5	0	65
Shortbread Sugar Free	1 (0.8 oz)	110	5	0	45
Strawberry Filled	1 (0.8 oz)	90	3	0	80
BP Gourmet					
Biscotti Fat Free Cinnamon Crunch	6 (1 oz)	110	0	0	75
Biscotti Fat Free Vanilla Crunch	4 (1 oz)	80	0	0	25
Chocolate Fudge Chip Sugar Free	5 (1 oz)	100	6	0	80
Dreams Chocolate	7 (1 oz)	120	3	0	35
Dreams Fat Free Chocolate Fudge	13 (1 oz)	100	0	0	35
Dreams Fat Free Vanilla	19 (1 oz)	100	0	0	35
Tangos Fat Free Chocolate Fudge Chip	4 (1 oz)	100	0	0	95
Bahlsen					
Afrika	8 (1.1 oz)	170	10	5	20
Butter Leaves	7 (1 oz)	140	7	15	50
Choco Leibniz	2 (1 oz)	140	7	5	50
Choco Star Dark Chocolate	3 (1.1 oz)	170	12	0	10
Choco Star Milk Chocolate	3 (1.1 oz)	180	12	<5	25
Chocolate Hearts	4 (1 oz)	160	9	5	25
Delice	6 (1 oz)	140	6	0	100
Deloba	4 (0.9 oz)	130	5	0	80
Hanover Waffelin	5 (1 oz)	160	10	0	35
Hit Chocolate Vanilla Filled	2 (1 oz)	140	8	0	75
Hit Vanilla Chocolate Filled	2 (1 oz)	140	7	0	65
Kipferl	4 (1 oz)	150	9	5	10
Leibniz	6 (1 oz)	130	4	10	125
Nuss Dessert	3 (1.1 oz)	180	11	10	60
Probiers	6 (1 oz)	150	6	0	60
Twingo	6 (1.1 oz)	170	11	0	15
Waffeletten	4 (1 oz)	160	9	<5	40
Baker's Harvest					
Cinnamon Grahams Low Fat	2 (0.9 oz)	110	2	0	120

FOOD	PORTION	CALS	FAT	CHOL	SOD
Graham Low Fat	2 (0.9 oz)	110	2	0	120
Iced Oatmeal	1 (0.6 oz)	70	3	0	65
Pecan Shortbread	1 (0.5 oz)	80	5	<5	55
Barbara's					
Animal Cookies Vanilla	8 (1 oz)	130	5	0	105
Chocolate Chip	1 (0.6 oz)	80	4	5	60
Double Dutch Chocolate	1 (0.6 oz)	80	4	5	60
Fat Free Homestyle Chewy Chocolate	2 (0.9 oz)	80	0	0	80
Fat Free Homestyle Chocolate Mint	2 (0.9 oz)	80	0	0	95
Fat Free Homestyle Nutt'n Crispies	2 (0.9 oz)	80	0	0	65
Fat Free Homestyle Oatmeal Raisin	2 (0.9 oz)	80	0	0	75
Fat Free Mini Carmel Apple	6 (1 oz)	110	0	0	125
Fat Free Mini Cocoa Mocha	6 (1 oz)	100	0	0	125
Fat Free Mini Double Chocolate	6 (1 oz)	100	0	0	135
Fat Free Mini Oatmeal Raisin	6 (1 oz)	110	0	0	105
Fig Bars Fat Free	1 (0.7 oz)	60	0	0	20
Fig Bars Fat Free Raspberry	1 (0.7 oz)	60	0	0	25
Fig Bars Fat Free Whole Wheat	1 (0.7 oz)	60	0	0	20
Fig Bars Fat Free Whole Wheat Apple Cinnamon	1 (0.7 oz)	60	0	0	20
Fig Bars Low Fat	1 (0.7 oz)	60	1	0	25
Fig Bars Low Fat Blueberry	1 (0.7 oz)	60	1	0	25
Old Fashioned Oatmeal	1 (0.6 oz)	70	3	5	65
Snackimals Chocolate Chip	8 (1 oz)	120	5	0	85
Snackimals Oatmeal Wheat Free	8 (1 oz)	120	5	0	75
Snackimals Vanilla	8 (1 oz)	120	5	0	55
Traditional Shortbread	1 (0.6 oz)	80	4	10	40
Barbara's Bakery					
Apple Cinnamon Bars Fat Free Whole Wheat	1 (0.7 oz)	60	0	0	20
Chocolate Chip	1 (0.6 oz)	80	4	5	60
Double Dutch Chocolate	1 (0.6 oz)	80	4	5	60
Fig Bars Fat Free Wheat Free	1 (0.7 oz)	60	0	0	20
Fig Bars Fat Free Whole Wheat	1 (0.7 oz)	60	0	0	20
Nature's Choice Coconut Almond	1 bar (1 oz)	120	5	0	10
Nature's Choice Expresso Bean	1 bar (1 oz)	120	3	0	10

FOOD	PORTION	CALS	FAT	CHOL	SOD
Barbara's Bakery (cont.)					
Nature's Choice Lemon Yogurt	1 bar (1 oz)	120	4	0	10
Nature's Choice Roasted Peanut	1 bar (1 oz)	130	5	0	50
Old Fashioned Oatmeal	1 (0.6 oz)	70	3	5	65
Raspberry Bars Fat Free Wheat Free	1 (0.7 oz)	60	0	0	25
Snackimals Chocolate Chip	8 (1 oz)	120	5	0	85
Snackimals Oatmeal Wheat Free	8 (1 oz)	120	5	0	75
Snackimals Vanilla	8 (1 oz)	120	5	0	55
Traditional Blueberry Low Fat	1 (0.7 oz)	60	1	0	25
Traditional Fig Low Fat	1 (0.7 oz)	60	1	0	25
Traditional Shortbread	1 (0.6 oz)	80	4	10	40
Bed & Breakfast					
Cranberry Orange Oatmeal	1 (0.8 oz)	110	5	10	75
Enrobed Shortbread	2 (1.4 oz)	190	9	15	125
Fruit Center Key Lime	2 (1.1 oz)	140	6	<5	55
Fruit Center Raspberry	2 (1.1 oz)	140	6	<5	55
Beigel's					
Black & White	1 (1 oz)	100	3	0	20
Breaktime					
Chocolate Chip	1 (0.3 oz)	37	2	0	37
Coconut	1 (0.3 oz)	35	1	0	15
Ginger	1 (0.3 oz)	34	1	0	<15
Oatmeal	1 (0.3 oz)	35	1	0	27
Sprinkles	1 (0.3 oz)	36	2	0	46
Brent & Sam's					
Chocolate Chip Pecan	2 (0.5 oz)	80	5	<5	60
Chocolate Chip Raspberry	2 (0.5 oz)	70	4	<5	60
Chocolate Chips	2 (0.5 oz)	70	4	<5	65
Key Lime White Chocolate	2 (0.5 oz)	70	4	<5	65
Oatmeal Raisin Pecan	2 (0.5 oz)	70	7	<5	70
Toffee Pecan	2 (0.5 oz)	80	5	5	75
White Chocolate Macadamia	2 (0.5 oz)	80	5	<5	65
Bud's Best					
Caco Creme	7 (1 oz)	140	6	0	110
Chocolate Chip	6 (1 oz)	140	6	0	65
French Vanilla	7 (1 oz)	150	6	0	70
Oatmeal	6 (1 oz)	130	5	0	65
Cadbury					
Fingers	3	85	4	2	30
Cafe					
Cinnamony Twists Chocolate Chip	1 (0.5 oz)	40	2	0	25
Sugar Free California Almond	4 (1 oz)	110	4	0	60
Twists Cinnamony	1 (0.3 oz)	40	2	0	25

FOOD	PORTION	CALS	FAT	CHOL	SOD
Carr's					
Ginger Lemon Cremes	2 (1 oz)	140	7	<5	105
Chortles					
Cookies	1/2 pkg. (1 oz)	125	3	0	109
Dare					
Blueberry Cheesecake	1 (0.6 oz)	90	5	4	56
Butter Shortbread	1 (0.5 oz)	63	4	6	45
Butter Creme	1 (0.6 oz)	85	4	2	96
Carrot Cake	1 (0.6 oz)	92	5	3	61
Chocolate Chip	1 (0.5 oz)	77	4	2	42
Chocolate Fudge	1 (0.7 oz)	97	5	1	36
Cinnamon Danish	1 (0.4 oz)	47	2	2	25
Coconut Creme	1 (0.7 oz)	99	5	1	42
French Creme	1 (0.5 oz)	80	5	1	21
Harvest From The Rain Forest	1 (0.5 oz)	70	4	2	39
Key Lime Creme	1 (0.6 oz)	86	4	0	69
Lemon Creme	1 (0.7 oz)	95	5	1	66
Maple Leaf Creme	1 (0.6 oz)	83	4	0	53
Maple Walnut Fudge	1 (0.7 oz)	99	5	0	36
Milk Chocolate Fudge	1 (0.7 oz)	99	5	1	32
Oatmeal Raisin	1 (0.4 oz)	59	3	4	22
Social Tea	1 (0.2 oz)	26	1	0	25
Sun Maid Raisin Oatmeal	1 (0.5 oz)	52	3	5	30
De Beukelaer					
Pirouline	8 (1 oz)	130	4	15	50
Pirouline Viennese Wafers	1 (1 oz)	150	7	30	25
Delacre					
Chocosprits	1 (0.6 oz)	90	5	9	50
Marquisettes	3 (0.9 oz)	140	7	5	45
Roules d'Or	4 (1 oz)	180	8	0	35
Dunkaroos					
Chocolate Chip w/ Chocolate Frosting	1 pkg (1 oz)	120	5	0	100
Cinnamon Graham w/ Vanilla Frosting & Sprinkles	1 pkg (1 oz)	130	5	0	75
Cookies'n Creme	1 pkg (1 oz)	120	5	0	120
Dutch Mill					
Chocolate Chip	3 (1.1 oz)	160	10	0	85
Coconut Macaroons	3 (1 oz)	120	7	0	115
Oatmeal Raisin	3 (1 oz)	130	6	0	75
Eddyleon					
Jelly Graham Raspberry	1 (0.9 oz)	134	8	2	44
Pudding Cookies	1 (0.9 oz)	134	6	2	44
Entenmann's					
Little Bites Chocolate Chip	8 (1.8 oz)	240	12	10	120
Soft Baked Chocolate Chip	1 (0.7 oz)	100	5	10	60
Soft Baked Double Chocolate Chip	1 (0.7 oz)	100	5	10	65

FOOD	PORTION	CALS	FAT	CHOL	SOD
Entenmann's (cont.)					
Soft Baked Milk Chocolate Chip	1 (0.7 oz)	100	5	10	60
Soft Baked Original Chocolate Chip	3 (1 oz)	150	7	10	90
Soft Baked White Chocolate Macadamia Nut	1 (0.7 oz)	100	6	10	65
Soft Baked Light Chocolatey Chip	2 (1 oz)	120	4	0	80
Soft Baked Light Oatmeal Raisin	2 (1 oz)	100	0	0	150
Estee					
Chocolate Chip	4	150	7	0	30
Coconut	4	140	6	0	25
Fig Bars	2	100	1	0	20
Fudge	4	150	7	0	45
Lemon Thins	4	140	6	0	25
Oatmeal Raisin	4	130	5	0	25
Sandwich Chocolate	3	160	6	0	60
Sandwich Original	3	160	6	0	45
Sandwich Peanut Butter	3	160	7	0	55
Sandwich Vanilla	3	160	5	0	35
Shortbread	4	130	4	0	150
Sugar Free Chocolate Chip	3	110	4	0	70
Sugar Free Chocolate Walnut	3	110	4	0	95
Sugar Free Coconut	3	110	4	0	110
Sugar Free Grahams Chocolate	2	110	2	0	110
Sugar Free Grahams Cinnamon	2	90	2	0	90
Sugar Free Grahams Old Fashion	2	90	2	0	115
Sugar Free Lemon	3	110	3	0	90
Sugar Free Wafer Banana Split	5	155	9	0	10
Sugar Free Wafer Chocolate	5	150	9	0	10
Sugar Free Wafer Chocolate Peanut Butter Caramel	5	150	8	0	45
Sugar Free Wafer Lemon Creme	5	150	8	0	10
Sugar Free Wafer Peanut Butter Creme	5	150	8	0	40
Sugar Free Wafer Vanilla	5	150	8	0	10
Sugar Free Wafer Vanilla Strawberry	5	150	8	0	10
Vanilla Thins	4	140	6	0	25
Falcone's					
Sorrentini	1 (1 oz)	100	4	10	55

FOOD	PORTION	CALS	FAT	CHOL	SOD
Famous Amos					
Butter Shortie	1 (0.5 oz)	80	5	10	65
Chocolate Chip	4 (1 oz)	140	7	0	105
Chocolate Chip & Pecan	4 (1 oz)	140	8	0	100
Chocolate Chip Toffee	4 (1 oz)	130	6	0	115
Chocolate Creme Sandwich	3 (1.2 oz)	140	6	0	90
Chunky Chocolate Chip	1 (0.5 oz)	70	4	0	80
Fat Free Fig Bar	2 (1 oz)	90	0	0	60
Fat Free Strawberry Fruit Bar	2 (1 oz)	90	0	0	50
Fig Bar	2 (1.1 oz)	120	3	0	150
Oatmeal Chocolate Chip Walnut	4 (1 oz)	140	7	0	120
Oatmeal Raisin	4 (1 oz)	130	6	5	135
Peanut Butter Chocolate Chunk	1 (0.5 oz)	80	5	0	70
Peanut Butter Creme Sandwich	3 (1.2 oz)	160	8	0	115
Pecan Shortie	1 (0.5 oz)	80	5	0	55
Vanilla Creme Sandwich	3 (1.2 oz)	160	7	0	85
Frookie					
Animal Frackers	14 (1 oz)	130	5	0	90
Chocolate Chip Wheat & Gluten Free	3 (1.1 oz)	140	5	0	100
Double Chocolate Wheat & Gluten Free	3 (1.1 oz)	130	4	0	105
Dream Creams Strawberry	4 (1 oz)	140	8	0	55
Dream Creams Vanilla	4 (1 oz)	140	8	0	55
Funky Monkeys Chocolate	16 (1 oz)	120	4	0	120
Funky Monkeys Vanilla	16 (1 oz)	120	4	0	120
Graham Cinnamon	2 (1 oz)	100	3	0	105
Graham Honey	2 (1 oz)	110	3	0	120
Lemon Wafers	8 (1 oz)	110	0	0	130
Old Fashioned Ginger Snaps	8 (1 oz)	120	2	0	110
Organic Chocolate Chip	3 (1.1 oz)	150	7	0	115
Organic Double Chocolate Chip	3 (1.1 oz)	140	6	0	95
Organic Iced Lemon	3 (1.3 oz)	165	6	0	115
Organic Oatmeal Raisin	3 (1.1 oz)	140	5	0	110
Peanut Butter Chunk Wheat & Gluten Free	3 (1.1 oz)	140	5	0	140
Sandwich Chocolate	2 (0.7 oz)	100	4	0	60
Sandwich Lemon	2 (0.7 oz)	100	4	0	60
Sandwich Peanut Butter	2 (0.7 oz)	100	4	0	60
Sandwich Vanilla	2 (0.7 oz)	100	4	0	60
Shortbread	5 (1 oz)	130	5	15	95
Vanilla Wafers	8 (1 oz)	110	0	0	120
General Henry					
Fruit Bars Apple	1 (0.6 oz)	60	1	0	70
Fruit Bars Blueberry	1 (0.6 oz)	60	1	0	75
Fruit Bars Fig	1 (0.6 oz)	60	1	0	70

FOOD	PORTION	CALS	FAT	CHOL	SOD
Girl Scout					
Apple Cinnamon Reduced Fat	3 (1 oz)	120	5	0	140
Do-si-dos	3 (1.2 oz)	170	8	0	105
Lemon Drops	3 (1.2 oz)	160	8	0	150
Samoas	2 (1 oz)	160	9	0	45
Striped Chocolate Chip	3 (1.2 oz)	180	10	0	100
Tagalongs	2 (0.9 oz)	150	10	0	85
Thin Mints	4 (1 oz)	140	8	0	80
Trefoils	5 (1.1 oz)	160	8	0	90
Golden Grahams Treats					
Chocolate Chunk	1 bar (0.8 oz)	90	3	0	110
Honey Graham	1 bar (0.8 oz)	90	2	0	120
King Size Chocolate Chunk	1 bar (1.6 oz)	190	5	0	220
King Size Honey Graham	1 bar (1.6 oz)	180	4	0	240
Gourmet					
Chocolate Chip	2 (1.1 oz)	160	9	15	85
Lemon Creme	2 (1.4 oz)	210	10	0	60
Oatmeal Raisin	2 (0.9 oz)	120	6	15	105
Peanut Butter Chip	2 (1 oz)	150	8	10	135
Raspberry Center	2 (1.1 oz)	140	5	10	60
Grandma's					
Chocolate Chip	1 (1.4 oz)	190	9	0	135
Fudge Chocolate Chip	1 (1.4 oz)	170	7	<5	160
Fudge Sandwich	3	180	5	0	200
Fudge Vanilla Sandwich	3	120	4	0	130
Mini Fudge	9	150	7	0	180
Mini Peanut Butter	9	150	7	0	140
Mini Vanilla	9	150	7	<5	85
Oatmeal Raisin	1 (1.4 oz)	160	6	5	250
Old Time Molasses	1 (1.4 oz)	160	4	<5	230
Peanut Butter	1 (1.4 oz)	190	9	5	200
Peanut Butter Chocolate Chip	1 (1.4 oz)	190	9	<5	170
Peanut Butter Sandwich	5	210	10	0	200
Rich N'Chewy	1 pkg	270	12	10	130
Vanilla Sandwich	3	180	5	0	160
Vanilla Sandwich	5	210	10	5	125
Handi-Snack					
Cookie Jammers Cookies & Fruit Spread	1 pkg (1.3 oz)	130	3	0	125
Health Valley					
Apple Spice	3	100	0	0	50
Apricot Delight	3	100	0	0	50
Biscotti Amaretto	2	120	3	0	50
Biscotti Chocolate	2	120	3	0	50
Biscotti Fruit & Nut	2	120	3	0	50
Cheesecake Bars Blueberry	1 bar	160	2	0	30
Cheesecake Bars Raspberry	1 bar	160	2	0	30

FOOD	PORTION	CALS	FAT	CHOL	SOD
Cheesecake Bars Strawberry	1 bar	160	2	0	30
Chips Double Chocolate	3	100	0	0	40
Chips Old Fashioned	3	100	0	0	40
Chips Original	3	100	0	0	40
Chocolate Fudge Center	2	70	0	0	25
Chocolate Sandwich Bars Bavarian Creme	1 bar	150	0	0	30
Chocolate Sandwich Bars Caramel Creme	1 bar	150	0	0	30
Chocolate Sandwich Bars Vanilla Creme	1 bar	150	0	0	30
Date Delight	3	100	0	0	50
Graham Amaranth	8	100	0	0	30
Graham Oat Bran	8	100	0	0	30
Graham Original Amaranth	6	120	3	0	80
Hawaiian Fruit	3	100	0	0	50
Jumbo Apple Raisin	1	80	0	0	35
Jumbo Raisin Raisin	1	80	0	0	35
Jumbo Raspberry	1	80	0	0	35
Marshmallow Bars Chocolate Chip	1	90	0	0	20
Marshmallow Bars Old Fashioned	1	90	0	0	20
Marshmallow Bars Tropical Fruit	1	90	0	0	20
Oat Bran Fruit Bars Raisin Cinnamon	1 bar	160	1	0	10
Raisin Oatmeal	3	100	0	0	50
Raspberry Fruit Center	1	70	0	0	20
Tarts Baked Apple Cinnamon	1	150	0	0	40
Tarts California Strawberry	1	150	0	0	40
Tarts Chocolate Fudge	1	150	0	0	50
Tarts Cranberry Apple	1	150	0	0	40
Tarts Mountain Blueberry	1	150	0	0	40
Tarts Red Raspberry	1	150	0	0	40
Tarts Sweet Red Cherry	1	150	0	0	40
Hellema					
Almond	1 pkg (0.6 oz)	90	5	0	35
Hershey					
Cripsy Rice Snacks Peanut Butter	1 (0.6 oz)	70	3	0	130
Joseph's					
Almond Sugar Free	2 (0.9 oz)	100	5	0	20
Chocolate Chip Sugar Free	2 (0.9 oz)	100	5	0	40
Chocolate Walnut Sugar Free	2 (0.9 oz)	100	6	0	40
Coconut Sugar Free	2 (0.9 oz)	105	5	0	40
Lemon Sugar Free	2 (0.9 oz)	95	4	0	30
Oatmeal Raisin Sugar Free	2 (0.9 oz)	100	5	0	40

FOOD	PORTION	CALS	FAT	CHOL	SOD
Joseph's (cont.)					
Peanut Butter Sugar Free	2 (0.9 oz)	95	5	0	40
Pecan Shortbread Sugar Free	2 (0.9 oz)	100	5	0	40
Keebler					
Animal Crackers Chocolate Chip	7 (1 oz)	130	5	0	120
Animal Crackers Ernie's	1 box	250	9	0	290
Animal Crackers Iced	6 (1.1 oz)	150	5	0	110
Animal Crackers Sprinkled	6 (1.1 oz)	150	5	0	105
Butter	5 (1.1 oz)	150	6	10	170
Chips Deluxe	1 (0.5 oz)	80	5	0	60
Chips Deluxe Chocolate Lovers	1 (0.6 oz)	90	5	5	80
Chips Deluxe Coconut	1 (0.5 oz)	80	5	0	50
Chips Deluxe Rainbow	1 (0.6 oz)	80	4	<5	45
Chips Deluxe Soft 'n Chewy	1 (0.6 oz)	80	4	5	60
Chips Deluxe w/ Peanut Butter Cups	1 (0.6 oz)	90	5	0	45
Classic Collection Chocolate Fudge Creme	1 (0.6 oz)	80	4	0	75
Classic Collection French Vanilla Creme	1 (0.6 oz)	80	4	0	65
Cookie Stix Butter	5 (1.2 oz)	160	6	10	150
Cookie Stix Chocolate Chip	4 (0.9 oz)	130	5	5	100
Cookie Stix Rainbow	5 (1.2 oz)	150	6	5	110
Danish Wedding	4 (0.9 oz)	120	5	0	80
Droxies	3 (1.1 oz)	140	6	0	95
Droxies Reduced Fat	3 (1.1 oz)	140	5	0	150
E.L. Fudge Butter w/ Fudge Filling	2 (0.9 oz)	120	6	<5	70
E.L. Fudge Fudge w/ Fudge Filling	2 (0.9 oz)	120	6	0	70
E.L. Fudge w/ Peanut Butter Filling	2 (0.9 oz)	120	6	0	150
Fudge Shoppe Deluxe Grahams	3 (1 oz)	140	7	0	105
Fudge Shoppe Double Fudge 'n Caramel	2 (1 oz)	140	7	0	65
Fudge Shoppe Fudge Sticks	3 (1 oz)	150	8	0	55
Fudge Shoppe Fudge Sticks Peanut Butter	3 (1 oz)	150	8	0	45
Fudge Shoppe Fudge Stripes	3 (1.1 oz)	160	8	0	140
Fudge Shoppe Fudge Stripes Reduced Fat	3 (1 oz)	140	5	0	120
Fudge Shoppe Grasshoppers	4 (1 oz)	150	7	0	70
Fudge Shoppe S'mores	3 (1.2 oz)	160	8	0	95
Ginger Snaps	5 (1.1 oz)	150	6	0	120

FOOD	PORTION	CALS	FAT	CHOL	SOD
Golden Fruit Cranberry	1 (0.7 oz)	80	2	0	55
Golden Fruit Raisin	1 (0.7 oz)	80	2	0	50
Graham Cinnamon Crisp	8 (1 oz)	140	5	0	170
Graham Cinnamon Crisp Low Fat	8 (1 oz)	110	2	0	190
Graham Honey	8 (1.1 oz)	150	6	0	140
Graham Honey Low Fat	8 (1.1 oz)	120	2	0	210
Graham Original Lemon Coolers	8 (1 oz)	130	3	0	135
	5 (1 oz)	140	6	0	100
Oatmeal Country Style	2 (0.8 oz)	120	5	0	115
Sandies Almond Shortbread	1 (0.5 oz)	80	5	5	50
Sandies Pecan Shortbread	1 (0.5 oz)	80	5	<5	75
Sandies Simply Shortbread	1 (0.5 oz)	80	5	10	70
Snack Size Chips Deluxe	1 pkg (2 oz)	300	16	5	170
Snack Size Chips Deluxe Chocolate Lovers	1 pkg (2 oz)	280	15	20	170
Snack Size Mini Fudge Stripes	1 pkg (2 oz)	280	14	0	150
Snack Size Rainbow Chips Deluxe	1 pkg (2 oz)	290	16	5	170
Snack Size Sandies w/ Pecans	1 pkg (2 oz)	300	17	10	190
Snackin' Grahams Cinnamon	21 (1 oz)	130	3	0	210
Snackin' Grahams Honey	23 (1 oz)	130	4	0	120
Soft Batch Chocolate Chip	1 (0.6 oz)	80	4	0	70
Soft Batch Homestyle Chocolate Chunk	1 (0.9 oz)	130	7	0	80
Soft Batch Homestyle Double Chocolate	1 (0.9 oz)	130	7	0	90
Soft Batch Homestyle Oatmeal Raisin	1 (0.9 oz)	130	5	0	150
Soft Batch Oatmeal Raisin	1 (0.5 oz)	70	3	0	65
Sugar Wafers Creme	3 (0.9 oz)	130	6	0	20
Sugar Wafers Lemon	3 (0.9 oz)	130	6	0	20
Sugar Wafers Peanut Butter	4 (1.1 oz)	170	9	0	75
Vanilla Wafers	8 (1.1 oz)	150	7	0	120
Vanilla Wafers Reduced Fat	8 (1.1 oz)	130	4	0	140
Vienna Fingers	2 (1 oz)	140	6	0	105
Vienna Fingers Lemon	2 (1 oz)	140	6	0	90
Knott's Berry Farm					
Shortbread Apricot	3 (1 oz)	120	5	4	70
Shortbread Boysenberry	3 (1 oz)	120	5	4	60
Shortbread Raspberry	3 (1 oz)	120	5	4	60
LU					
Le Bastogne	2 (0.8 oz)	120	5	0	50
Le Chocolatiers	3 (1 oz)	150	8	0	10
Le Dore	4 (1 oz)	140	6	<5	55
Le Fondant	4 (1.1 oz)	170	10	0	5
Le Palmier	4 (1.2 oz)	180	10	0	140
Le Petit Beurre	4 (1.2 oz)	150	4	10	180

FOOD	PORTION	CALS	FAT	CHOL	SOD
LU (cont.)					
Le Petit Ecolier Dark Chocolate	2 (0.9 oz)	130	6	5	55
Le Petit Ecolier Hazelnut Milk Chocolate	2 (0.9 oz)	130	7	5	55
Le Petit Ecolier Milk Chocolate	2 (0.9 oz)	130	6	5	55
Le Pim's Orange	2 (0.9 oz)	90	3	5	25
Le Pim's Raspberry	2 (0.9 oz)	90	3	5	25
Le Raisin Dore	4 (1.2 oz)	160	7	20	130
Le Truffe Coconut	4 (1.2 oz)	190	12	0	15
Le Truffe Praline Chocolate	4 (1.2 oz)	170	9	0	15
Les Varietes	3 (0.9 oz)	140	7	5	35
La Choy					
Fortune	4 (1 oz)	112	tr	0	11
Lance					
Apple Bar Fat Free	1 (1.75 oz)	160	0	0	80
Apple Oatmeal Bar	1 (1.8 oz)	190	6	10	180
Big Town Banana	1 pkg (2 oz)	250	10	0	160
Big Town Chocolate	1 pkg (2 oz)	250	8	0	160
Big Town Vanilla	1 pkg (2 oz)	250	11	0	120
Choc-O-Lunch	1 pkg (1.5 oz)	200	8	0	190
Choc-O-Mint	1 pkg (1 1/4 oz)	190	9	0	100
Coated Graham	1 pkg (1.3 oz)	190	8	0	95
Fig Bar	1 (1.75 oz)	180	4	0	150
Fudge Chocolate Chip	1 (2 oz)	130	5	<5	75
Gourmet Chocolate Chip	1 (2 oz)	130	6	5	75
Lem-O-Lunch	1 pkg (3.4 oz)	240	11	0	150
Lemon Nekot	1 pkg (1.5 oz)	210	10	0	125
Nut-O-Lunch	1 pkg (3.3 oz)	240	11	0	150
Oatmeal	1 (2 oz)	130	6	0	90
Oatmeal Creme	1 (2 oz)	240	10	0	220
Peanut Butter	1 (2 oz)	140	8	<5	65
Peanut Butter Creme Wafer	1 pkg (1.5 oz)	230	12	0	80
Van-O-Lunch	1 pkg (1.5 oz)	210	8	0	130
Larzaroni					
Arancelli	8 (1 oz)	160	8	8	36
Calypso	3 (1 oz)	150	8	0	30
Limonelli	5 (1 oz)	140	8	5	30
Malaika	5 (1 oz)	158	9	17	36
Nanette	4 (1.2 oz)	170	9	<5	30
Okla	3 (1 oz)	186	10	6	43
Oskar	10 (1 oz)	150	9	0	10
Samba	5 (1 oz)	160	10	0	150
Velieri	3 (0.9 oz)	120	5	10	60
Linden's					
Lemon	1 (1 oz)	120	5	10	135

FOOD	PORTION	CALS	FAT	CHOL	SOD
Little Debbie					
Apple Flips	1 (1.2 oz)	150	5	5	115
Caramel Bars	1 (1.2 oz)	160	8	0	85
Cherry Cordials	1 (1.3 oz)	170	8	0	95
Coconut Rounds	1 (1.2 oz)	150	7	0	90
Cookie Wreaths	1 (0.6 oz)	100	5	0	60
Easter Puffs	1 (1.2 oz)	140	6	0	65
Fig Bars	1 (1.5 oz)	150	4	0	110
Fudge Delights	1 (1.1 oz)	110	2	0	170
Fudge Rounds	1 (1.2 oz)	140	6	0	85
German Chocolate Ring	1 (1 oz)	140	8	0	65
Ginger	1 (0.7 oz)	90	3	5	60
Jelly Creme Pies	1 (1.2 oz)	160	7	0	160
Marshmallow Crispy Bar	1 (1.3 oz)	140	4	0	170
Marshmallow Supremes	1 (1.1 oz)	130	5	0	65
Marshmallow Pie Banana	1 pkg (1.5 oz)	180	6	0	110
Marshmallow Pie Chocolate	1 (1.4 oz)	160	6	0	95
Nutty Bar	1 (2 oz)	310	18	0	110
Oatmeal Raisin	1 (1.3 oz)	160	7	0	170
Oatmeal Creme Pie	1 (1.3 oz)	170	7	0	190
Oatmeal Delights	1 (1.1 oz)	110	2	0	135
Oatmeal Lights	1 (1.3 oz)	130	3	0	180
Peanut Butter Bars	1 (1.9 oz)	270	15	0	140
Peanut Butter & Jelly Oatmeal Pie	1 (1.1 oz)	130	5	0	100
Peanut Clusters	1 (1.4 oz)	190	11	0	120
Pumpkin Delights	1 (1.2 oz)	150	5	5	140
Raisin Creme Pie	1 (1.2 oz)	140	5	0	120
Star Crunch	1 (1.1 oz)	140	6	0	70
Sugar Free Chocolate Chip	3 (1.1 oz)	140	7	0	100
Sugar Free Oatmeal	6 (1.1 oz)	120	4	0	130
Yo-Yo's	1 (1.2 oz)	130	6	0	125
Milk Lunch Brand					
New England Biscuits	4 (1.1 oz)	140	5	<5	220
MoonPie					
Chocolate	1 (2.75 oz)	330	10	0	256
Mini Banana	1 (1.2 oz)	152	5	0	120
Mini Chocolate	1 (1.2 oz)	152	5	0	120
Mini Vanilla	1 (1.2 oz)	152	5	0	120
Mother's					
Almond Shortbread	3	180	11	0	115
Checkerboard Wafers	8	150	8	0	40
Chocolate Chip	2	160	8	10	105
Chocolate Chip Angel	3	180	9	0	70
Chocolate Chip Parade	4	130	5	0	100
Circus Animals	6	140	6	0	55
Classic Assortments	2	140	7	0	105

FOOD	PORTION	CALS	FAT	CHOL	SOD
Mother's (cont.)					
Cocadas	5	150	7	5	140
Cookie Parade	4	140	7	0	95
Dinosaur Grrrahams	2	130	3	0	130
Double Fudge	2	180	9	0	110
English Tea	2	180	7	0	100
Flaky Flix Fudge	2	140	7	0	50
Flaky Flix Vanilla	2	140	8	0	40
Gaucho Peanut Butter	2	190	10	0	200
Iced Oatmeal	2	130	4	0	160
Iced Raisin	2	180	8	0	110
MLB Double Header Duplex	3	170	8	5	130
Macaroon	2	150	8	0	80
Marias	3	170	6	5	150
Oatmeal	2	110	5	0	150
Oatmeal Chocolate Chip	2	120	5	0	140
Oatmeal Raisin	5	150	7	5	125
Oatmeal Walnut Chocolate Chip	2	130	6	0	135
Rainbow Wafers	8	150	8	0	40
Striped Shortbread	3	170	8	0	75
Sugar	2	140	6	0	75
Taffy	2	180	8	0	160
Triplet Assortment	2	140	7	0	112
Vanilla Wafers	6	150	6	4	85
Wallops Boysenberry	1	80	2	0	40
Wallops Honey Crust Fig	1	80	2	0	55
Wallops Honey Graham Fig	1	80	2	0	55
Wallops Mixed Berry	1	80	2	0	40
Wallops Peach Apricot	1	80	2	0	40
Wallops Raspberry	1	80	2	0	40
Wallops Strawberry	1	80	2	0	40
Walnut Fudge	2	130	7	0	90
Zoo Pals	14	140	5	0	120
Mrs. Alison's					
Coconut Bar	2 (1 oz)	130	6	0	85
Creme Wafers	5 (1.1 oz)	170	10	0	35
Duplex Sandwich	3 (1 oz)	130	5	0	105
Fudge Fingers	3 (1 oz)	160	10	0	20
Ginger Snaps	4 (1 oz)	130	3	<2	170
Jelly Tops	5 (1 oz)	140	7	0	45
Lemon Creme	3 (1 oz)	130	5	0	115
Macaroons	2 (1 oz)	140	7	0	95
Pecan	2 (1 oz)	140	7	0	75
Shortbread	5 (1 oz)	120	5	0	100
Vanilla Sandwich	3 (1 oz)	130	5	0	115

FOOD	PORTION	CALS	FAT	CHOL	SOD
Murray's					
Sugar Free Double Fudge	3 (1.2 oz)	140	6	0	110
Sugar Free Ginger Snap	6 (1 oz)	110	4	0	100
Sugar Free Peanut Butter	6 (1 oz)	130	7	0	85
Sugar Free Vanilla Sandwich Creme	3 (1 oz)	120	5	0	65
Sugar Free Vanilla Wafers	9 (1.1 oz)	120	4	0	85
Nabisco					
Barnum's Animal Crackers	10 (1 oz)	130	4	0	150
Barnum's Animal Crackers Chocolate	10 (1 oz)	130	4	0	160
Biscos Sugar Wafers	8 (1 oz)	140	6	0	40
Cafe Cremes Cappuccino	2 (1.1 oz)	160	8	0	130
Cafe Cremes Vanilla	2 (1.1 oz)	160	7	0	130
Cafe Cremes Vanilla Fudge	2 (1.1 oz)	200	10	0	140
Cameo	2 (1 oz)	130	5	0	105
Chips Ahoy!	3 (1.1 oz)	160	8	0	105
Chips Ahoy! Chewy	3 (1.3 oz)	170	8	0	125
Chips Ahoy! Chunky	1 (0.5 oz)	80	4	5	35
Chips Ahoy! Munch Size	6 (1.1 oz)	160	8	0	150
Chips Ahoy! Reduced Fat	3 (1.1 oz)	140	5	0	150
Family Favorites Iced Oatmeal	1 (0.6 oz)	80	3	0	55
Family Favorites Oatmeal	1 (0.6 oz)	80	3	0	65
Famous Chocolate Wafers	5 (1.1 oz)	140	4	<5	230
Grahams	4 (1 oz)	120	3	0	180
Honey Maid Chocolate	8 (1 oz)	120	3	0	170
Honey Maid Cinnamon Grahams	8 (1 oz)	120	3	0	180
Honey Maid Honey Grahams	8 (1 oz)	120	3	0	180
Honey Maid Low Fat Cinnamon Grahams	8 (1 oz)	110	2	0	170
Honey Maid Low Fat Grahams	8 (1 oz)	110	2	0	200
Honey Maid Oatmeal Crunch	8 (1 oz)	120	3	0	140
Lorna Doone	4 (1 oz)	140	7	5	130
Mallomars	2 (0.9 oz)	120	5	0	35
Marshmallow Twirls	1 (1 oz)	130	6	0	75
Mystic Mint	1 (0.5 oz)	90	5	0	65
Newton Fat Free Fig	2 (1 oz)	90	0	0	115
Newtons Fig	2 (1.1 oz)	110	3	0	125
Newtons Fat Free Apple	2 (1 oz)	90	0	0	65
Newtons Fat Free Cobblers Apple Cinnamon	1 (0.8 oz)	70	0	0	40
Newtons Fat Free Cobblers Peach Apricot	1 (0.8 oz)	70	0	0	55
Newtons Fat Free Cranberry	2 (1 oz)	100	0	0	95
Newtons Fat Free Raspberry	2 (1 oz)	100	0	0	115
Newtons Fat Free Strawberry	2 (1 oz)	90	0	0	95
Nilla Wafers	8 (1.1 oz)	140	5	<5	100

FOOD	PORTION	CALS	FAT	CHOL	SOD
Nabisco (cont.)					
Nilla Wafers Chocolate Reduced Fat	8 (1 oz)	110	2	0	120
Nilla Wafers Reduced Fat	8 (1 oz)	120	2	0	105
Nutter Butter Bites	10 (1 oz)	150	7	<5	125
Nutter Butter Chocolate Peanut Butter Sandwich	2 (1 oz)	130	5	0	140
Nutter Butter Peanut Butter Sandwich	2 (1 oz)	130	6	<5	110
Old Fashioned Ginger Snaps	4 (1 oz)	120	3	0	230
Oreo	3 (1.2 oz)	160	7	0	220
Oreo Double Stuff	2 (1 oz)	140	7	0	150
Oreo Reduced Fat	3 (1.1 oz)	130	4	0	190
Oreo Halloween	2 (1 oz)	140	7	0	115
Pecanz	1 (0.5 oz)	90	5	<5	50
Pinwheels Chocolate Marshmallow	1 (1 oz)	130	5	0	35
Rugrats Chocolate Frosted	8 (1.1 oz)	150	5	0	110
Rugrats Vanilla Frosted	8 (1.1 oz)	150	6	0	105
Social Tea	6 (1 oz)	120	4	5	115
Sweet Crispers Chocolate	18 (1.1 oz)	130	3	0	190
Sweet Crispers Chocolate Chip	18 (1.1 oz)	130	3	0	160
Teddy Grahams Chocolate	24 (1 oz)	130	5	0	170
Teddy Grahams Chocolately Chip	24 (1 oz)	130	5	0	135
Teddy Grahams Cinnamon	24 (1 oz)	130	4	0	150
Teddy Grahams Honey	24 (1 oz)	130	4	0	150
Nestle					
Flipz Crunchy Graham White Fudge Chocolate	8 (1 oz)	140	6	0	85
Newman's Own					
Fig Newman's Organic	2 (1.3 oz)	120	0	0	140
Nonni's					
Biscotti Cioccalati	1 (1 oz)	130	5	5	50
Biscotti Decadence	1 (1.1 oz)	130	5	5	55
Biscotti Original	1 (1 oz)	100	4	5	50
Biscotti Paradiso	1 (1.1 oz)	130	6	5	60
NutraBalance					
Fibre Oatmeal Raisin	1 (0.7 oz)	80	4	0	85
Protein Fortified	1 (2 oz)	260	14	10	180
ReNeph Spice	1 (2 oz)	210	7	0	230
Old Brussels					
Ginger Crisps	2 (0.9 oz)	140	4	0	115
Old London					
Coffee Toppers Chocolate Creme	3 (0.5 oz)	70	3	0	75
Coffee Toppers Vanilla Creme	3 (0.5 oz)	70	4	0	80

FOOD	PORTION	CALS	FAT	CHOL	SOD
Olde World					
Pizzelle Almond	3 (1 oz)	90	4	45	15
Pizzelle Anise	3 (1 oz)	90	4	45	15
Pizzelle Chocolate	3 (1 oz)	100	5	45	15
Pizzelle Lemon	3 (1 oz)	90	4	45	15
Pizzelle Vanilla	3 (1 oz)	90	4	45	15
Otis Spunkmeyer					
Butter Sugar	1 med (1.3 oz)	160	8	15	140
Butter Sugar	1 (2 oz)	250	12	20	210
Carnival	1 med (1.3 oz)	170	7	10	80
Chocolate Chip	1 med (1.3 oz)	170	8	10	120
Chocolate Chip	1 bite size (0.75 oz)	100	5	5	70
Chocolate Chip	1 (2 oz)	250	11	15	210
Chocolate Chip Pecan	1 med (1.3 oz)	170	9	10	110
Chocolate Chip Walnut	1 med (1.3 oz)	180	9	10	105
Chocolate Chip Walnut	1 bite size (0.75 oz)	100	5	5	60
Chocolate Chip Walnut	1 (2 oz)	270	14	15	160
Double Chocolate Chip	1 med (1.3 oz)	180	9	10	130
Double Chocolate Chip	1 bite size (0.75 oz)	100	5	5	75
Oatmeal Raisin	1 bite size (0.75 oz)	90	4	5	75
Oatmeal Raisin	1 med (1.3 oz)	160	7	10	130
Otis Express Chocolate Chunk	1 (2 oz)	280	13	20	190
Otis Express Double Chocolate Chip	1 (2 oz)	270	14	15	200
Otis Express Oatmeal Raisin	1 (2 oz)	240	10	15	200
Otis Express Peanut Butter	1 (2 oz)	270	15	15	250
Peanut Butter	1 med (1.3 oz)	180	10	10	160
Pinnacle Checkpoint Chocolate Almond Coconut	1 (2.4 oz)	320	18	25	230
Pinnacle Mach One Mocha Chocolate Chunk	1 (2.4 oz)	300	13	20	230
Pinnacle Passport Peanut Butter Chocolate Chunk	1 (2.4 oz)	300	13	25	250
Pinnacle Ripcord Rocky Road	1 (2.4 oz)	310	15	15	230
Pinnacle Takeoff Triple Chocolate	1 (2.4 oz)	300	14	20	180
Pinnacle Transatlantic Turtle	1 (2.4 oz)	310	16	20	250
Travel Lite Low Fat Apple Cinnamon	1 (1.3 oz)	130	2	0	90
Travel Lite Low Fat Chocolate Chip	1 (1.3 oz)	130	2	0	110
Travel Lite Low Fat Ginger Spice	1 (1.3 oz)	130	2	0	90
Travel Lite Low Fat Oatmeal Rum Raisin	1 (1.3 oz)	130	2	0	90
White Chocolate Macadamia Nut	1 med (1.3 oz)	180	10	10	110

FOOD	PORTION	CALS	FAT	CHOL	SOD
Otis Spunkmeyer (cont.)					
White Chocolate Macadamia Nut	1 (2 oz)	280	15	20	170
Pally					
Butter	5 (1 oz)	140	3	1	170
Carnival	5 (1 oz)	130	3	0	130
Cinnamon Biscuit	5 (1 oz)	130	3	0	130
Mariel Biscuit	6 (1 oz)	150	4	0	140
Tea Biscuits	5 (1 oz)	150	4	0	170
Pamela's					
Pecan Shortbread Rice Flour	1 (0.8 oz)	130	8	20	65
Parmalat					
Grisbi Lemon	1 (0.6 oz)	90	6	5	0
Peek Freans					
Arrowroot	4 (1.2 oz)	150	5	0	80
Assorted Creme	1 (1 oz)	130	6	<5	50
Dream Puffs	2 (0.9 oz)	110	4	0	50
Fruit Creme	2 (0.9 oz)	130	5	0	35
Ginger Crisp	4 (1.2 oz)	150	4	0	65
Nice	4 (1.2 oz)	160	6	0	100
Petit Beret Creme Caramel	2 (0.8 oz)	110	5	0	120
Petit Beret Fudge Truffle	2 (0.8 oz)	110	5	0	100
Petit Beurre	4 (1 oz)	130	4	tr	115
Rich Tea	4 (1.2 oz)	160	5	0	150
Shortcake	2 (0.9 oz)	140	7	20	70
Traditional Oatmeal	1 (0.7 oz)	90	3	0	100
Tropical Cremes Calypso Lime	2 (0.9 oz)	130	5	0	15
Pepperidge Farm					
Biscotti Almond	1 (0.7 oz)	90	4	5	65
Biscotti Chocolate Hazelnut	1 (0.7 oz)	90	5	15	80
Biscotti Cranberry Pistachio	1 (0.7 oz)	90	3	5	65
Bordeaux	4	130	5	10	95
Brussels	3	150	7	5	65
Chantilly Raspberry	2 (1 oz)	120	3	0	115
Chessman	3	120	8	20	80
Chocoate Chunk Soft Baked Double Chocolate	1 (0.9 oz)	130	7	0	60
Chocolate Chunk Chesapeake	1 (0.7 oz)	140	8	10	80
Chocolate Chunk Minis Nantucket	4 (1 oz)	150	8	10	70
Chocolate Chunk Minis Sausalito	4 (1 oz)	160	9	10	70
Chocolate Chunk Montauk	1 (0.9 oz)	130	7	10	90
Chocolate Chunk Nantucket	1 (0.9 oz)	140	7	10	80
Chocolate Chunk Sausalito	1 (0.7 oz)	140	8	10	80

FOOD	PORTION	CALS	FAT	CHOL	SOD
Chocolate Chunk Soft Baked	1	130	6	10	80
Chocolate Chunk Soft Baked Milk Chocolate Macademia	1	130	7	10	75
Chocolate Chunk Soft Baked Reduced Fat	1	110	5	15	85
Chocolate Chunk Soft Baked White Chocolate Pecan	1	120	5	5	65
Chocolate Chunk Tahoe	1 (0.9 oz)	130	8	10	90
Fruitful Strawberry Cup	3	140	5	10	105
Geneva	3	160	9	0	95
Ginger Man	4 (1 oz)	130	4	10	100
Lemon Nut Crunch	3	170	9	15	60
Lido	1	90	5	<5	40
Milano Endless Chocolate	3	180	10	<5	85
Milano Milk Chocolate	3	170	9	10	110
Milano Double Chocolate	2 (0.7 oz)	140	8	10	70
Milano Mint	2	130	7	<5	65
Pirouettes Chocolate Laced	5 (1.1 oz)	180	10	5	90
Pirouettes Traditional	5 (1.2 oz)	170	9	5	90
Shortbread	2	140	7	10	105
Soft Baked Oatmeal Raisin	1 (0.9 oz)	130	7	10	75
Soft Baked Reduced Fat Oatmeal Raisin	1 (0.9 oz)	100	3	10	85
Spritzers Cool Key Lime	6 (1.1 oz)	140	7	<5	60
Spritzers Ripe Red Raspberry	5 (1.1 oz)	140	7	<5	60
Spritzers Zesty Lemon	5 (1.1 oz)	140	7	<5	60
Verona Strawberry	3 (1.1 oz)	140	5	10	105
Ralston					
Cinnamon Grahams Low Fat	2 (0.9 oz)	110	2	0	120
Real Torino					
Lady Fingers	3 (1 oz)	110	1	5	70
Reko					
Pizzelle Maple	5 (1 oz)	150	6	15	20
Pizzelle Vanilla	1 (6 g)	30	1	3	4
Royal					
Apple Bars	1 (1.1 oz)	100	2	0	65
Apple Cake	1 (1.1 oz)	110	3	0	50
Brownie Rounds	1 (1.1 oz)	130	6	0	135
Chocolate Chip	1 (1.1 oz)	140	6	0	120
Devilfood	1 (1 oz)	110	5	0	110
Fig Bars	1 (1.1 oz)	100	2	0	65
Oatmeal	1 (1.1 oz)	130	6	0	140
Raisin	1 (1 oz)	110	5	0	115
Strawberry Bars	1 (1.1 oz)	100	2	0	65

FOOD	PORTION	CALS	FAT	CHOL	SOD
Salerno					
Mini Butter	25 (1 oz)	180	6	15	125
Mini Dinosaur Chocolate Graham	16 (1.1 oz)	140	5	0	125
Scooter Pie	1 (1.2 oz)	140	5	0	80
Santa Fe Farms					
Chocolate Chocolate Chip Fat Free	2 (1 oz)	60	0	0	90
Chocolate Mint Fat Free	2 (1 oz)	60	0	0	90
Ginger Fat Free	2 (1 oz)	70	0	0	95
Sargento					
MooTown Snackers Honey Graham Sticks & Vanilla Creme w/ Sprinkles	1 pkg (1 oz)	140	7	0	50
MooTown Snackers Vanilla Sticks & Chocolate Fudge Creme	1 pkg (1 oz)	130	6	0	50
Savion					
Chocolate Biscuits	5 (1 oz)	120	3	0	45
Tea Biscuits	5 (1 oz)	120	3	0	80
Tea Biscuits Vanilla	5 (1 oz)	120	3	0	80
Scotto's					
Biscotti Fat Free French Vanilla	4 (1 oz)	80	0	0	25
Season					
Hamantashen Poppy	1 (1 oz)	150	7	7	60
Hamantashen Apricot	1 (1 oz)	150	7	7	60
Simple Pleasures					
Almond	1 (0.3 oz)	37	2	0	9
Cinnamon Snaps	1 (0.2 oz)	31	1	0	27
Digestive	1 (0.3 oz)	46	2	0	34
Encore Tea Cookie	1 (0.2 oz)	29	1	0	32
Lemon Social Tea Spice	1 (0.2 oz)	29	1	0	32
Snaps	1 (0.3 oz)	34	1	0	56
SnackWell's					
Bite Size Chocolate Chip	13 (1 oz)	130	4	0	160
Bite Size Double Chocolate Chip	13 (1 oz)	130	4	0	190
Bite Size Peanut Butter	13 (1 oz)	120	4	0	210
Caramel Delights	1 (0.6 oz)	70	2	0	35
Chocolate Sandwich	2 (0.8 oz)	110	3	0	210
Creme Sandwich	2 (0.9 oz)	110	3	0	130
Fat Free Devil's Food	1 (0.5 oz)	50	0	0	30
Golden Devil's Food	1 (0.5 oz)	50	1	0	25
Mint Creme	2 (0.9 oz)	110	4	0	70
Oatmeal Raisin	2 (0.9 oz)	110	3	<5	130
Stella D'Oro					
Almond Toast Mandel	2 (1 oz)	110	3	30	85

FOOD	PORTION	CALS	FAT	CHOL	SOD
Angel Wings	2 (0.9 oz)	140	9	<5	80
Angelica	1 (0.8 oz)	100	4	15	45
Anginetti	4 (1.1 oz)	140	4	40	10
Anisette Sponge	2 (0.9 oz)	90	1	40	80
Anisette Toast	3 (1.2 oz)	130	1	35	150
Biscotti Almond	1 (0.8 oz)	100	3	10	55
Biscotti Chocolate Almond	1 (0.8 oz)	90	3	10	55
Biscotti Chocolate Chunk	1 (0.8 oz)	90	3	10	60
Biscotti Hazelnut	1 (0.8 oz)	100	4	10	60
Biscottini Cashews	1 (0.7 oz)	110	6	5	50
Breakfast Treats	1 (0.8 oz)	100	3	10	80
Breakfast Treats Chocolate	1 (0.8 oz)	100	4	10	70
Breakfast Treats Viennese Cinnamon	1 (0.8 oz)	100	3	10	65
Chinese Dessert Cookies	1 (1.2 oz)	170	9	5	90
Chocolate Castelets	2 (1 oz)	130	6	<5	55
Egg Jumbo	2 (0.8 oz)	90	1	30	60
Fruit Slices Fat Free	1 (0.6 oz)	50	0	0	45
Kichel Low Sodium	21 (1 oz)	150	9	80	25
Lady Stella Assortment	3 (1 oz)	130	5	5	55
Margherite Chocolate	2 (1.1 oz)	140	6	10	75
Margherite Vanilla	2 (1.1 oz)	140	5	15	90
Roman Egg Biscuits	1 (1.2 oz)	140	5	20	125
Sesame Regina	3 (1.1 oz)	150	6	10	85
Swiss Fudge	2 (0.9 oz)	130	7	5	55
Stieffenhofer					
Choco Minis	4 (1 oz)	160	8	15	40
Snaky	3 (1 oz)	160	8	0	20
Streit's					
Wafers	3 (1 oz)	160	9	0	35
Suissette					
Swiss Chocolate Hearts	4 (1 oz)	170	10	5	40
Swiss Delight	4 (1 oz)	160	9	5	35
Swiss Praline	4 (1 oz)	150	9	15	15
Sunshine					
All American Butter	5 (1.1 oz)	140	6	<5	135
All American Lemon Coolers	5 (1 oz)	140	6	0	100
All American Mini Chip-A-Roos	5 (1.1 oz)	160	8	0	140
Animal Crackers	14 (1.1 oz)	140	4	0	125
Ginger Snaps	7 (1 oz)	130	5	0	150
Golden Fruit Cranberry	1 (0.7 oz)	80	2	0	55
Golden Fruit Raisin	1 (0.7 oz)	80	2	0	50
Hydrox	3 (1.1 oz)	150	7	0	125
Hydrox Reduced Fat	3 (1.1 oz)	140	5	0	150
Oatmeal Country Style	2 (0.8 oz)	120	5	0	115
Sugar Wafers Peanut Butter Creme	4 (1.1 oz)	170	9	0	75

FOOD	PORTION	CALS	FAT	CHOL	SOD
Sunshine (cont.)					
Sugar Wafers Vanilla Creme	3 (0.9 oz)	130	6	0	30
Vanilla Wafers	7 (1.1 oz)	150	7	3	110
Vienna Fingers	2 (1 oz)	140	6	0	105
Vienna Fingers Lemon	2 (1 oz)	140	6	0	90
Vienna Fingers Reduced Fat	2 (1 oz)	130	5	0	105
Sweet Rewards					
Fat Free Blueberry w/ Drizzle	1 bar (1.3 oz)	120	0	0	80
Fat Free Double Fudge Supreme	1 bar (1.3 oz)	100	0	0	90
Fat Free Raspberry	1 bar (1.3 oz)	120	0	0	80
Fat Free Strawberry w/ Drizzle	1 bar (1.3 oz)	120	0	0	80
Low Fat Chocolate Chip	1 bar (1.1 oz)	110	2	0	115
Sweet'N Low					
Sugar Free Amaretto Biscotti	4 (1 oz)	120	6	10	180
Sugar Free Chocolate Chip	4 (1 oz)	135	8	10	35
Sugar Free Cinnamon Graham	7 (1 oz)	120	6	15	90
Sugar Free Morning Crunch Bars	2 (1 oz)	120	6	10	150
Sugar Free Vanilla Wafers	7 (1 oz)	120	6	15	80
Sweetzels					
Chocolate Chip	7 (1 oz)	160	9	5	70
Ginger Snaps	4 (1.2 oz)	140	3	0	120
Vanilla Wafers	7 (1.1 oz)	137	5	0	94
Tastykake					
Chocolate Chip	1 (1.4 oz)	180	7	10	160
Chocolate Chip Bar	1 (2 oz)	270	12	10	125
Chocolate Fudge Iced	1 (1.4 oz)	170	7	55	190
Fudge Bar	1 (2 oz)	250	10	5	140
Lemon Bar	1 (2 oz)	260	10	5	125
Oatmeal Raisin Bar	1 (2 oz)	260	10	15	230
Oatmeal Raisin Boxed	3 (0.4 oz)	130	6	5	70
Oatmeal Raisin Iced	1 (1.4 oz)	170	6	25	150
Strawberry Bar	1 (2 oz)	260	10	5	125
Sugar Boxed	3 (0.4 oz)	120	6	10	85
The Source					
Barry's Raspberry Palmiers	1 (0.7 oz)	80	3	0	50
Tom's					
Animal Crackers	1/2 pkg (1 oz)	120	2	0	140
Big Cookie Chocolate Chip	1 pkg (2.75 oz)	340	16	0	280
Big Cookie Peanut Butter Chocolate Chip	1 pkg (2 oz)	280	15	0	180
Chocolate Chip	1 pkg (2 oz)	280	15	0	180
Confetti Chip	1 pkg (2 oz)	300	13	0	140
Fat Free Apple Bar	1 pkg (1.75 oz)	160	0	0	250
Fat Free Fig Bar	1 pkg (1.75 oz)	160	0	0	180
Vanilla Wafers	1/2 pkg (1 oz)	130	5	0	100

FOOD	PORTION	CALS	FAT	CHOL	SOD
Twix					
Bars Chocolate Caramel	1 (0.9 oz)	140	7	0	55
Voortman					
Almonette	2 (1 oz)	150	8	0	65
Chocolate Chip	1 (0.7 oz)	100	5	0	45
Chocolate Wafers Sugar Free	3 (1 oz)	160	11	0	30
Coconut Delight	1 (0.6 oz)	90	5	0	25
Peanut Delight	1 (0.9 oz)	130	7	<5	90
Strawberry Wafers Sugar Free	3 (1 oz)	160	11	0	30
Sugar	1 (0.6 oz)	80	4	0	45
Turnovers Blueberry	1 (0.9 oz)	100	3	<5	50
Turnovers Cherry	1 (0.9 oz)	100	3	<5	50
Turnovers Strawberry	1 (0.9 oz)	100	3	<5	50
Vanilla Wafers Sugar Free	3 (1 oz)	160	11	0	30
Windmill	1 (0.7 oz)	90	4	0	100
Walkers					
Shortbread Triangles	2 (0.7 oz)	100	6	15	65
Weight Watchers					
Apple Raisin Bar	1 (0.75 oz)	70	2	0	60
Chocolate Chip	2 (1.06 oz)	140	5	0	90
Chocolate Sandwich	2 (1.06)	140	4	0	160
Fruit Filled Fig	1 (0.7 oz)	70	0	0	50
Fruit Filled Raspberry	1 (0.7 oz)	70	0	0	45
Oatmeal Raisin	2 (1.06 oz)	120	2	0	90
Vanilla Sandwich	2 (1.06 oz)	140	3	0	80
White Eagle Bakery					
Chruscik	2 (1 oz)	140	8	45	95
refrigerated					
chocolate chip	1 (0.42 oz)	59	3	3	28
chocolate chip unbaked	1 oz	126	6	7	59
oatmeal	1 (0.4 oz)	56	3	3	39
oatmeal raisin	1 (0.4 oz)	56	3	3	39
peanut butter	1 (0.4 oz)	60	3	4	52
peanut butter dough	1 oz	130	7	8	112
sugar	1 (0.42 oz)	58	3	4	56
sugar dough	1 oz	124	6	8	120
Pillsbury					
Bunny	2	130	7	<5	100
Chocolate Chip	1 (1 oz)	130	6	<5	85
Chocolate Chip Reduced Fat	1 (1 oz)	110	3	<5	85
Chocolate Chip w/ Walnuts	1 (1 oz)	140	7	<5	90
Chocolate Chunk	1 (1 oz)	130	6	<5	90
Christmas Tree	2	130	7	<5	100
Double Chocolate	1 (1 oz)	130	6	<5	90
Flag	2	130	7	<5	100
Frosty	2	130	7	<5	100
M&M's	1 (1 oz)	130	6	<5	75
Oatmeal Chocolate Chip	1 (1 oz)	120	6	<5	95

FOOD	PORTION	CALS	FAT	CHOL	SOD
Pillsbury (cont.)					
One Step Pan Chocolate Chip	1/8 pan (1 oz)	130	6	<5	100
One Step Pan M&M's	1/8 pan (1 oz)	130	6	<5	85
Peanut Butter	1 (1 oz)	120	6	<5	130
Pumpkin	2	130	7	<5	100
Reeses	1 (1 oz)	130	6	<5	105
Shamrock	2	130	7	<5	100
Sugar	2	130	3	<5	125
Sugar Holiday Red & Green	2	130	6	<5	125
Valentine	2	130	7	<5	100
White Chocolate Chunk	1 (1 oz)	130	6	<5	100
Toll House					
Brownie Dough	1/12 pkg (1.5 oz)	180	7	15	160
take-out					
black & white	1 lg (3 oz)	302	9	58	72
finikia	1 (1.2 oz)	171	5	27	26
koulourakia butter cookie twist	1 (0.9 oz)	113	6	32	59
CORIANDER					
leaf dried	1 tsp	2	tr	0	1
leaf fresh	1/4 cup	1	tr	0	1
seed	1 tsp	5	tr	0	1
CORN					
(*see also* BRAN, CEREAL, CORNMEAL)					
canned					
Green Giant					
Cream Style	1/2 cup (4.5 oz)	100	1	0	430
Mexicorn	1/3 cup (2.7 oz)	60	0	0	430
Niblets	1/3 cup (2.7 oz)	70	0	0	230
Niblets 50% Less Sodium	1/3 cup (2.7 oz)	60	0	0	115
Niblets Extra Sweet	1/3 cup (2.6 oz)	50	1	0	200
Niblets No Added Sugar or Salt	1/3 cup (2.7 oz)	60	0	0	0
White Shoepeg	1/3 cup	80	1	0	220
Whole Sweet	1/2 cup (4.3 oz)	80	1	0	360
Whole Sweet 50% Less Sodium	1/2 cup (4.2 oz)	80	1	0	180
dried					
Goya					
Giant White	1/3 cup (1.6 oz)	160	2	0	10
fresh					
on-the-cob w/ butter cooked	1 ear	155	3	6	30
frozen					
Birds Eye					
Baby Corn Blend	2/3 cup (2.9 oz)	60	1	0	15
Baby Gold & White	2/3 cup (3.3 oz)	80	1	0	10
In Butter Sauce	1/2 cup (4.6 oz)	110	3	5	230

FOOD	PORTION	CALS	FAT	CHOL	SOD
Green Giant					
Butter Sauce Niblets	2/3 cup (4.3 oz)	130	3	<5	350
Butter Sauce Shoepeg White	3/4 cup (4 oz)	120	3	<5	320
Cream Corn	1/2 cup (4.1 oz)	110	1	0	330
Extra Sweet Niblets	2/3 cup (3.1 oz)	70	1	0	0
Harvest Fresh Niblets	2/3 cup (3.4 oz)	80	1	0	60
Harvest Fresh Shoepeg White	1/2 cup (2.6 oz)	70	1	0	45
Niblets	2/3 cup (2.9 oz)	80	1	0	5
On The Cob Extra Sweet	1 ear (4.4 oz)	120	2	0	0
On The Cob Nibblers	1 ear (2.1 oz)	70	1	0	0
On The Cob Niblets	1 ear (5 oz)	160	2	0	10
Select Extra Sweet White	2/3 cup (2.9 oz)	50	1	0	0
Select Shoepeg White	3/4 cup (3.2 oz)	100	1	0	0
Stouffer's					
Souffle	1/2 cup (6 oz)	170	7	65	490
CORN CHIPS					
(*see* CHIPS)					
CORNISH HENS					
(*see* CHICKEN)					
CORNMEAL					
(*see also* POLENTA)					
corn grits cooked	1 cup	146	tr	0	0
yellow self-rising	1 cup (4.3 oz)	407	4	0	1521
Albers					
White	3 tbsp	110	0	0	0
Yellow	3 tbsp	110	0	0	0
take-out					
hush puppies	1 (0.75 oz)	74	3	10	147
CORNSTARCH					
cornstarch	1 cup (4.5 oz)	488	tr	0	12
Armour					
Cream Cornstarch	1 tbsp (0.4 oz)	40	0	0	0
COTTAGE CHEESE					
Breakstone's					
2% Fat Large Curd	1/2 cup (4.2 oz)	90	3	15	390
2% Fat Small Curd	1/2 cup (4.2 oz)	90	3	15	390
4% Fat Large Curd	1/2 cup (4.2 oz)	120	5	25	400
4% Fat Small Curd	1/2 cup (4.2 oz)	120	5	25	400
Cottage Doubles Peach	1 pkg (5.5 oz)	140	3	15	390
Dry Curd	1/4 cup (1.9 oz)	45	0	<5	30
Free	1/2 cup (4.4 oz)	80	0	5	440
Snack 2% Fat Small Curd	1 pkg (4 oz)	90	2	15	370
Snack 4% Fat Small Curd	1 pkg (4 oz)	110	5	25	380
Snack Free	1 pkg (4 oz)	70	0	5	400
Horizon Organic					
Cottage Cheese	1/2 cup (3.9 oz)	110	5	15	340

FOOD	PORTION	CALS	FAT	CHOL	SOD
Knudsen					
1.5% Fat Small Curd Pineapple	1/2 cup (4.6 oz)	120	2	10	330
2% Fat Small Curd	1/2 cup (4.2 oz)	100	3	15	400
4% Fat Large Curd	1/2 cup (4.5 oz)	130	5	30	330
4% Fat Small Curd	1/2 cup (4.3 oz)	120	5	25	400
Free	1/2 cup (4.2 oz)	80	0	5	380
On The Go! 1.5% Fat Peach	1 pkg (4 oz)	110	2	10	300
On The Go! 1.5% Fat Pineapple	1 pkg (4 oz)	110	2	10	300
On The Go! 1.5% Fat Strawberry	1 pkg (4 oz)	110	2	10	290
On The Go! 1.5% Fat Tropical Fruit	1 pkg (4 oz)	110	2	10	300
On The Go! 2% Fat	1 pkg (4 oz)	90	2	15	370
On The Go! Free	1 pkg (4 oz)	70	0	5	350
Light N'Lively					
1% Fat	1/2 cup (4 oz)	80	1	10	370
1% Fat Garden Salad	1/2 cup (4.2 oz)	80	2	10	390
1% Fat Peach & Pineapple	1/2 cup (4.3 oz)	110	1	10	340
Fat Free	1/2 cup (4.4 oz)	80	0	5	440
COTTONSEED					
kernels roasted	1 tbsp	51	4	0	3
COUSCOUS					
cooked	1 cup (5.5 oz)	176	tr	0	8
dry	1 cup (6.1 oz)	650	1	0	17
Melting Pot					
Calypso Cranberry	1 cup	200	0	0	220
Lentil Curry	1 cup	170	0	0	290
Lucky Seven	1 cup	190	1	0	300
Mango Salsa	1 cup	190	0	0	270
Roasted Garlic	1 cup	170	0	0	370
Sesame Ginger	1 cup	180	1	0	350
Sun-Dried Tomatoes	1 cup	190	1	0	230
Wild Mushroom	1 cup	190	0	0	370
COWPEAS					
catjang dried cooked	1 cup	200	1	0	32
common canned	1 cup	184	1	0	718
frozen cooked	1/2 cup	112	tr	0	5
leafy tips chopped cooked	1 cup	12	tr	0	3
CRAB					
canned					
blue	3 oz	84	1	76	283
blue	1 cup	133	2	120	5
fresh					
alaska king cooked	1 leg (4.7 oz)	129	2	72	1436
alaska king cooked	3 oz	82	1	45	911
blue cooked	3 oz	87	2	85	237
blue cooked	1 cup	138	2	135	376
queen steamed	3 oz	98	1	60	587

FOOD	PORTION	CALS	FAT	CHOL	SOD
take-out					
baked	1 (3.8 oz)	160	2	184	550
cake	1 (2 oz)	160	10	82	492
soft-shell fried	1 (4.4 oz)	334	18	45	1118
CRACKER CRUMBS					
cracker meal	1 cup (4 oz)	440	2	0	32
Baker's Harvest					
Graham	1/3 cup (1 oz)	130	4	0	110
Kellogg's					
Corn Flake Crumbs	2 tbsp (0.4 oz)	40	0	0	105
CRACKERS					
(*see also* CRACKER CRUMBS)					
Ak-mak					
100% Whole Wheat	5 (1 oz)	116	2	0	214
Armenian Cracker Bread	1 sheet (1 oz)	100	2	0	200
Armenian Cracker Bread Whole Wheat	1 sheet (1 oz)	116	2	0	214
Round Cracker Bread No Seeds	1 (1 oz)	100	1	0	170
Round Cracker Bread Seeded	1 (1 oz)	100	2	0	200
Round Cracker Bread Whole Wheat	1 (1 oz)	116	2	0	214
Austin					
Cracker Sandwich Cheese On Cheese	6 (1.3 oz)	170	7	0	310
Cracker Sandwich Cheese Peanut Butter	6 (1.3 oz)	170	7	0	320
Cracker Sandwich Toasty Peanut Butter	6 (1.3 oz)	170	7	0	340
Cracker Sandwich Whole Wheat Cheese	6 (1.3 oz)	170	7	0	280
Baker's Harvest					
Cheese	23 (1 oz)	150	6	0	370
Cheese Reduced Fat	29 (1 oz)	130	4	0	310
Snackers Reduced Fat	10 (1.1 oz)	140	4	0	260
Wheat Snacks Reduced Fat	16 (1.1 oz)	140	4	0	220
Woven Wheats	7 (1.1 oz)	140	5	0	170
Woven Wheats Reduced Fat	8 (1.1 oz)	130	3	0	180
Barbara's					
Cheese Bites	26 (1 oz)	120	2	0	290
French Onion	3	60	1	0	140
Rite Lite Rounds	5 (0.5 oz)	55	tr	0	150
Roasted Garlic & Herb	3	60	1	0	140
Sundried Tomato & Basil	3	60	1	0	140
Toasted Sesame	3	60	2	0	135
Wheatines All Flavors	1 lg sq (0.5 oz)	50	2	0	110

FOOD	PORTION	CALS	FAT	CHOL	SOD
Barbara's Bakery					
Cheese Bites	26 (1 oz)	120	2	0	290
Right Lite Rounds Original	5 (0.5 oz)	55	5	0	150
Rite Lite Rounds Savory Poppy	5 (0.5 oz)	70	2	0	135
Rite Lite Rounds Tamari Sesame	5 (0.5 oz)	70	2	0	160
Wheatines All Flavors	1 lg sq (0.5 oz)	50	2	0	110
Blue Diamond					
Nut Thins Almond	16 (1 oz)	130	5	0	75
Nut Thins Hazelnut	16 (1 oz)	120	4	0	75
Nut Thins Pecan	16 (1 oz)	130	5	0	75
Cheetos					
Bacon Cheddar	1 pkg	190	9	<5	410
Cheddar Cheese	1 pkg	210	11	<5	340
Golden Toast	1 pkg	240	14	5	440
Cheez It					
Big	13 (1 oz)	150	8	0	230
Big Reduced Fat	15 (1 oz)	140	5	0	280
Heads & Tails	37 (1 oz)	140	6	0	330
Hot & Spicy	26 (1 oz)	150	8	0	300
Low Sodium	27 (1 oz)	160	8	0	70
Nacho	28 (1 oz)	150	7	0	280
Original	27 (1 oz)	160	8	0	240
Party Mix	1/2 cup (1 oz)	140	5	0	270
Party Mix Nacho	1/2 cup (1 oz)	130	5	0	330
Party Mix Reduced Fat	1/2 cup (1 oz)	130	3	0	300
Peanut Butter	1 pkg (1.3 oz)	190	10	0	400
Reduced Fat	29 (1 oz)	140	5	0	280
Snack Mix	1/2 cup (1 oz)	130	5	0	330
Snack Mix Big Crunch	3/4 cup (1 oz)	110	6	0	360
Snack Mix Double Cheese	3/4 cup (1 oz)	110	5	0	450
White Cheddar	26 (1 oz)	150	7	<5	280
Courtney's					
Sun-Dried Tomato Organic	4 (0.5 oz)	60	1	0	130
Dare					
Breton	1 (5 g)	21	1	0	40
Breton 50% Less Salt	1 (5 g)	21	1	0	15
Breton Garden Vegetable	1 (5 g)	20	1	0	34
Breton Light	1 (5 g)	20	1	0	39
Breton Sesame	1 (5 g)	22	1	0	40
Breton Minis	20 (0.6 oz)	89	4	0	169
Breton Minis Cheddar Cheese	20 (0.6 oz)	87	4	3	211
Breton Minis Garden Vegetable	20 (0.6 oz)	87	4	0	144
Cabaret	1 (5 g)	23	1	0	45
Vivant Italian Bruschetta	1 (5 g)	22	1	0	39

FOOD	PORTION	CALS	FAT	CHOL	SOD
Doritos					
Jalapeno Cheese	1 pkg	230	14	<5	450
Nacho Cheddar	1 pkg	240	14	<5	340
Estee					
Sugar Free Cracked Pepper	18	120	2	0	200
Sugar Free Golden	10	130	2	0	200
Sugar Free Wheat	17	100	2	0	200
Frito Lay					
Cheddar Snacks	1 pkg	200	10	<5	530
Frookie					
Cheddar	17 (1 oz)	140	4	0	420
Cracked Pepper	8 (0.7 oz)	70	0	0	85
Garden Vegetable	13 (1 oz)	130	4	0	380
Garlic & Herb	8 (0.7 oz)	70	0	0	170
Pizza	17 (1 oz)	130	3	0	420
Snack & Party	10 (1 oz)	140	5	0	260
Water Crackers	8 (0.7 oz)	70	0	0	135
Wheat & Onion	12 (1 oz)	120	4	0	400
Wheat & Rye	13 (1 oz)	120	4	0	380
Health Valley					
Healthy Pizza Garlic & Herb	6	50	0	0	140
Healthy Pizza Italiano	6	50	0	0	140
Healthy Pizza Zesty Cheese	6	50	0	0	140
Low Fat Mild Jalapeno	6	60	2	0	90
Low Fat Mild Ranch	6	60	2	0	90
Low Fat Roasted Garlic	6	60	2	0	90
Original Oat Bran	6	120	3	0	80
Original Rice Bran	6	110	3	0	70
Whole Wheat	5	50	0	0	80
Whole Wheat Cheese	5	50	0	0	100
Whole Wheat Herb	5	50	0	0	100
Whole Wheat No Salt Vegetable	5	50	0	0	15
Whole Wheat Onion	5	50	0	0	80
Whole Wheat Vegetable	5	50	0	0	80
Keebler					
Club 33% Reduced Fat	5 (0.6 oz)	70	2	0	200
Club 50% Reduced Sodium	4 (0.5 oz)	70	3	0	80
Club Orignal	4 (0.5 oz)	70	3	0	160
Elfin	23 (1 oz)	130	2	0	140
Export Soda	3 (0.5 oz)	60	2	0	80
Harvest Bakery Multigrain	2 (0.6 oz)	70	3	0	80
Munch'ems Cheddar	39	140	5	0	320
Munch'ems Cheddar	30 (1 oz)	130	4	0	320
Munch'ems Chili Cheese	28 (1.1 oz)	130	4	0	470
Munch'ems Mexquite BBQ	40 (1 oz)	140	5	0	290
Munch'ems Ranch	40	140	5	0	260

FOOD	PORTION	CALS	FAT	CHOL	SOD
Keebler (cont.)					
Munch'ems Ranch	33 (1 oz)	130	4	0	310
Munch'ems Salsa	28 (1.1 oz)	130	4	0	260
Munch'ems Seasoned Original	30 (1 oz)	130	5	0	350
Munch'ems Sour Cream & Onion	39 (1 oz)	140	5	0	280
Munch'ems Sour Cream & Onion 55% Reduced Fat	33 (1 oz)	130	4	0	390
Paks Cheese & Peanut Butter	1 pkg	190	9	<5	420
Paks Club & Cheddar	1 pkg	190	11	10	320
Paks Toast & Peanut Butter	1 pkg	190	9	0	300
Paks Wheat & Cheddar	1 pkg (1.3 oz)	180	10	5	300
Toasteds Buttercrisp	5 (0.5 oz)	80	4	0	150
Toasteds Buttercrisp	9 (1 oz)	140	7	<5	280
Toasteds Medley	9 (1 oz)	140	6	0	270
Toasteds Onion	9 (1 oz)	140	6	0	310
Toasteds Sesame	5 (0.5 oz)	80	4	0	160
Toasteds Sesame	9 (1 oz)	140	6	0	320
Toasteds Sesame Reduced Fat	10 (1 oz)	120	3	0	310
Toasteds Wheat	5 (0.5 oz)	80	3	0	160
Toasteds Wheat	9 (1 oz)	140	6	0	270
Toasteds Wheat Reduced Fat	5 (0.5 oz)	60	2	0	160
Toasteds Wheat Reduced Fat	10 (1 oz)	120	3	0	300
Town House	5 (0.5 oz)	80	5	0	150
Town House 50% Reduced Fat	5 (0.5 oz)	70	2	0	180
Town House 50% Reduced Sodium	5 (0.5 oz)	80	5	0	75
Town House Reduced Fat	6 (0.6 oz)	70	2	0	180
Town House Wheat	5 (0.6 oz)	80	4	0	140
Wheatables Honey Wheat	12 (1 oz)	140	6	0	200
Wheatables Original	12 (1 oz)	140	6	0	210
Wheatables Seven Grain	12 (1 oz)	140	6	0	250
Zesta Saltine 50% Reduced Sodium	5 (0.5 oz)	60	2	0	95
Zesta Saltine Fat Free	5 (0.5 oz)	50	0	0	150
Zesta Saltine Original	5 (0.5 oz)	60	2	0	190
Zesta Saltine Unsalted Top	5 (0.5 oz)	70	2	0	90
Zesta Soup & Oyster	42 (0.5 oz)	80	3	0	160
Lance					
Bonnie	6 (1 1/8 oz)	160	7	10	160
Captain Wafers w/ Cream Cheese & Chives	1 pkg (1.3 oz)	190	9	0	250

FOOD	PORTION	CALS	FAT	CHOL	SOD
Cheese-On-Wheat	1 pkg (1.3 oz)	190	10	<5	280
Cranberry Bar Fat Free	1 (1.75 oz)	160	0	0	55
Lanchee	1 pkg (1 1/4 oz)	190	11	0	120
Malt	1 pkg (1 1/4 oz)	190	10	0	130
Nekot	1 pkg (1.5 oz)	210	10	0	130
Nip-Chee	1 pkg (1.3 oz)	190	10	<5	330
Peanut Butter Wheat	1 pkg (1.3 oz)	190	11	0	240
Rye-Chee	1 pkg (1.4 oz)	210	11	<5	340
Sour Dough w/ Cheddar & Sour Cream	1 pkg (1.6 oz)	240	15	5	430
Toastchee	1 pkg (1.4 oz)	200	12	0	260
Toasty	1 pkg (1 1/4 oz)	190	11	0	220
Wheat Italian	3/4 cup (1.4 oz)	200	11	0	430
Wheat Pizza	3/4 cup (1.4 oz)	200	10	0	390
Little Debbie					
Cheese Crackers With Peanut Butter	1 (0.9 oz)	140	8	0	210
Cheese On Cheese Crackers	1 (0.9 oz)	140	8	<5	220
Cream Cheese & Chive	1 (0.9 oz)	140	7	0	220
Toasty Crackers With Peanut Butter	1 (0.9 oz)	140	7	0	210
Wheat Crackers With Cheddar Cheese	1 (0.9 oz)	140	8	<5	230
Nabisco					
Royal Lunch	1 (0.4 oz)	60	2	0	70
Zwieback	1 (8 g)	35	1	0	10
No-No					
Flatbreads Tortilla Corn Low Fat Sugar Free Everything	3 (1 oz)	95	1	0	140
Partners					
Walla Walla Sweet Onion Preservative Free	0.5 oz	65	3	3	60
Pepperidge Farm					
Butter Thins	4 (0.5 oz)	70	3	10	95
English Water Biscuits	4 (0.5 oz)	70	2	0	95
Goldfish Cheddar	55	140	6	10	250
Goldfish Cheddar 30% Less Sodium	60 (1.1 oz)	150	6	10	175
Goldfish Cheese Trio	58	140	6	<5	280
Goldfish Original	55	140	6	0	230
Goldfish Parmesan Cheese	60	140	5	0	300
Goldfish Pizza Flavored	55 (1 oz)	140	6	0	160
Goldfish Pretzel	43 (1 oz)	120	3	0	430
Goldfish Toasted Wheat	41	150	7	0	280
Hearty Wheat	3 (0.6 oz)	80	4	0	100
Sesame	3 (0.5 oz)	70	3	0	95
Snack Mix Fat Free Goldfish	2/3 cup (0.9 oz)	90	0	0	380

FOOD	PORTION	CALS	FAT	CHOL	SOD
Peter Pan					
Cheese Peanut Butter	1 pkg	210	10	0	350
Toast Peanut Butter	1 pkg	210	11	0	280
Premium					
Saltine Multigrain	5 (0.5 oz)	60	2	0	150
Ralston					
Cheese	23 (1 oz)	150	6	0	370
Cheese Reduced Fat	29 (1 oz)	130	4	0	310
Saltines Fat Free	5 (0.5 oz)	60	0	0	135
Snackers Reduced Fat	10 (1.1 oz)	140	4	0	260
Wheat Snacks Reduced Fat	16 (1.1 oz)	140	4	0	220
Woven Wheats	7 (1.1 oz)	140	5	0	170
Woven Wheats Reduced Fat	8 (1.1 oz)	130	3	0	180
RedOval Farms					
Stoned Wheat Thins Cracked Pepper	4 (0.6 oz)	70	3	0	190
Savory Thins					
Toasted Onion & Garlic	15 (1 oz)	110	1	0	90
SnackWell's					
Salsa Cheddar	32 (1 oz)	120	2	0	340
Sunshine					
Hi Ho	4 (0.5 oz)	70	4	0	130
Hi Ho Reduced Fat	5 (0.5 oz)	70	3	0	140
Krispy	5 (0.5 oz)	60	2	0	180
Krispy Fat Free	5 (0.5 oz)	50	0	0	150
Krispy Mild Cheddar	5 (0.5 oz)	60	2	0	180
Krispy Soup & Oyster	17 (0.5 oz)	60	2	0	200
Krispy Unsalted Tops	5 (0.5 oz)	60	2	0	120
Krispy Whole Wheat	5 (0.5 oz)	60	2	0	130
Venus					
Fat Free Cracked Pepper	11 (0.5 oz)	60	0	0	80
Fat Free Garden Vegetable	5 (0.5 oz)	60	0	0	80
Fat Free Garlic & Herb	11 (0.5 oz)	60	0	0	90
Fat Free Multi-Grain	5 (0.5 oz)	60	0	0	100
Fat Free Spicy Chili	10 (0.5 oz)	60	0	0	100
Fat Free Toasted Onion	5 (0.5 oz)	60	0	0	120
Fat Free Toasted Wheat	5 (0.5 oz)	60	0	0	140
Fat Free Tomato & Basil	10 (0.5 oz)	60	0	0	100
Fat Free Zesty Italian	10 (0.5 oz)	60	0	0	120
Garden Vegetable	6 (1 oz)	150	8	0	230
Honey Wheat	1 oz	140	5	0	200
Low Fat Cracker Bread	5 (0.5 oz)	60	2	0	105
Low Fat Water Crackers	4 (0.5 oz)	60	1	0	75
Sesame & Flaxseed	1 oz	130	3	0	240
Soup Original	0.5 oz	60	2	0	90
Toasted Wheat	6 (1 oz)	150	7	0	240
Wine Cheese Caviar Original	0.5 oz	60	2	0	90

FOOD	PORTION	CALS	FAT	CHOL	SOD
Wine Cheese Caviar Pepper & Poppy	0.5 oz	60	2	0	90
Wasa					
Crisp	3 (0.5 oz)	50	0	0	100
Crisp'N Light Sourdough Rye	3 (0.6 oz)	60	0	0	120
Crisp'N Light Wheat	2 (0.5 oz)	50	0	0	100
Crispbread Cinnamon Toast	1 (0.6 oz)	60	1	0	65
Crispbread Fiber Rye	1 (0.4 oz)	30	1	0	60
Crispbread Gluten & Wheat Free Corn	1 (0.4 oz)	40	1	0	90
Crispbread Hearty Rye	1 (0.5 oz)	45	0	0	40
Crispbread Light Rye	1 (0.3 oz)	25	0	0	40
Crispbread Multi Grain	1 (0.5 oz)	45	0	0	85
Crispbread Organic Rye	1 (0.3 oz)	25	0	0	50
Crispbread Sodium Free Rye	1 (0.3 oz)	30	0	0	0
Crispbread Sourdough Rye	1 (0.4 oz)	35	0	0	55
Crispbread Toasted Wheat	1 (0.5 oz)	50	2	0	85
Crispbread Whole Wheat	1 (0.5 oz)	50	1	0	55
Wortz					
Cheese	23 (1 oz)	150	6	0	370
Saltines Fat Free	5 (0.5 oz)	60	0	0	135
Wheat Snacks Reduced Fat	16 (1.1 oz)	140	4	0	220
Woven Wheats	7 (1.1 oz)	140	5	0	170
CRANBERRIES					
fresh chopped	1 cup	54	tr	0	1
Ocean Spray					
Craisins	1/3 cup (1.4 oz)	130	0	0	0
Cran*Fruit Cranberry Orange	1/4 cup	120	0	0	35
Cranberry Sauce Jellied	1/4 cup	110	0	0	35
Fresh	2 oz	25	0	0	0
Whole Berry Sauce	1/4 cup	110	0	0	35
CRANBERRY BEANS					
canned	1 cup	216	1	0	863
dried cooked	1 cup	240	1	0	1
CRANBERRY JUICE					
Crystal Light					
Cranberry Breeze Drink	1 serv (8 oz)	5	0	0	20
Cranberry Breeze Drink Mix as prep	1 serv (8 oz)	5	0	0	0
Everfresh					
Cranberry Cocktail	1 can (8 oz)	140	0	0	0
Mott's					
Cocktail	8 oz	150	0	0	5
Nantucket Nectars					
Cocktail	8 oz	140	0	0	5

FOOD	PORTION	CALS	FAT	CHOL	SOD
Ocean Spray					
Cocktail	8 oz	140	0	0	35
Cocktail Reduced Calorie	8 oz	50	0	0	35
Lightstyle Cranberry Juice Cocktail	8 oz	40	0	0	75
Tropicana					
Twister Ruby Red	1 bottle (10 oz)	160	0	0	40
Veryfine					
Cocktail	1 bottle (10 oz)	180	0	0	30
Wellfleet Farms					
Cranberry	8 oz	130	0	0	35
CRAYFISH					
(*see also* LOBSTER)					
cooked	3 oz	97	1	151	58
CREAM					
(*see also* SOUR CREAM, SOUR CREAM SUBSTITUTES, WHIPPED TOPPINGS)					
liquid					
Land O'Lakes					
Fat Free Half & Half	2 tbsp (1 oz)	20	0	0	30
Half & Half	2 tbsp (1 oz)	40	4	15	20
Heavy Whipping	1 tbsp (0.5 oz)	50	6	20	10
Organic Valley					
Half & Half	2 tbsp (1 oz)	40	3	15	15
whipped					
heavy whipping	1 cup (4.1 oz)	411	44	163	89
light whipping	1 cup (4.2 oz)	345	37	132	82
CREAM CHEESE					
Alpine Lace					
Reduced Fat Roasted Garlic & Herbs	1 tsp (1 oz)	60	4	10	190
Reduced Fat Sundried Tomato & Basil	2 tsp (1 oz)	70	5	15	300
Boar's Head					
Cream Cheese	2 tbsp (1 oz)	100	10	30	100
Breakstone's					
Temp-Tee Whipped	2 tbsp (0.8 oz)	80	8	25	70
Galaxy					
Slices	1 slice (1 oz)	50	3	10	190
Horizon Organic					
Spreadable	2 tbsp	100	10	30	100
Organic Valley					
Cream Cheese	1 oz	100	9	30	100
Philadelphia					
Free	1 oz	30	0	<5	140
Regular	1 oz	100	10	30	90
Soft	2 tbsp (1 oz)	100	10	30	100
Soft Apple Cinnamon	2 tbsp (1.1 oz)	100	8	25	100

FOOD	PORTION	CALS	FAT	CHOL	SOD
Soft Cheesecake	2 tbsp (1 oz)	110	9	25	95
Soft Chives & Onions	2 tbsp (1.1 oz)	110	10	30	135
Soft Garden Vegetable	2 tbsp (1.1 oz)	110	11	30	170
Soft Honey Nut	2 tbsp (1.1 oz)	110	10	30	150
Soft Pineapple	2 tbsp (1.1 oz)	100	9	25	100
Soft Salmon	3 tbsp (1.1 oz)	100	9	30	200
Soft Strawberry	2 tbsp (1.1 oz)	100	9	25	100
Soft Free	2 tbsp (1.2 oz)	30	0	<5	200
Soft Free Garden Vegetable	2 tbsp (1.2 oz)	30	0	<5	220
Soft Free Strawberry	2 tbsp (1.2 oz)	45	0	<5	180
Soft Light	2 tbsp (1.1 oz)	70	5	15	150
Soft Light Jalapeno	2 tbsp (1.1 oz)	60	5	15	210
Soft Light Raspberry	2 tbsp (1.1 oz)	70	5	15	125
Soft Light Roasted Garlic	2 tbsp (1.1 oz)	70	5	15	180
Whipped	2 tbsp (0.7 oz)	70	7	25	85
Whipped Chives	2 tbsp (0.7 oz)	70	6	20	130
Whipped Smoked Salmon	2 tbsp (0.7 oz)	70	6	20	140
With Chives	1 oz	90	9	30	135
CREAM OF TARTAR					
cream of tartar	1 tsp	8	0	0	2
CREPES					
Frieda's					
Ready-To-Use	2 (0.8 oz)	50	1	5	90
CRESS					
(*see also* WATERCRESS)					
garden cooked	1/2 cup	16	tr	0	5
garden raw	1/2 cup	8	tr	0	4
CROAKER					
atlantic breaded & fried	3 oz	188	11	71	296
CROISSANT					
take-out					
w/ egg & cheese	1 (4.5 oz)	368	25	216	551
w/ egg cheese & bacon	1 (4.5 oz)	413	28	215	889
w/ egg cheese & ham	1 (5.3 oz)	474	34	213	1081
w/ egg cheese & sausage	1 (5.6 oz)	523	38	216	1115
CROUTONS					
plain	1 cup (1 oz)	122	2	0	209
Pepperidge Farm					
Garlic	6 (0.2 oz)	30	1	0	80
Homestyle	6 (0.2 oz)	30	1	0	80
Sourdough	6 (0.2 oz)	35	2	0	70
Up Country Naturals					
Organic Whole Wheat Garlic & Herb	1/4 cup (0.3 oz)	35	2	0	110
CUCUMBER					
fresh	1 (11 oz)	38	tr	0	6
fresh sliced	1/2 cup (1.8 oz)	7	tr	0	1

FOOD	PORTION	CALS	FAT	CHOL	SOD
take-out					
cucumber salad	3.5 oz	50	tr	0	480
kimchee	1/2 cup (1.8 oz)	36	2	0	173
tzatziki	1/2 cup (3.4 oz)	72	6	5	197
CUMIN					
seed	1 tsp	8	tr	0	4
CURRANTS					
black fresh	1/2 cup	36	tr	0	1
zante dried	1/2 cup	204	tr	0	6
CUSK					
fillet baked	3 oz	106	1	50	38
CUSTARD					
mix					
Jell-O					
Americana Custard Dessert as prep w/ 2% milk	1/2 cup (5 oz)	140	3	10	190
Flan as prep w/ 2% milk	1/2 cup (5.1 oz)	140	3	10	65
ready-to-eat					
Kozy Shack					
Flan	1 pkg (4 oz)	150	4	40	90
Swiss Miss					
Egg Custard	1 pkg (4 oz)	153	5	4	138
take-out					
baked	1/2 cup (5 oz)	148	7	123	109
flan	1/2 cup (5.4 oz)	220	6	140	86
CUTTLEFISH					
steamed	3 oz	134	1	190	632
DANDELION GREENS					
fresh cooked	1/2 cup	17	tr	0	23
raw chopped	1/2 cup	13	tr	0	21
DANISH PASTRY					
ready-to-eat					
Dolly Madison					
Danish Rollers	3 (2.8 oz)	290	10	0	130
Tastykake					
Cheese	1 (3 oz)	290	14	20	290
Lemon	1 (3 oz)	290	14	20	280
Raspberry	1 (3 oz)	290	14	20	260
take-out					
almond	1 (4 1/4 in) (2.3 oz)	280	16	30	236
cheese	1 (3.2 oz)	353	25	20	319
cinnamon	1 (3.1 oz)	349	17	27	326
cinnamon nut	1 (4 1/4 in) (2.3 oz)	280	16	30	236
fruit	1 (3.3 oz)	335	16	19	333
raisin nut	1 (4 1/4 in) (2.3 oz)	280	16	30	236
DATES					
Calavo					
Dried Pitted	5-6 (1.4 oz)	120	0	0	0

FOOD	PORTION	CALS	FAT	CHOL	SOD
California Redi-Date					
Deglet Noor Dried	5-6 (1.4 oz)	120	0	0	0
Dromedary					
Chopped Dried	1/4 cup	130	0	0	0
DEER					
(*see* VENISON)					
DELI MEATS/COLD CUTS					
(*see also* BEEF, CHICKEN, HAM, MEAT SUBSTITUTES, TURKEY)					
headcheese pork	1 oz	60	5	23	356
mortadella beef & pork	1 oz	88	7	16	353
olive loaf pork	1 oz	67	5	11	421
pickle & pimiento loaf pork	1 oz	74	6	10	394
Boar's Head					
Bologna Beef	2 oz	150	13	35	520
Bologna Garlic	2 oz	150	13	35	530
Bologna Lowered Sodium	2 oz	150	13	30	410
Bologna Pork & Beef	2 oz	150	13	35	530
Braunschweiger Lite	2 oz	120	8	50	450
Head Cheese	2 oz	90	5	65	420
Liverwurst Strassburger	2 oz	170	15	85	560
Olive Loaf	2 oz	130	12	20	630
Pastrami	2 oz	90	4	30	620
Prosciutto	1 oz	60	3	15	770
Red Pastrami	2 oz	90	4	30	620
Salami Beef	2 oz	120	9	25	470
Salami Cooked	2 oz	130	11	40	550
Salami Genoa	2 oz	180	14	55	970
Salami Hard	1 oz	110	9	25	490
Spiced Ham	2 oz	120	10	30	570
Carl Buddig					
Beef	1 pkg (2.5 oz)	100	5	50	1020
Corned Beef	1 pkg (2.5 oz)	100	5	50	980
Pastrami	1 pkg (2.5 oz)	100	5	50	750
Hormel					
Liverwurst Spread	4 tbsp (2 oz)	130	10	70	650
Pepperoni Chunk	1 oz	140	13	35	470
Pepperoni Sliced	15 slices (1 oz)	140	13	35	470
Pepperoni Twin	1 oz	140	13	35	500
Pillow Pack Genoa Salami	2 oz	160	18	50	940
Pillow Pack Pepperoni	16 slices (1 oz)	140	13	35	470
Jordan's					
Healthy Trim 95% Fat Free Macaroni & Cheese Loaf	2 slices (1.6 oz)	50	2	15	290
Healthy Trim 95% Fat Free Olive Loaf	2 slices (1.6 oz)	50	2	15	290
Healthy Trim 95% Fat Free Pickle & Pepper Loaf	2 slices (1.6 oz)	50	2	15	290

FOOD	PORTION	CALS	FAT	CHOL	SOD
Jordan's (cont.)					
Healthy Trim 97% Fat Free Corned Beef	2 slices (1.6 oz)	45	2	30	290
Healthy Trim Low Fat Cooked Salami	3 slices (2 oz)	70	3	25	360
Healthy Trim Low Fat German Brand Bologna	3 slices (2 oz)	70	3	25	360
Oscar Mayer					
Bologna	1 slice (1 oz)	90	8	30	290
Bologna Beef	1 slice (1 oz)	90	8	20	310
Bologna Garlic	1 slice (1.4 oz)	110	12	40	420
Bologna Wisconsin Made Ring	2 oz	180	16	35	460
Braunschweiger Spread	2 oz	190	17	90	630
Braunschweiger	1 slice (1 oz)	100	9	40	320
Free Bologna	1 slice (1 oz)	20	0	5	280
Light Bologna	1 slice (1 oz)	60	4	15	310
Light Bologna Beef	1 slice (1 oz)	60	4	15	310
Liver Cheese	1 slice (1.3 oz)	120	10	80	420
Luncheon Loaf Spiced	1 slice (1 oz)	70	5	20	340
Old Fashioned Loaf	1 slice (1 oz)	70	5	15	330
Olive Loaf	1 slice (1 oz)	70	6	20	370
Pepperoni	15 slices (1 oz)	140	13	25	550
Salami Cotto	1 slice (1 oz)	70	5	25	280
Salami Cotto Beef	1 slice (1 oz)	60	5	25	370
Salami For Beer	1 slice (1.6 oz)	110	9	30	580
Salami Hard	3 slices (1 oz)	100	9	25	510
Sandwich Spread	2 oz	130	10	25	460
Summer Sausage	2 slices (1.6 oz)	140	13	40	650
Summer Sausage Beef	2 slices (1.6 oz)	140	12	35	640
Spam					
Less Salt	2 oz	170	16	40	560
Lite	2 oz	110	8	45	560
Original	2 oz	170	16	40	750
Smoked	2 oz	170	16	40	750

DIETING AIDS

(*see* NUTRITION SUPPLEMENTS)

DILL

seed	1 tsp	6	tr	0	tr
sprigs fresh	1 cup	4	tr	0	5
sprigs fresh	5	0	tr	0	1
weed dry	1 tsp	3	tr	0	2

DINNER

(*see also* ASIAN FOOD, PASTA DISHES, POT PIES, SPANISH FOOD)

frozen

Amy's Organic

Whole Meals Country Dinner	1 pkg (11 oz)	380	12	15	570

FOOD	PORTION	CALS	FAT	CHOL	SOD
Armour					
Classics Veal Parmigiana	1 meal (11.25 oz)	400	22	65	1050
Birds Eye					
Chicken Voila Garlic	2 cups (6.2 oz)	260	11	25	540
Chicken Voila Teriyaki	2 1/3 cups (6.1 oz)	230	6	15	610
Chicken Voila Alfredo	1 cup (6.1 oz)	230	8	20	660
Easy Recipe Meal Starter Cacciatore as prep	1 serv	280	8	69	336
Easy Recipe Meal Starter Orange Glaze Chicken as prep	1 serv	280	8	69	336
Easy Recipe Meal Starter Southwestern	1 serv	280	8	69	336
Easy Recipe Meal Starter Sweet & Sour as prep	1 serv	280	8	69	336
Green Giant					
Create A Meal Broccoli Stir Fry as prep	1 1/3 cups (9.9 oz)	290	13	60	1160
Create A Meal Cheese & Herb Primavera as prep	1 1/4 cups (10 oz)	330	11	65	920
Create A Meal Garlic Herb as prep	1 1/4 cups (10 oz)	340	14	145	670
Create A Meal Hearty Vegetable Stew as prep	1 1/4 cups (10 oz)	280	9	55	1000
Create A Meal Lemon Herb as prep	1 1/2 cups (10 oz)	360	11	65	830
Create A Meal Mushroom & Wine as prep	1 1/4 cups (10 oz)	390	16	75	910
Create A Meal Vegetable Almond Stir Fry as prep	1 1/3 cups (10 oz)	320	11	65	1190
Lean Cuisine					
Cafe Classics Baked Chicken	1 pkg (8.6 oz)	240	5	30	550
Cafe Classics Baked Fish	1 pkg (9 oz)	290	6	40	590
Cafe Classics Beef Peppercorn	1 pkg (8.75 oz)	260	7	25	590
Cafe Classics Beef Portobello	1 pkg (9 oz)	220	7	35	590
Cafe Classics Beef Pot Roast	1 pkg (9 oz)	210	6	30	570
Cafe Classics Chicken Carbonara	1 pkg (9 oz)	280	7	30	560
Cafe Classics Chicken Medallions w/ Creamy Cheese Sauce	1 pkg (9.37 oz)	300	7	35	690
Cafe Classics Chicken Mediterranean	1 pkg (10.5 oz)	260	4	20	690
Cafe Classics Chicken & Vegetables	1 pkg (10.5 oz)	240	5	30	690
Cafe Classics Chicken In Peanut Sauce	1 pkg (9 oz)	260	6	30	690

FOOD	PORTION	CALS	FAT	CHOL	SOD
Lean Cuisine (cont.)					
Cafe Classics Chicken In Wine Sauce	1 pkg (8.1 oz)	220	5	45	690
Cafe Classics Chicken L'Orange	1 pkg (9 oz)	230	2	40	300
Cafe Classics Chicken Parmesan	1 pkg (10.9 oz)	300	6	35	600
Cafe Classics Chicken Piccata	1 pkg (9 oz)	300	9	30	590
Cafe Classics Chicken w/ Basil Cream Sauce	1 pkg (8.5 oz)	260	7	35	650
Cafe Classics Country Vegetables & Beef	1 pkg (9 oz)	210	4	25	590
Cafe Classics Fiesta Chicken	1 pkg (9.25 oz)	270	5	30	690
Cafe Classics Glazed Chicken	1 pkg (8.5 oz)	240	6	55	480
Cafe Classics Glazed Turkey Tenderloins	1 pkg (9 oz)	260	5	25	640
Cafe Classics Grilled Chicken	1 pkg (9.4 oz)	250	5	40	690
Cafe Classics Grilled Chicken Salsa	1 pkg (8.9 oz)	270	7	45	570
Cafe Classics Herb Roasted Chicken	1 pkg (8 oz)	190	4	35	690
Cafe Classics Honey Mustard Chicken	1 pkg (8 oz)	270	4	35	690
Cafe Classics Honey Roasted Chicken	1 pkg (8.5 oz)	270	6	25	550
Cafe Classics Honey Roasted Pork	1 serv (9.5 oz)	250	6	45	590
Cafe Classics Meatloaf w/ Whipped Potatoes	1 pkg (9.4 oz)	260	7	45	600
Cafe Classics Oriental Beef	1 pkg (9.25 oz)	210	4	25	530
Cafe Classics Oven Roasted Beef	1 pkg (9.25 oz)	260	8	50	590
Cafe Classics Roasted Turkey Breast	1 pkg (9.75 oz)	270	2	25	590
Cafe Classics Salisbury Steak	1 pkg (9.5 oz)	280	8	60	590
Cafe Classics Sirlion Beef Peppercorn	1 pkg (8.75 oz)	220	7	35	580
Cafe Classics Southern Beef Tips	1 pkg (8.75 oz)	270	6	35	480
Everday Favorites Vegetable Lasagna	1 pkg (10.5 oz)	260	7	20	590
Everyday Favorites Chicken Florentine	1 pkg (8 oz)	220	5	25	640
Everyday Favorites Chicken Chow Mein	1 pkg (9 oz)	240	4	35	590
Everyday Favorites Homestyle Turkey	1 pkg (9.4 oz)	240	5	40	590

FOOD	PORTION	CALS	FAT	CHOL	SOD
Everyday Favorites Hunan Beef & Broccoli	1 pkg (8.5 oz)	240	4	20	690
Everyday Favorites Mandarin Chicken	1 pkg (9 oz)	260	5	35	570
Everyday Favorites Roasted Chicken	1 pkg (8.1 oz)	260	7	20	640
Everyday Favorites Stuffed Cabbage	1 pkg (9.5 oz)	210	8	20	590
Hearty Portions Cheese & Spinach Manicotti	1 serv	370	8	35	850
Hearty Portions Chicken & Barbecue Sauce	1 serv	370	6	40	840
Hearty Portions Homestyle Beef Stroganoff	1 serv	350	9	30	850
Hearty Portions Jumbo Rigatoni w/ Meatballs	1 serv	440	9	35	820
Hearty Portions Oriental Glazed Chicken	1 serv	370	2	35	850
Hearty Portions Roasted Chicken w/ Mushrooms	1 serv	330	4	40	740
Skillet Sensations Beef Teriyaki & Rice	1 serv	280	3	25	700
Skillet Sensations Chicken Primavera	1 serv	320	5	30	790
Skillet Sensations Chicken Oriental	1 serv	280	3	15	790
Skillet Sensations Fiesta Beef & Rice	1 serv	300	4	25	760
Skillet Sensations Garlic Chicken	1 serv	340	5	20	730
Skillet Sensations Herb Chicken & Roasted Potatoes	1 serv	270	5	40	790
Skillet Sensations Roasted Turkey	1 serv	220	2	25	790
Skillet Sensations Savory Beef & Vegetables	1 serv	290	7	35	1440
Skillet Sensations Three Cheese Chicken	1 serv	370	10	50	820
Marie Callenders					
Complete Skillet Meal Herb Chicken	1 serv	270	6	50	1100
Stouffer's					
Baked Chicken Breast w/ Mashed Potatoes	1 serv (12.2 oz)	330	14	60	1070
Beef Stroganoff	1 pkg (9.75 oz)	390	20	85	1100
Chicken A La King	1 pkg (9.5 oz)	350	13	40	800
Creamed Chicken	1 pkg (6.5 oz)	260	19	80	680

FOOD	PORTION	CALS	FAT	CHOL	SOD
Stouffer's (cont.)					
Creamed Chipped Beef	1/2 cup (5.5 oz)	160	11	40	690
Creamy Chicken & Broccoli	1 pkg (8.9 oz)	320	15	60	820
Escalloped Chicken & Noodles	1 pkg (10 oz)	430	27	50	1120
Fish w/ Macaroni & Cheese	1 serv (9.5 oz)	460	20	55	970
Glazed Chicken w/ Rice	1 serv (11.8 oz)	290	6	45	810
Green Pepper Steak	1 pkg (10.5 oz)	330	9	35	650
Homestyle Beef Pot Roast & Browned Potatoes	1 pkg (8.9 oz)	250	8	35	780
Homestyle Fish Filet w/ Macaroni & Cheese	1 pkg (9 oz)	430	21	70	930
Homestyle Fried Chicken & Whipped Potatoes	1 pkg (7.5 oz)	310	12	45	680
Homestyle Meatloaf & Whipped Potatoes	1 pkg (9.9 oz)	330	16	70	850
Homestyle Roast Turkey w/ Gravy Stuffing & Whipped Potatoes	1 pkg (9.6 oz)	320	13	50	950
Homestyle Salisbury Steak & Gravy & Macaroni & Cheese	1 pkg (9.6 oz)	350	16	70	1290
Homestyle Baked Chicken & Gravy & Whipped Potatoes	1 pkg (8.9 oz)	270	12	75	750
Meatloaf	1 serv (5.5 oz)	210	12	60	520
Meatloaf w/ Whipped Potatoes	1 serv (11.5 oz)	380	18	70	950
Stuffed Pepper	1 pkg (10 oz)	200	5	20	820
Swedish Meatballs	1 pkg (10.25 oz)	480	24	60	960
Swanson					
Beef Pot Roast	1 pkg (14 oz)	320	8	35	1200
Chicken Parmigiana w/ Spaghetti	1 pkg (11 oz)	380	17	25	700
Turkey Breast	1 pkg (11.7 oz)	330	6	40	1290
Tamarind Tree					
Alu Chole	1 pkg (9.2 oz)	350	6	0	620
Channa Dal Masala	1 pkg (9.2 oz)	340	5	0	700
Dal Makhini	1 pkg (9.2 oz)	330	6	5	670
Dhingri Mutter	1 pkg (9.2 oz)	290	5	0	680
Navratan Korma	1 pkg (9.2 oz)	430	15	5	700
Palak Paneer	1 pkg (9.2 oz)	380	15	35	640
Saag Chole	1 pkg (9.2 oz)	370	10	0	800
Vegetable Jalfrazi	1 pkg (9.2 oz)	310	6	0	600
Tyson					
BBQ Chicken Potato & Vegetable Medley	1 pkg (14.7 oz)	560	21	30	1190
Blackened Chicken Spanish Rice & Corn	1 pkg (8.8 oz)	260	5	30	480

FOOD	PORTION	CALS	FAT	CHOL	SOD
Chicken Primavera	1 pkg (11.3 oz)	350	6	30	610
Chicken Divan Candied Carrots & Pasta	1 pkg (9.8 oz)	370	15	50	530
Chicken Francais Sliced Potatoes & Green Beans	1 pkg (8.8 oz)	260	10	45	790
Chicken Kiev Rice Pilaf & Broccoli Carrots	1 pkg (9.1 oz)	440	25	85	900
Chicken Marsala Carrots & Red Potatoes	1 pkg (8.8 oz)	180	5	30	520
Chicken Mesquite Corn & Pea Medley & Au Gratin Potatoes	1 pkg (8.8 oz)	320	8	25	780
Chicken Picatta	1 pkg (8.8 oz)	190	6	35	500
Chicken w/ Broccoli & Cheese Carrots & Pasta	1 pkg (8.8 oz)	270	12	40	690
Chicken w/ Mushroom Sauce Rice Pilaf & Candied Carrots	1 pkg (8.8 oz)	220	6	30	510
Chicken w/ Tabasco BBQ Sauce	1 pkg (8.8 oz)	260	7	25	610
Fried Chicken & Gravy w/ Mashed Potatoes & Corn	1 pkg (10.8 oz)	360	15	30	840
Grilled Chicken Corn O'Brien & Ranch Beans	1 pkg (8.8 oz)	230	4	30	590
Grilled Italian Chicken Pasta & Vegetable Medley	1 pkg (8.8 oz)	190	4	30	440
Honey Dijon Chicken Pasta & Pea Medley	1 pkg (11.3 oz)	340	7	25	900
Roasted Chicken w/ Garlic Sauce Pasta & Vegetable Medley	1 pkg (8.8 oz)	210	7	25	460
Weight Watchers					
Smart Ones Grilled Salisbury Steak	1 pkg (8.5 oz)	250	9	40	620
Smart Ones Chicken Mirabella	1 pkg (9.2 oz)	180	2	20	480
Smart Ones Fiesta Chicken	1 pkg (8.5 oz)	210	2	25	570
Smart Ones Honey Mustard Chicken	1 pkg (8.5 oz)	200	2	30	370
Smart Ones Lemon Herb Chicken Piccata	1 pkg (8.5 oz)	190	2	25	460
Smart Ones Pepper Steak	1 pkg (10 oz)	240	5	35	690
Smart Ones Risotto w/ Cheese & Mushrooms	1 pkg (10 oz)	290	7	20	540
Smart Ones Roast Turkey Medallions & Mushrooms	1 pkg (8.5 oz)	180	2	20	530
Smart Ones Shrimp Marinara	1 pkg (9 oz)	180	2	40	570

FOOD	PORTION	CALS	FAT	CHOL	SOD
Weight Watchers (cont.)					
Smart Ones Stuffed Turkey Breast	1 pkg (10 oz)	260	7	30	680
Smart Ones Swedish Meatballs	1 pkg (9 oz)	280	70	30	690
Yves					
Veggie Country Stew	1 pkg (10.5 oz)	170	0	0	1020
ready-to-eat					
Tyson					
Beef Stir Fry	1 pkg (14 oz)	430	5	45	1560
Chicken Stir Fry Kit	2 3/4 cups (14 oz)	430	5	45	1700
DIP					
Breakstone's					
Bacon & Onion	2 tbsp (1.1 oz)	60	5	20	180
Chesapeake Clam	2 tbsp (1.1 oz)	50	4	20	180
Free Creamy Salsa	2 tbsp (1.1 oz)	20	0	<5	240
Free French Onion	2 tbsp (1.1 oz)	25	0	<5	260
Free Ranch	2 tbsp (1.1 oz)	25	0	<5	330
French Onion	2 tbsp (1.1 oz)	50	5	20	160
Toasted Onion	2 tbsp (1.1 oz)	50	5	20	170
Cheez Whiz					
Medium Cheese & Salsa	2 tbsp (1.2 oz)	100	8	20	490
Mild Cheese & Salsa	2 tbsp (1.2 oz)	100	8	20	490
Chi-Chi's					
Fiesta Bean	2 tbsp (0.9 oz)	35	2	0	140
Fiesta Cheese	2 tbsp (0.9 oz)	40	3	10	270
Fritos					
Bean	2 tbsp (1.2 oz)	40	1	0	140
Chili Cheese	1.2 oz	45	3	<5	310
French Onion	2 tbsp (1.1 oz)	60	5	15	230
Hot Bean	2 tbsp (1.2 oz)	40	1	0	170
Jalapeno & Cheddar Cheese	2 tbsp (1.2 oz)	50	4	5	300
Guiltless Gourmet					
Black Bean Mild	2 tbsp (1 oz)	30	0	0	100
Black Bean Spicy	2 tbsp (1 oz)	30	0	0	100
Knudsen					
Free Creamy Salsa	2 tbsp (1.1 oz)	20	0	<5	240
Free French Onion	2 tbsp (1.1 oz)	25	0	<5	260
Free Ranch	2 tbsp (1.1 oz)	25	0	<5	330
Kraft					
Avocado	2 tbsp (1.1 oz)	60	4	0	240
Bacon & Horseradish	2 tbsp (1.1 oz)	60	5	0	220
Clam	2 tbsp (1.1 oz)	60	4	0	250
Free French Onion	2 tbsp (1.1 oz)	25	0	<5	260
Free Ranch	2 tbsp (1.1 oz)	25	0	<5	330
Free Salsa	2 tbsp (1.1 oz)	20	0	<5	240
French Onion	2 tbsp (1.1 oz)	60	4	0	230

FOOD	PORTION	CALS	FAT	CHOL	SOD
Green Onion	2 tbsp (1.1 oz)	60	4	0	190
Jalapeno Cheese	2 tbsp (1.1 oz)	60	4	0	260
Premium Sour Cream	2 tbsp (1.1 oz)	50	4	20	180
Premium Sour Cream Bacon & Horseradish	2 tbsp (1.1 oz)	60	5	15	240
Premium Sour Cream Bacon & Onion	2 tbsp (1.1 oz)	60	5	20	180
Premium Sour Cream Creamy Onion	2 tbsp (1.1 oz)	45	4	15	160
Premium Sour Cream French Onion	2 tbsp (1.1 oz)	45	4	15	160
Premium Sour Cream Ranch	2 tbsp (1.1 oz)	50	4	15	230
Ranch	2 tbsp (1.1 oz)	60	5	0	210
Ruffles					
French Onion	2 tbsp	70	5	0	240
Ranch	2 tbsp (1.2 oz)	70	6	0	300
Snyder's Of Hanover					
Microwavable Hot Nacho Cheese	2 tbsp	48	3	3	270
Microwavable Mild Cheese	2 tbsp	45	3	5	250
Mustard Pretzel	2 tbsp	60	2	0	0
Sour Cream & Onion	2 tbsp	60	5	15	220
Taco Bell					
Fat Free Black Bean	2 tbsp (1.2 oz)	30	0	0	220
Salsa Con Queso Medium	2 tbsp (1.2 oz)	45	3	<5	270
Salsa Con Queso Mild	2 tbsp (1.2 oz)	45	3	<5	270
Tyson					
Bleu Cheese For Dipping Wings	2 tbsp (1.4 oz)	140	14	25	370
Utz					
Fat Free Sour Cream & Onion	2 tbsp (1.1 oz)	30	0	0	210
Jalapeno & Cheddar	2 tbsp (1 oz)	30	3	0	250
Low Fat Desert Garden	2 tbsp (1.1 oz)	40	2	0	210
Low Fat Salsa Con Queso	2 tbsp (1 oz)	40	2	0	240
Mild Cheddar	2 tbsp (1 oz)	45	3	5	250
Sour Cream & Onion	2 tbsp (1 oz)	60	5	15	220
DOCK					
raw chopped	1/2 cup	15	tr	0	3
DOLPHINFISH					
fresh baked	3 oz	93	1	80	96
DOUGHNUTS					
(see also doughnut shops in Part 2)					
Dolly Madison					
Chocolate Frosted	1 (1.1 oz)	140	8	5	130
Donut Gems Chocolate	4 (2 oz)	260	15	10	230
Donut Gems Crunch	3 (2 oz)	220	10	10	250
Donut Gems Powdered	4 (2 oz)	230	11	15	260
English Cruller	1 (2 oz)	250	14	30	190

FOOD	PORTION	CALS	FAT	CHOL	SOD
Dolly Madison (cont.)					
Glazed Whirl	1 (1.6 oz)	210	11	25	150
Glazed Yeast	1 (1.5 oz)	190	9	10	130
Old Fashioned	1 (2.1 oz)	280	16	20	360
Plain	1 (1.2 oz)	140	7	10	190
Powdered	1 (1 oz)	120	6	10	140
Dutch Mill					
Cider	1 (2.1 oz)	240	10	15	220
Cinnamon	1 (1.8 oz)	210	11	15	250
Donut Holes Double-Dipped Chocolate	3 (1.4 oz)	220	16	5	140
Donut Holes Shootin' Stars	3 (1.4 oz)	190	10	5	110
Double-Dipped Chocolate	1 (2.1 oz)	280	17	15	360
Glazed	1 (2.1 oz)	250	12	15	220
Glazed Chocolate	1 (2.4 oz)	270	11	15	380
Plain	1 (1.8 oz)	210	12	15	270
Sugared	1 (1.8 oz)	220	11	15	260
Hostess					
Blueberry	1 (1.7 oz)	210	13	10	120
Donettes Crumb	3 (1.5 oz)	170	8	10	190
Donettes Frosted	3 (1.5 oz)	200	12	10	170
Donettes Powdered	3 (1.5 oz)	180	9	10	190
Frosted	1 (1.4 oz)	180	11	5	170
O's Raspberry Filled	1 (2.2 oz)	230	10	5	230
Old Fashioned Glazed	1 (2.1 oz)	260	13	25	220
Plain	1 (1.1 oz)	140	7	10	190
Powdered	1 (1.3 oz)	150	8	10	180
Little Debbie					
Donut Sticks	1 (1.6 oz)	210	12	10	150
Mini Powdered	1 pkg (2.5 oz)	290	14	10	290
Tastykake					
Mini Plain Glaze	1 pkg (2.5 oz)	260	11	25	330
Mini Powdered Sugar	1 pkg (2.5 oz)	260	12	30	360
Mini Rich Frosted	1 pkg (3 oz)	370	22	25	340
Tom's					
Chocolate Gem	1 pkg (2.5 oz)	320	18	10	430
Dunkin' Sticks	1 pkg (2.5 oz)	370	22	10	300
Powdered Gems	1 pkg (2.5 oz)	320	18	10	430
DRESSING					
(*see* STUFFING/DRESSING)					
DRINK MIXERS					
(*see also* SODA, WATER)					
Daily's					
Bloody Mary Original	1 serv (6 oz)	50	0	0	1040
Margarita Daiquiri Strawberry	1 serv (4 oz)	180	0	0	65
Margarita Green Demon	1 serv (3 oz)	80	0	0	45
Pina Colada	1 serv (3 oz)	160	2	0	115

FOOD	PORTION	CALS	FAT	CHOL	SOD
Tabasco					
Bloody Mary Mix	1 serv (8.4 oz)	56	tr	0	1548
Bloody Mary Mix Extra Spicy	1 serv (8.4 oz)	58	tr	0	1645
DRUM					
freshwater baked	3 oz	130	5	70	82
DUCK					
w/ skin w/ bone leg roasted	3 oz	184	10	97	94
w/ skin w/o bone breast roasted	3 oz	172	9	116	71
w/o skin roasted	1 cup (4.9 oz)	281	16	125	91
Grimaud Farms					
Muscovy Duck Confit	1 serv (3 oz)	170	10	95	140
DUMPLING					
Health Is Wealth					
Potstickers Chicken Free	2 (1.6 oz)	80	4	0	300
Potstickers Pork Free	2 (1.6 oz)	80	4	0	300
Potstickers Vegetable	2 (1.6 oz)	90	3	0	190
Steamed Dumpling	2 (1.6 oz)	50	2	0	310
Pepperidge Farm					
Apple	1 (3 oz)	230	11	0	180
Peach	1 (3 oz)	320	11	0	150
DURIAN					
fresh	3 1/2 oz	141	2	0	1
EDAMAME					
(*see* SOYBEANS)					
EEL					
fresh cooked	3 oz	200	13	137	55
EGG					
(*see also* EGG DISHES, EGG SUBSTITUTES)					
chicken					
hard cooked	1	77	5	213	62
hard cooked chopped	1 cup	210	14	578	169
poached	1	74	5	212	140
raw	1	75	5	213	63
white only	1	17	0	0	55
EggsPlus					
Fresh	1 (1.8 oz)	70	5	215	65
Horizon Organic					
Medium	1 (1.5 oz)	70	4	190	55
Organic Valley					
Brown Extra Large	1 (2.2 oz)	90	6	225	330
Brown Large	1 (2 oz)	80	6	200	380
Brown Medium	1 (1.8 oz)	70	5	175	260
other poultry					
duck preserved hard core	1 (1.8 oz)	80	6	220	350
duck preserved soft core	1 (1.8 oz)	80	6	220	350
duck raw	1 (2.5 oz)	130	10	619	102
duck salted	1 (1.9 oz)	100	7	195	320

FOOD	PORTION	CALS	FAT	CHOL	SOD
EGG DISHES					
frozen					
Weight Watchers					
Handy Ham & Cheese Omelet	1 (4 oz)	220	5	30	440
take-out					
deviled	2 halves	145	13	280	180
omelette plain	1 serv (3.5 oz)	172	13	350	245
scrambled plain	2 (3.3 oz)	199	15	400	211
scrambled w/ whole milk & margarine	1 serv	365	27	774	616
sunny side up	1	91	7	211	162
EGG ROLLS					
(*see also* ASIAN FOOD)					
egg roll wrapper fresh	1	83	tr	3	162
Health Is Wealth					
Broccoli	1 (3 oz)	150	5	5	560
Oriental Vegetable	1 (3 oz)	160	4	0	390
Oriental Chicken Free	1 (3 oz)	120	4	0	390
Pizza	1 (3 oz)	200	9	0	470
Spinach	1 (3 oz)	180	8	0	300
Spring Rolls	1 (1.6 oz)	70	2	0	200
Veggie	1 (3 oz)	130	4	0	550
Worthington					
Vegetarian Egg Rolls	1 (3 oz)	180	8	0	380
take-out					
lobster	1 (4.8 oz)	270	7	0	460
meat & shrimp	1 (4.8 oz)	320	12	10	470
pork & shrimp	1 (5 oz)	300	10	15	890
shrimp	1 (3 oz)	170	5	<5	420
spicy pork	1 (3 oz)	200	9	5	410
vegetable	1 (3 oz)	170	4	0	520
EGG SUBSTITUTES					
Egg Beaters					
Eggs Substitute	1/4 cup	25	0	0	80
Morningstar Farms					
Better'n Eggs	1/4 cup (2 oz)	20	0	0	90
Breakfast Sandwich Bagel Scramblers Pattie Cheese	1 (5.9 oz)	320	5	10	900
Breakfast Sandwich English Muffin Scramblers Pattie	1 (5.1 oz)	240	3	5	700
Breakfast Sandwich English Muffin Scramblers Pattie Cheese	1 (6 oz)	280	3	10	1000
Scramblers	1/4 cup (2 oz)	35	0	0	95
EGGNOG					
eggnog	1 qt	1368	76	596	553
Oberweis					
Egg Nog	1/2 cup	240	15	40	70

FOOD	PORTION	CALS	FAT	CHOL	SOD
EGGPLANT					
canned					
Progresso					
Caponata	2 tbsp (1 oz)	25	2	0	130
fresh					
cubed cooked	1/2 cup	13	tr	0	2
take-out					
baba ghannouj	1/4 cup	55	4	0	95
caponata	2 tbsp (1 oz)	30	2	0	115
iman bayildi eggplant w/ onion & tomato	1 serv (15.6 oz)	345	28	0	552
indian eggplant runi	1 serv	180	14	0	228
papoutsakis little shoes	1 serv (15.5 oz)	245	16	40	751
ELDERBERRY JUICE					
elderberry	3 1/2 oz	38	0	0	1
ELK					
roasted	3 oz	124	2	62	52
ENDIVE					
fresh	3 1/2 oz	9	tr	0	53
raw chopped	1/2 cup	4	tr	0	6
ENERGY BARS					
(*see also* CEREAL BARS, ENERGY DRINKS, NUTRITION SUPPLEMENTS)					
Benecol					
Chocolate Crisp	1 bar (1.2 oz)	130	3	5	60
Chocolate Crisp	1 bar (1.2 oz)	130	3	5	60
Peanut Crisp	1 bar (1.2 oz)	140	4	5	105
Better Bar					
Chocolate Coated Caramel Pecan	1 bar (1.8 oz)	180	4	0	35
Chocolate Coated Peanut	1 bar (1.8 oz)	180	4	0	35
Yogurt Coated Raspberry	1 bar (1.8 oz)	180	3	0	35
Breakthru					
Organic Chocolate Fudge	1 bar (2.1 oz)	230	3	0	120
Organic Cinnamon Crunch	1 bar (2.1 oz)	220	3	0	160
Organic Honey Graham	1 bar (2.1 oz)	220	3	0	160
Organic Mocha Fudge	1 bar (2.1 oz)	230	3	0	120
Clif Bar					
Apricot	1 bar (2.4 oz)	220	3	0	90
Carrot Cake	1 bar (2.4 oz)	240	4	0	150
Chocolate Brownie	1 bar (2.4 oz)	240	4	0	150
Chocolate Almond Fudge	1 bar (2.4 oz)	230	5	0	140
Chocolate Chip	1 bar (2.4 oz)	240	4	0	170
Chocolate Chip Peanut Crunch	1 bar (2.4 oz)	240	5	0	290
Cookies'N Cream	1 bar (2.4 oz)	230	4	0	180
Cranberry Apple Cherry	1 bar (2.4 oz)	220	2	0	135
Crunchy Peanut Butter	1 bar (2.4 oz)	240	5	0	290
GingerSnap	1 bar (2.4 oz)	230	4	0	140

FOOD	PORTION	CALS	FAT	CHOL	SOD
Ensure					
Honey Graham Crunch	1 bar (2.23 oz)	130	3	<5	115
Extend					
Chocolate Chip Crunch	1 bar (1.4 oz)	160	3	0	80
Peanut Butter Crunch	1 bar (1.4 oz)	160	3	0	85
GeniSoy					
Soy Protein Chocolate	1 bar (2.2 oz)	210	0	0	190
Soy Protein Chocolate Coated	1 bar (2.2 oz)	220	4	0	190
HeartBar					
Cranberry	1 bar (1.8 oz)	190	3	0	95
Original	1 bar (1.76 oz)	180	3	0	140
Jenny Craig					
Meal Bar Chocolate Peanut	1 bar (2 oz)	220	5	0	240
Meal Bar Lemon Meringue	1 bar (2 oz)	210	5	0	130
Meal Bar Milk Chocolate	1 bar (2 oz)	210	5	0	180
Meal Bar Oatmeal Raisin	1 bar (1.97 oz)	210	3	0	75
Meal Bar Yogurt Peanut	1 bar (2 oz)	220	5	0	270
Kashi					
GoLean Chocolate Peanut Butter	1 (2.7 oz)	280	6	0	150
GoLean Honey Vanilla Yogurt	1 (2.7 oz)	280	4	0	70
GoLean Strawberry Vanilla Yogurt	1 (2.7 oz)	280	4	0	75
Luna					
Chai Tea	1 bar (1.7 oz)	180	4	0	125
Sesame Raisin Crunch	1 bar (1.7 oz)	170	3	0	125
Toasted Nuts 'n Cranberry	1 bar (1.7 oz)	170	3	0	130
Tropical Crisp	1 bar (1.7 oz)	180	4	0	135
NiteBite					
Chocolate Fudge	1 bar (0.9 oz)	100	4	5	40
Peanut Butter	1 bar (0.9 oz)	100	4	5	80
Nutiva					
Flaxseed & Raisin Organic	1 bar (1.4 oz)	280	19	0	10
Hempseed Bar Organic	1 bar (1.4 oz)	210	14	0	5
Odwalla Bar!					
Peanut Crunch	1 bar (2.2 oz)	260	7	0	180
PowerBar					
Apple Cinnamon	1 bar (2.3 oz)	230	3	0	90
Banana	1 bar (2.3 oz)	230	2	0	90
Chocolate	1 bar (2.3 oz)	230	2	0	90
Essentials Chocolate	1 bar (1.9 oz)	180	4	0	105
Harvest Blueberry	1 bar (2.3 oz)	240	4	0	80
Harvest Strawberry	1 bar (2.3 oz)	240	4	0	80
Malt-Nut	1 bar (2.3 oz)	230	3	0	90
Mocha	1 bar (2.3 oz)	230	3	0	90
Oatmeal Raisin	1 bar (2.3 oz)	230	3	0	120
Peanut Butter	1 bar (2.3 oz)	230	3	0	110

FOOD	PORTION	CALS	FAT	CHOL	SOD
Power Gel Strawberry Banana	1 pkg	110	0	0	50
Vanilla Crisp	1 bar (2.3 oz)	230	3	0	90
Wild Berry	1 bar (2.3 oz)	230	3	0	90
Slim-Fast					
Crispy Peanut Caramel	1 bar	120	4	<5	80
Dutch Chocolate	1 bar	140	5	5	80
Meal On-The-Go Apple Cobbler	1 bar	220	5	<5	150
Meal On-The-Go Chocolate Cookie Dough	1 bar	220	5	<5	180
Meal On-The-Go Honey Peanut	1 bar	220	5	<5	160
Meal On-The-Go Milk Chocolate Peanut	1 bar	220	5	<5	120
Meal On-The-Go Oatmeal Raisin	1 bar	220	5	<5	100
Meal On-The-Go Rich Chocolate Brownie	1 bar	220	5	<5	150
Meal On-The-Go Toasted Oat & Spice	1 bar	220	5	<5	140
Peanut Butter	1 bar	150	5	5	80
Peanut Butter Crunch	1 bar	130	4	0	80
Rich Chewy Caramel	1 bar	120	4	5	65
Sweet Success					
Chewy Chocolate Brownie	1 bar (1.2 oz)	120	4	3	35
Think!					
Apple Spice	1 bar (2 oz)	205	3	62	36
Chocolate Almond Coconut Raisin	1 bar (2 oz)	243	7	9	160
Chocolate Fruit Harvest	1 bar (2 oz)	217	3	38	42
ZonePerfect					
Honey Peanut	1 bar (1.8 oz)	200	7	0	150
ENERGY DRINKS					
(*see also* ENERGY BARS, ICED TEA, NUTRITION SUPPLEMENTS, SODA, WATER)					
California Joe					
All Natural Protein Drink Mix as prep	1 serv (8 oz)	165	4	0	166
Calorie Shed					
Shake Fat Free No Sugar Caramel Ripple	1/2 cup (4 fl oz)	70	0	5	45
Shake Fat Free No Sugar Chocolate	1/2 cup (4 fl oz)	70	0	5	45
Shake Fat Free No Sugar Marshmellow Nougat	1/2 cup (4 fl oz)	70	0	5	45
GeniSoy					
Soy Protein Shake Chocolate	1 scoop (1.2 oz)	120	0	0	170
Soy Protein Shake Vanilla	1 scoop (1.2 oz)	130	0	0	180

FOOD	PORTION	CALS	FAT	CHOL	SOD
Hansen's					
D-Stress	1 can (8.2 oz)	110	0	0	25
Healthy Pleasures					
Chocolate Irish Cream	1 bottle (10.5 oz)	260	2	6	320
Kashi					
GoLean Shake Man	1 pkg (2.5 oz)	260	1	0	135
GoLean Shake Woman	1 pkg (2.5 oz)	250	2	0	120
Nancy Grey's					
Shake Hi-Protein Black Raspberry	1 cup (8 fl oz)	340	16	65	160
Shake Hi-Protein Chocolate	1 cup (8 fl oz)	340	15	60	140
Shake Hi-Protein Vanilla	1 cup (8 fl oz)	340	16	65	160
Nantucket Nectars					
Super Nectars Ginkgo Mango	8 oz	150	0	0	15
Super Nectars Green Angel	8 oz	140	0	0	15
Super Nectars Protein Smoothie	8 oz	170	1	0	45
Super Nectars Red Guarana Tea	8 oz	110	0	0	5
Super Nectars Vital C	8 oz	130	0	0	10
NutraShake					
Citrus	1 pkg (4 oz)	200	0	0	30
Citrus Free	1 serv (4 oz)	200	0	0	110
Vanilla	1 serv (8 oz)	400	12	36	120
Vanilla No Added Sugar	1 serv (4 oz)	200	8	18	75
Pounds Off					
Dark Chocolate Ectasy	1 can (11 oz)	200	3	0	220
French Vanilla	1 can (11 oz)	220	3	0	460
Red Bull					
Energy Drink	1 can (8.3 oz)	113	0	0	215
Slim-Fast					
Chocolate as prep w/ fat free milk	1 serv	190	1	9	240
Chocolate Malt as prep w/ fat free milk	1 serv	190	1	8	250
JumpStart Chocolate as prep w/ fat free milk	1 serv	240	2	14	280
JumpStart Vanilla as prep w/ fat free milk	1 serv	240	2	9	300
Strawberry as prep w/ fat free milk	1 serv	190	1	9	260
Vanilla as prep w/ fat free milk	1 serv	190	1	9	260
SoBe					
Adrenaline Rush	1 can (8.3 oz)	140	0	0	60
Drive	8 oz	120	0	0	15
Edge	8 oz	110	0	0	15

FOOD	PORTION	CALS	FAT	CHOL	SOD
Elixir 3C Strawberry Carrot	8 oz	90	0	0	15
Jing Essentials	1 bottle (14 oz)	140	0	0	35
Jing Essentials Citrus Soy Blend	1 bottle (14 oz)	170	1	0	70
Karma	8 oz	120	0	0	5
Lean Sugar Free Metabolic Enhancer Diet Green Tea	8 oz	5	0	0	15
Lean Sugar Free Metabolic Enhancer Diet Orange Carrot	8 oz	10	0	0	15
Lizard Lightning Orange Mango	8 oz	130	0	0	20
Qi Essential Berry Soy Blend	1 bottle (14 oz)	170	1	0	70
Qi Essentials	1 bottle (14 oz)	140	0	0	35
Shen Essentials	1 bottle (14 oz)	140	0	0	35
Shen Essentials Peach Soy Blend	1 bottle (14 oz)	170	1	0	70
Tsunami Orange Cream	8 oz	110	0	0	20
Sweet Success					
Creamy Milk Chocolate	1 can	200	3	4	230
Creamy Milk Chocolate as prep w/ skim milk	1 serv	180	1	6	240
The Pumper					
Body Building MilkShake Chocolate	1 serv (13.5 oz)	390	2	5	260
Body Building MilkShake Banana	1 serv (13.5 oz)	390	2	10	230
TwinLab					
Ultra Fuel	1 bottle (16 oz)	400	0	0	55
Ultra Slim-Fast					
Cafe Mocha as prep w/ fat free milk	1 serv	200	2	9	240
Chocolate Fudge as prep w/ fat free milk	1 serv	200	3	9	230
Chocolate Malt as prep w/ fat free milk	1 serv	200	2	9	230
Chocolate Royale as prep w/ fat free milk	1 serv	200	2	9	260
Fruit Juice Mixable as prep w/ juice	1 serv	200	1	5	210
Milk Chocolate as prep w/ fat free milk	1 serv	210	2	8	270
Ready-To-Drink Cappuccino Delight	1 serv	220	2	5	240
Ready-To-Drink Apple Cranberry Raspberry	1 serv	220	2	10	160
Ready-To-Drink Chocolate Royale	1 serv	220	3	5	220

FOOD	PORTION	CALS	FAT	CHOL	SOD
Ultra Slim-Fast (cont.)					
Ready-To-Drink Creamy Milk Chocolate	1 serv	220	3	5	220
Ready-To-Drink Dark Chocolate Fudge	1 serv	220	3	5	300
Ready-To-Drink Orange Strawberry Banana	1 serv	220	2	10	160
Ready-To-Drink Orange Pineapple	1 serv	220	2	10	200
Ready-To-Drink Strawberries N' Cream	1 serv	220	3	5	220
Strawberry as prep w/ fat free milk	1 serv	200	1	9	250
Vanilla as prep w/ fat free milk	1 serv	200	1	9	260
ENGLISH MUFFIN					
frozen					
Weight Watchers					
Sandwich	1 (4 oz)	210	5	20	420
ready-to-eat					
crumpets	1 (1.5 oz)	80	0	0	270
plain toasted	1	133	1	0	262
Milton's					
Multi-Grain	1 (2 oz)	150	1	0	180
Wonder					
Cinnamon Raisin	1 (2.1 oz)	140	2	0	260
Original	1 (2 oz)	130	1	0	290
Sourdough	1 (2 oz)	130	1	0	290
take-out					
w/ butter	1 (2.2 oz)	189	6	13	386
w/ cheese & sausage	1 (4 oz)	393	24	59	1036
w/ egg cheese & canadian bacon	1 (4.8 oz)	289	13	234	729
w/ egg cheese & sausage	1 (5.8 oz)	487	31	274	1135
EPAZOTE					
fresh	1 tbsp (1 g)	tr	0	0	tr
fresh sprig	1 (2 g)	1	tr	0	1
EPPAW					
raw	1/2 cup	75	1	0	6
FALAFEL					
take-out					
falafel	1 (1.2 oz)	57	3	0	50
FAST FOODS					
(*see individual names in Part 2*)					
FAT					
(*see also* BUTTER, BUTTER BLENDS, BUTTER SUBSTITUTES, MARGARINE, OIL)					
beef cooked	1 oz	193	20	27	12
beef tallow	1 tbsp (13 g)	115	13	14	0
duck	1 tbsp (13 g)	115	13	13	0

FOOD	PORTION	CALS	FAT	CHOL	SOD
lamb new zealand raw	1 oz	182	19	25	6
lard	1 cup (205 g)	1849	205	195	tr
lard	1 tbsp (13 g)	115	13	12	0
pork backfat	1 oz	230	25	16	3
pork cooked	1 oz	178	18	26	10
salt pork	1 oz	212	23	25	404
Crisco					
Shortening	1 tbsp (0.4 oz)	110	12	0	0
FAT SUBSTITUTES					
Soy Is Us					
Fat Not! Organic	3 tbsp	66	1	0	3
FAVA BEANS					
Progresso					
Fava Beans	1/2 cup (4.6 oz)	110	1	0	250
FEIJOA					
fresh	1 (1.75 oz)	25	tr	0	2
puree	1 cup	119	2	0	7
FENNEL					
fresh bulb	1 (8.2 oz)	72	tr	0	122
fresh sliced	1 cup	27	tr	0	45
seed	1 tsp	7	tr	0	2
FENUGREEK					
seed	1 tsp	12	tr	0	2
FIDDLEHEAD FERNS					
fresh	3.5 oz	34	tr	0	1
FIGS					
canned					
in heavy syrup	3	75	tr	0	1
in light syrup	3	58	tr	0	1
water pack	3	42	tr	0	1
dried					
cooked	1/2 cup	140	1	0	6
whole	10	477	2	0	20
fresh					
fig	1 med	50	tr	0	1
FIREWEED					
leaves chopped	1 cup (0.8 oz)	24	1	0	8
FISH					
(*see also individual fish names,* FISH SUBSTITUTES, SUSHI)					
frozen					
sticks	1 stick (1 oz)	76	3	31	163
Gorton's					
Baked Au Gratin	1 piece (4.6 oz)	130	5	50	400
Baked Broccoli Cheddar	1 piece (4.6 oz)	130	5	50	310
Baked Primavera	1 piece (4.6 oz)	120	5	50	340
Batter Dipped Portions	1 piece (2.5 oz)	170	11	20	390
Crunchy Golden Fillets Breaded	2 (3.8 oz)	250	14	35	480

FOOD	PORTION	CALS	FAT	CHOL	SOD
Gorton's (cont.)					
Crunchy Golden Sticks	6 (3.8 oz)	250	13	30	340
Garlic & Herb	2 pieces (3.6 oz)	220	11	30	670
Garlic Butter Crumb	1 piece (4.6 oz)	170	9	55	350
Grilled Cajun Blackened	1 piece (3.8 oz)	120	6	60	240
Grilled Garlic Butter	1 piece (3.8 oz)	120	6	60	200
Grilled Italian Herb	1 piece (3.8 oz)	130	6	60	330
Grilled Lemon Butter	1 piece (3.8 oz)	120	6	60	380
Grilled Lemon Pepper	1 piece (3.8 oz)	120	6	60	160
Parmesan	2 pieces (3.6 oz)	260	15	30	650
Ranch	1 piece (3.6 oz)	240	13	30	650
Southern Fried Country Style	2 pieces (3.6 oz)	230	14	30	660
Tenders	3.5 pieces (4 oz)	250	14	30	530
Tenders Extra Crunchy	3.5 pieces (4 oz)	270	12	30	640
Mrs. Paul's					
Seafood Platter Combination	9 oz	600	33	85	408
take-out					
jamaican brown fish stew	1 serv	426	22	84	419
FISH SUBSTITUTES					
Loma Linda					
Ocean Platter not prep	1/3 cup (0.9 oz)	90	1	0	450
Worthington					
Fillets	2 (3 oz)	180	10	0	750
Tuno	1/2 cup (1.9 oz)	80	6	0	290
FLAXSEED					
Bite Me					
Flax Bar	1 bar (1.8 oz)	242	11	0	79
FLOUNDER					
fresh					
cooked	1 fillet (4.5 oz)	148	2	86	133
cooked	3 oz	99	1	58	89
take-out					
battered & fried	3.2 oz	211	11	31	484
breaded & fried	3.2 oz	211	11	31	484
FLOUR					
potato	1 cup (6.3 oz)	628	1	0	61
white cake unsifted	1 cup (4.8 oz)	496	1	0	3
All Trump					
Flour	1/4 cup (1 oz)	100	0	0	0
Betty Crocker					
Softasilk Velvet Cake Flour	1/4 cup (1 oz)	100	0	0	0
General Mills					
Wondra	1/4 cup (1 oz)	100	0	0	0
Gold Medal					
All Purpose	1/4 cup (1 oz)	100	0	0	0
Better For Bread	1/4 cup (1 oz)	100	0	0	0
Better For Bread Wheat Blend	1/4 cup (1 oz)	110	1	0	0

FOOD	PORTION	CALS	FAT	CHOL	SOD
Self Rising	1/4 cup (1 oz)	100	0	0	400
Supreme Hygluten	1/4 cup (1 oz)	100	0	0	0
Unbleached	1/4 cup (1 oz)	100	0	0	0
La Pina					
Flour	1/4 cup (1 oz)	100	0	0	0
Red Band					
All Purpose	1/4 cup (1 oz)	100	0	0	0
Bread	1/4 cup (1 oz)	100	0	0	0
Self-Rising	1/4 cup (1 oz)	100	0	0	400
Robin Hood					
All Purpose	1/4 cup (1 oz)	100	0	0	0
Self-Rising	1/4 cup (1 oz)	100	0	0	0
Unbleached	1/4 cup (1 oz)	100	0	0	0
Whole Wheat	1/4 cup (1 oz)	90	1	0	0
FRANKFURTER					
(*see* HOT DOG)					
FRENCH BEANS					
dried cooked	1 cup	228	1	0	11
FRENCH FRIES					
(*see* POTATO)					
FRENCH TOAST					
frozen					
french toast	1 slice (2 oz)	126	4	48	292
take-out					
sticks	5 (4.9 oz)	513	29	75	499
w/ butter	2 slices (4.7 oz)	356	19	116	513
FROSTING					
(*see* CAKE ICING)					
FRUCTOSE					
Estee					
Fructose	1 tsp	15	0	0	0
Packet	1 pkg	10	0	0	0
FRUIT DRINKS					
(*see also individual fruit names,* LEMONADE)					
mix					
Crystal Light					
Fruit Punch as prep	1 serv (8 oz)	5	0	0	0
Lemon-Lime Drink as prep	1 serv (8 oz)	5	0	0	0
Passion Fruit Pineapple Drink as prep	1 serv (8 oz)	5	0	0	0
Pineapple Orange Drink as prep	1 serv (8 oz)	5	0	0	0
Strawberry Orange Banana as prep	1 serv (8 oz)	5	0	0	0
Strawberry Kiwi as prep	1 serv (8 oz)	5	0	0	0
Watermelon Strawberry as prep	1 serv (8 oz)	5	0	0	0

FOOD	PORTION	CALS	FAT	CHOL	SOD
Kool-Aid					
Cherry as prep	1 serv (8 oz)	60	0	0	0
Grape Berry Splash Drink as prep	1 serv (8 oz)	70	0	0	0
Grape Berry Splash Drink as prep w/ sugar	1 serv (8 oz)	100	0	0	0
Kickin' Kiwi Lime Drink as prep	1 serv (8 oz)	60	0	0	0
Kickin' Kiwi Lime Drink as prep w/ sugar	1 serv (8 oz)	100	0	0	10
Lemon-Lime Drink as prep w/ sugar	1 serv (8 oz)	100	0	0	5
Man-O-Mango Berry Drink as prep	1 serv (8 oz)	60	0	0	0
Man-O-Mango Berry Drink as prep w/ sugar	1 serv (8 oz)	100	0	0	0
Oh Yeah Orange Pineapple Drink as prep	1 serv (8 oz)	60	0	0	0
Oh Yeah Orange Pineapple Drink as prep w/ sugar	1 serv (8 oz)	100	0	0	0
Pina-Pineapple Drink as prep	1 serv (8 oz)	60	0	0	0
Pina-Pineapple Drink as prep w/ sugar	1 serv (8 oz)	100	0	0	0
Roarin' Raspberry Cranberry Drink as prep	1 serv (8 oz)	70	0	0	20
Roarin' Raspberry Cranberry Drink as prep w/ sugar	1 serv (8 oz)	100	0	0	10
Slammin' Strawberry Kiwi Drink as prep	1 serv (8 oz)	70	0	0	15
Slammin' Strawberry Kiwi Drink as prep w/ sugar	1 serv (8 oz)	100	0	0	15
Strawberry Raspberry Drink as prep	1 serv (8 oz)	60	0	0	0
Strawberry Raspberry Drink as prep w/ sugar	1 serv (8 oz)	100	0	0	0
Sugar Free Tropical Punch as prep	1 serv (8 oz)	5	0	0	10
Tropical Punch as prep	1 serv (8 oz)	60	0	0	0
Tropical Punch as prep w/ sugar	1 serv (8 oz)	100	0	0	15
Watermelon Cherry Drink as prep	1 serv (8 oz)	60	0	0	0
Watermelon Cherry Drink as prep w/ sugar	1 serv (8 oz)	100	0	0	10
Tang					
Orange Pineapple as prep	1 serv (8 oz)	100	0	0	45

FOOD	PORTION	CALS	FAT	CHOL	SOD
ready-to-drink					
Apple & Eve					
Apple Cranberry	8 oz	120	0	0	20
Capri Sun					
Fruit Punch	1 pkg (7 oz)	100	0	0	20
Maui Punch	1 pkg (7 oz)	100	0	0	20
Mountain Cooler	1 pkg (7 oz)	90	0	0	25
Pacific Cooler	1 pkg (7 oz)	100	0	0	20
Red Berry	1 pkg (7 oz)	100	0	0	20
Safari Punch	1 pkg (7 oz)	100	0	0	20
Strawberry Kiwi Drink	1 pkg (7 oz)	100	0	0	20
Surfer Cooler Drink	1 pkg (7 oz)	100	0	0	20
Citrus Squeeze					
California Punch	8 oz	130	0	0	85
Florida Punch	8 oz	120	0	0	100
Coco Lopez					
Mango Kiwi	8 oz	130	0	0	0
Crystal Light					
Fruit Punch	1 serv (8 oz)	5	0	0	20
Kiwi Strawberry	1 serv (8 oz)	5	0	0	20
Orange Strawberry Banana Drink	1 serv (8 oz)	5	0	0	20
Dole					
Apple Berry Burst	8 oz	120	0	0	20
Cranberry Apple	8 oz	120	0	0	35
Fruit Fiesta	8 oz	140	0	0	20
Fruit Punch	1 carton (10 oz)	160	0	0	25
Mountain Cherry	8 oz	150	0	0	30
Orange Peach Mango	8 oz	120	0	0	35
Orange Strawberry Banana	8 oz	120	0	0	30
Orchard Peach	8 oz	140	0	0	35
Pineapple Orange	8 oz	120	0	0	20
Pineapple Orange Strawberry	8 oz	130	0	0	20
Tropical Fruit	8 oz	160	0	0	30
Everfresh					
Cranberry-Apple Drink	1 can (8 oz)	120	0	0	0
Grape-Strawberry	1 can (8 oz)	120	0	0	0
Kiwi-Strawberry	1 can (8 oz)	120	0	0	0
Mandarin Orange Mango Drink	1 can (8 oz)	120	0	0	0
Orange Banana Strawberry Drink	1 can (8 oz)	120	0	0	19
Tropical Fruit Punch	1 can (8 oz)	120	0	0	0
Wild Blackberry Lime Drink	1 can (8 oz)	120	0	0	0
Fresh Samantha					
Banana Strawberry	1 cup (8 oz)	130	0	0	24
Carrot Orange	1 cup (8 oz)	100	0	0	24
Desperately Seeking C	1 cup (8 oz)	110	0	0	0
The Big Bang	1 cup (8 oz)	100	0	0	0

FOOD	PORTION	CALS	FAT	CHOL	SOD
Fruitopia					
Fruit Integration	8 oz	110	0	0	80
Guzzler					
Citrus Punch	8 oz	140	0	0	10
Island Punch	8 oz	140	0	0	30
Juicy Juice					
Apple Grape	1 box (8.45 oz)	140	0	0	15
Berry	1 box (8.45 oz)	130	0	0	15
Punch	1 box (4.23 oz)	70	0	0	10
Punch	1 box (8.45 oz)	140	0	0	15
Tropical	1 box (8.45 oz)	140	0	0	15
Kool-Aid					
Bursts Great Bluedini	1 (7 oz)	100	0	0	30
Bursts Kickin' Kiwi Lime	1 (7 oz)	100	0	0	30
Bursts Oh Yeah Orange Pineapple	1 (7 oz)	100	0	0	30
Bursts Slammin' Strawberry Kiwi	1 (7 oz)	100	0	0	30
Bursts Tropical Punch	1 (7 oz)	100	0	0	30
Splash Grape Berry Punch	1 serv (8 oz)	120	0	0	35
Splash Kiwi Strawberry Drink	1 serv (8 oz)	110	0	0	35
Splash Tropical Punch	1 serv (8 oz)	120	0	0	35
Mauna La'i					
Island Guava	8 oz	130	0	0	35
Paradise Passion	8 oz	130	0	0	35
Mott's					
Berry	1 box (8 oz)	100	0	0	10
Fruit Punch	8 oz	130	0	0	0
Fruit Punch	1 box (8 oz)	110	0	0	15
Nantucket Nectars					
Apple Raspberry	8 oz	140	0	0	10
California Melonberry	8 oz	110	0	0	15
Cranberry Apple	8 oz	140	0	0	5
Fruit Punch	8 oz	130	0	0	5
Kiwi Berry	8 oz	120	0	0	5
Orange Passionfruit	8 oz	120	0	0	15
Orange Mango	8 oz	130	0	0	5
Pineapple Orange Banana	8 oz	140	0	0	15
Pineapple Orange Guava	8 oz	120	0	0	0
Watermelon Strawberry	8 oz	120	0	0	5
Oberweis					
Fruit Punch	8 oz	120	0	0	5
Ocean Spray					
Cran*Blueberry	8 oz	160	0	0	35
Cran*Cherry	8 oz	160	0	0	35
Cran*Currant	8 oz	140	0	0	35
Cran*Grape	8 oz	170	0	0	35
Cran*Mango	8 oz	130	0	0	35

FOOD	PORTION	CALS	FAT	CHOL	SOD
Cran*Raspberry	8 oz	140	0	0	35
Cran*Raspberry Reduced Calorie	8 oz	50	0	0	35
Cran*Strawberry	8 oz	140	0	0	35
Cran*Tangerine	8 oz	130	0	0	35
Cranapple	8 oz	160	0	0	35
Cranapple Reduced Calorie	8 oz	50	0	0	35
Cranicot	8 oz	160	0	0	35
Crazy Kiwi Passion	8 oz	130	0	0	35
Fruit Punch	8 oz	130	0	0	35
Kiwi Strawberry	8 oz	120	0	0	35
Lightstyle Cran*Grape	8 oz	40	0	0	75
Lightstyle Cran*Mango	8 oz	40	0	0	75
Lightstyle Cran*Raspberry	8 oz	40	0	0	35
Mandarin Magic	8 oz	120	0	0	35
Ruby Red & Tangerine Grapefruit	8 oz	130	0	0	35
Ruby Red & Mango	8 oz	130	0	0	35
Shasta Plus					
Apple-Strawberry	1 can (11.5 oz)	160	0	0	45
Fruit Punch	1 can (11.5 oz)	160	0	0	45
Pineapple-Cherry	1 can (11.5 oz)	160	0	0	45
Snapple					
Cranberry Raspberry	8 oz	120	0	0	10
Diet Cranberry Raspberry	8 oz	10	0	0	10
Fruit Punch	8 oz	110	0	0	10
Kiwi Strawberry	8 oz	110	0	0	10
Squeezit					
Berry B. Wild	1 bottle (7 oz)	110	0	0	0
Blue Raspberry	1 bottle (7 oz)	110	0	0	0
Cherry Cola	1 bottle (7 oz)	110	0	0	0
Chucklin' Cherry	1 bottle (7 oz)	110	0	0	0
Green Apple	1 bottle (7 oz)	110	0	0	0
Grumpy Grape	1 bottle (7 oz)	110	0	0	0
Lemon Lime	1 bottle (7 oz)	110	0	0	0
Rockin' Red Puncher	1 bottle (7 oz)	110	0	0	0
Smarty Arty Orange	1 bottle (7 oz)	110	0	0	45
Strawberry	1 bottle (7 oz)	110	0	0	0
Tropical Punch	1 bottle (7 oz)	110	0	0	0
Watermelon	1 bottle (7 oz)	110	0	0	0
Tropicana					
Berry Punch	8 oz	130	0	0	15
Citrus Punch	8 oz	140	0	0	15
Fruit Punch	8 oz	130	0	0	15
Tangerine Orange Juice	8 oz	110	0	0	0
Tropics Orange Strawberry Banana	8 oz	110	0	0	5
Tropics Orange Kiwi Passion	8 oz	100	0	0	15

FOOD	PORTION	CALS	FAT	CHOL	SOD
Tropicana (cont.)					
Tropics Orange Peach Mango	8 oz	110	0	0	15
Tropics Orange Pineapple	8 oz	110	0	0	15
Twister Apple Raspberry Blackberry	1 bottle (10 oz)	160	1	0	20
Twister Citrus Punch	1 bottle (10 oz)	180	0	0	15
Twister Cranberry Punch	1 bottle (10 oz)	170	0	0	20
Twister Fruit Punch	1 bottle (10 oz)	170	0	0	40
Twister Light Orange Strawberry Banana	1 bottle (10 oz)	45	0	0	25
Twister Orange Cranberry	1 bottle (10 oz)	160	0	0	60
Twister Orange Strawberry Banana	1 bottle (10 oz)	160	0	0	60
Twister Ruby Red Tangerine	1 bottle (10 oz)	160	0	0	25
Twister Strawberry Kiwi	1 bottle (10 oz)	160	0	0	25
V8					
Splash Berry Blend	8 oz	110	0	0	40
Veryfine					
Apple Cranberry	1 bottle (10 oz)	190	0	0	10
Apple Quenchers Black Cherry White Grape	8 oz	120	0	0	10
Apple Quenchers Cranberry Tangerine	8 oz	120	0	0	10
Apple Quenchers Peach Kiwi	8 oz	130	0	0	25
Apple Quenchers Peach Plum	8 oz	130	0	0	25
Apple Quenchers Pear Passionfruit	8 oz	120	0	0	15
Apple Quenchers Raspberry Cherry	8 oz	120	0	0	25
Apple Quenchers Raspberry Lime	8 oz	120	0	0	25
Apple Quenchers Strawberry Banana	8 oz	120	0	0	20
Chillers Arctic Mango Tangerine	8 oz	110	0	0	5
Chillers Freezing Fruit Punch	8 oz	130	0	0	20
Chillers Lemon Lime Blizzard	8 oz	120	0	0	5
Chillers Shivering Strawberry Melon	1 can (11.5 oz)	160	0	0	10
Chillers Tropical Freeze	8 oz	120	0	0	10
Cranberry Raspberry	8 oz	160	0	0	10
Fruit Punch	1 bottle (10 oz)	170	0	0	25
Juice-Ups Berry	8 oz	140	0	0	15
Juice-Ups Fruit Punch	8 oz	140	0	0	15
Juice-Ups Orange Punch	8 oz	140	0	0	15
Orange Strawberry	8 oz	120	0	0	30
Papaya Punch	1 bottle (10 oz)	160	0	0	25
Pineapple Orange	1 bottle (10 oz)	160	0	0	20

FOOD	PORTION	CALS	FAT	CHOL	SOD
Strawberry Banana	1 can (11.5 oz)	160	0	0	15
Strawberry Banana Punch	1 can (11.5 oz)	190	0	0	30
Wellfleet Farms					
Cranberry & Georgia Peach	8 oz	140	0	0	35
Cranberry & Granny Smith Apple	8 oz	130	0	0	35
Cranberry & Key Lime	8 oz	140	0	0	35
FRUIT MIXED					
(see also individual fruit names)					
canned					
Del Monte					
Orchard Select California Mixed	1/2 cup (4.4 oz)	80	0	0	10
Tropical Fruit Salad	1/2 cup (4.4 oz)	80	0	0	10
Dole					
FruitBowls Tropical Fruit	1 pkg (4 oz)	60	0	0	10
Mott's					
Fruitsations Banana	1 pkg (4 oz)	90	0	0	0
Fruitsations Cherry	1 pkg (4 oz)	70	0	0	0
Fruitsations Mango Peach	1 pkg (4 oz)	70	0	0	0
Fruitsations Mixed Berry	1 pkg (4 oz)	90	0	0	0
Fruitsations Pear	1 pkg (4 oz)	90	0	0	0
Fruitsations Strawberry	1 pkg (4 oz)	80	0	0	10
Fruitsations Tropical Fruit	1 pkg (4 oz)	70	0	0	0
Ocean Spray					
Cran*Fruit Cranberry Raspberry	1/4 cup	120	0	0	35
Cran*Fruit Cranberry Strawberry	1/4 cup	120	0	0	35
White House					
Apple Banana Sauce	1 pkg (4 oz)	100	0	0	25
Apple Mixed Berry Sauce	1 pkg (4 oz)	110	0	0	25
Apple Peach Sauce	1 pkg (4 oz)	100	0	0	20
dried					
mixed	11 oz pkg	712	1	0	52
Paradise					
Old English Fruit & Peel Mix	1 tbsp (0.8 oz)	70	0	0	15
Sun-Maid					
Tropical Medley	1/4 cup (1.4 oz)	130	0	0	10
frozen					
Birds Eye					
Mixed Fruit	1/2 cup (4.4 oz)	90	0	0	5
FRUIT SNACKS					
Betty Crocker					
Fruit By The Foot All Flavors	1 roll (0.9 oz)	80	2	0	50
Fruit Gushers All Flavors	1 pkg (0.9 oz)	90	1	0	40
Fruit Roll-Ups All Flavors	1 (0.5 oz)	50	1	0	55
Fruit String Thing All Flavors	1 pkg (0.7 oz)	80	1	0	45

FOOD	PORTION	CALS	FAT	CHOL	SOD
Favorite Brands					
Cherry Fruit Snack	1 pkg (0.9 oz)	80	0	0	15
Creepy Crawler Fruit Snack	1 pkg (0.9 oz)	80	0	0	15
Dinosaur Fruit Snack	1 pkg (0.9 oz)	80	0	0	15
Grape Fruit Snack	1 pkg (0.9 oz)	80	0	0	15
Space Alien Fruit Snack	1 pkg (0.9 oz)	80	0	0	15
Sports Fruit Snack	1 pkg (0.9 oz)	80	0	0	15
Strawberry Fruit Snack	1 pkg (0.9 oz)	80	0	0	15
Teenage Mutant Ninja Turtle Fruit Snack	1 pkg (0.9 oz)	80	0	0	15
Troll Fruit Snack	1 pkg (0.9 oz)	80	0	0	15
Zoo Animal Fruit Snack	1 pkg (0.9 oz)	80	0	0	15
General Mills					
Fruit Snacks All Flavors	1 pkg (0.9 oz)	80	0	0	50
Health Valley					
Bakes Apple	1 bar	70	0	0	30
Bakes Date	1 bar	70	0	0	30
Bakes Raisin	1 bar	70	0	0	30
Fruit Bars Apple	1	140	0	0	0
Fruit Bars Apricot	1	140	0	0	5
Fruit Bars Date	1	140	0	0	5
Fruit Bars Raisin	1	140	0	0	5
Seneca					
Apple Chips	12 chips (1 oz)	140	7	0	15
Sensible Foods					
Crackin' Fruit Cherry Berry	1 pkg (0.6 oz)	51	0	0	85
Crackin' Fruit Tropical Fruit	1 pkg (0.6 oz)	65	1	0	61
Sunbelt					
Fruit Jammers	1 pkg (1 oz)	100	1	0	15
Sunkist					
100% Fruit Roll All Flavors	1 (0.5 oz)	50	0	0	10
Weight Watchers					
Apple & Cinnamon	1 pkg (0.5 oz)	50	0	0	125
Apple Chips	1 pkg (0.75 oz)	70	0	0	125
Peach & Strawberry	1 pkg (0.5 oz)	50	0	0	125
GARBANZOS					
(*see* CHICKPEAS)					
GARLIC					
clove	1	4	tr	0	1
powder	1 tsp	9	tr	0	1
Dorot					
Frozen Crushed Cubes	1 cube (4 g)	5	0	0	40
GEFILTE FISH					
sweet	1 piece (1.5 oz)	35	1	12	220

FOOD	PORTION	CALS	FAT	CHOL	SOD
GELATIN					
mix					
Jell-O					
1-2-3-Brand Strawberry as prep	2/3 cup (5.2 oz)	130	2	0	50
Apricot as prep	1/2 cup (5 oz)	80	0	0	80
Berry Black as prep	1/2 cup (5 oz)	80	0	0	80
Berry Blue as prep	1/2 cup (5 oz)	80	0	0	80
Black Cherry as prep	1/2 cup (5 oz)	80	0	0	80
Cherry as prep	1/2 cup (5 oz)	80	0	0	100
Cranberry Raspberry as prep	1/2 cup (5 oz)	80	0	0	75
Cranberry Strawberry as prep	1/2 cup (5 oz)	80	0	0	75
Cranberry as prep	1/2 cup (5 oz)	80	0	0	75
Grape as prep	1/2 cup (5 oz)	80	0	0	80
Lemon as prep	1/2 cup (5 oz)	80	0	0	120
Lime as prep	1/2 cup (5 oz)	80	0	0	90
Mango as prep	1/2 cup (5 oz)	80	0	0	80
Mixed Fruit as prep	1/2 cup (5 oz)	80	0	0	80
Orange as prep	1/2 cup (5 oz)	80	0	0	80
Peach as prep	1/2 cup (5 oz)	80	0	0	80
Peach Passion Fruit as prep	1/2 cup (5 oz)	80	0	0	80
Pineapple as prep	1/2 cup (5 oz)	80	0	0	80
Raspberry as prep	1/2 cup (5 oz)	80	0	0	80
Sparkling White Grape as prep	1/2 cup (5 oz)	80	0	0	80
Strawberry Banana as prep	1/2 cup (5 oz)	80	0	0	80
Strawberry Kiwi as prep	1/2 cup (5 oz)	80	0	0	80
Strawberry as prep	1/2 cup (5 oz)	80	0	0	90
Sugar Free Cherry as prep	1/2 cup (4.2 oz)	10	0	0	70
Sugar Free Cranberry as prep	1/2 cup (4.2 oz)	10	0	0	80
Sugar Free Lemon	1/2 cup (4.2 oz)	10	0	0	55
Sugar Free Lime as prep	1/2 cup (4.2 oz)	10	0	0	60
Sugar Free Mixed Fruit as prep	1/2 cup (4.2 oz)	10	0	0	50
Sugar Free Orange as prep	1/2 cup (4.2 oz)	10	0	0	65
Sugar Free Raspberry as prep	1/2 cup (4.2 oz)	10	0	0	55
Sugar Free Strawberry Banana as prep	1/2 cup (4.2 oz)	10	0	0	50
Sugar Free Strawberry as prep	1/2 cup (4.2 oz)	10	0	0	55
Sugar Free Strawberry Kiwi as prep	1/2 cup (4.2 oz)	10	0	0	60
Sugar Free Watermelon as prep	1/2 cup (4.2 oz)	10	0	0	55
Watermelon as prep	1/2 cup (5 oz)	80	0	0	80
Wild Strawberry as prep	1/2 cup (5 oz)	80	0	0	120

FOOD	PORTION	CALS	FAT	CHOL	SOD
ready-to-eat					
Handi-Snacks					
Gels Blue Raspberry	1 serv (4 oz)	80	0	0	45
Gels Cherry	1 serv (4 oz)	80	0	0	45
Gels Orange	1 serv (3.5 oz)	80	0	0	45
Gels Strawberry	1 serv (3.5 oz)	80	0	0	40
Hunt's					
Snack Pack Juicy Gels Mixed Fruit	1 (4 oz)	100	0	0	42
Snack Pack Gels Cherry	1 serv (3.5 oz)	100	0	0	42
Snack Pack Gels Raspberry Berry	1 serv (3.5 oz)	100	0	0	42
Snack Pack Gels Strawberry	1 serv (3.5 oz)	100	0	0	42
Snack Pack Gels Strawberry Orange	1 serv (3.5 oz)	100	0	0	42
Jell-O					
Berry Black	1 serv (3.5 oz)	70	0	0	40
Berry Blue	1 serv (3.5 oz)	70	0	0	40
Cherry	1 serv (3.5 oz)	70	0	0	40
Orange	1 serv (3.5 oz)	70	0	0	40
Orange Strawberry Banana	1 serv (3.5 oz)	70	0	0	40
Raspberry	1 serv (3.5 oz)	70	0	0	40
Rhymin' Lymon	1 serv (3.5 oz)	70	0	0	40
Strawberry	1 serv (3.5 oz)	70	0	0	40
Strawberry Kiwi	1 serv (3.5 oz)	10	0	0	45
Sugar Free Orange	1 serv (3.2 oz)	10	0	0	45
Sugar Free Raspberry	1 serv (3.2 oz)	10	0	0	45
Sugar Free Strawberry	1 serv (3.2 oz)	10	0	0	45
Tropical Berry	1 serv (3.5 oz)	10	0	0	45
Tropical Fruit Punch	1 serv (3.5 oz)	70	0	0	40
Wild Watermelon	1 serv (3.5 oz)	70	0	0	40
Kozy Shack					
Gel Treat Cherry	1 pkg (4 oz)	100	0	0	25
Gel Treat Lemon Lime	1 pkg (4 oz)	100	0	0	25
Gel Treat Orange	1 pkg (4 oz)	100	0	0	25
Gel Treat Strawberry	1 pkg (4 oz)	100	0	0	25
Gel Treat Sugar Free Orange	1 pkg (4 oz)	10	0	0	25
Gel Treat Sugar Free Strawberry	1 pkg (4 oz)	10	0	0	25
Swiss Miss					
Gels Berry Strawberry	1 pkg (3.5 oz)	79	0	0	38
Gels Berry Lemon	1 pkg (3.5 oz)	79	0	0	38
Gels Raspberry Orange	1 pkg (3.5 oz)	79	0	0	38
Gels Strawberry Raspberry	1 pkg (3.5 oz)	79	0	0	38
GIBLETS					
capon simmered	1 cup (5 oz)	238	8	629	80
chicken floured & fried	1 cup (5 oz)	402	19	647	164
chicken simmered	1 cup (5 oz)	228	7	570	85
turkey simmered	1 cup (5 oz)	243	7	606	85

FOOD	PORTION	CALS	FAT	CHOL	SOD
GINGER					
ground	1 tsp (1.8 g)	6	tr	0	1
root fresh	5 slices	8	tr	0	1
root fresh sliced	1/4 cup	17	tr	0	3
GINKGO NUTS					
canned	1 oz	32	tr	0	87
dried	1 oz	99	tr	0	4
raw	1 oz	52	tr	0	1
GIZZARDS					
chicken simmered	1 cup (5 oz)	222	5	281	97
turkey simmered	1 cup (5 oz)	236	6	336	79
Shady Brook					
Turkey	4 oz	130	4	180	90
GOAT					
roasted	3 oz	122	3	64	73
GOOSE					
w/ skin roasted	6.6 oz	574	41	172	132
w/o skin roasted	5 oz	340	18	138	108
GOOSEBERRIES					
canned in light syrup	1/2 cup	93	tr	0	3
fresh	1 cup	67	1	0	1
GRANOLA					
(*see* CEREAL, CEREAL BARS)					
GRAPE JUICE					
Capri Sun					
Drink	1 pkg (7 oz)	100	0	0	20
Daily					
Drink	8 oz	110	0	0	30
Everfresh					
Juice	1 can (8 oz)	150	0	0	10
Juicy Juice					
Drink	1 box (8.45 oz)	140	0	0	15
Drink	1 box (4.23 oz)	70	0	0	10
Kool-Aid					
Bursts Grape Drink	1 (7 oz)	100	0	0	30
Drink as prep w/ sugar	1 serv (8 oz)	100	0	0	10
Drink Mix as prep	1 serv (8 oz)	60	0	0	0
Sugar Free Drink Mix as prep	1 serv (8 oz)	5	0	0	0
Mott's					
100% Juice	1 box (8 oz)	130	0	0	15
Grape Juice	8 oz	130	0	0	10
Nantucket Nectars					
100% Juice	8 oz	160	0	0	20
Grapeade	8 oz	130	0	0	5
Shasta Plus					
Grape Drink	1 can (11.5 oz)	160	0	0	45

FOOD	PORTION	CALS	FAT	CHOL	SOD
Veryfine					
100% Juice	1 bottle (10 oz)	200	0	0	35
Chillers Glacial Grape	1 can (11.5 oz)	160	0	0	10
Grape Drink	1 bottle (10 oz)	160	0	0	10
Juice-Ups	8 oz	130	0	0	10
Welch's					
100% White	8 oz	160	0	0	20
GRAPE LEAVES					
canned	1 (4 g)	3	tr	0	114
fresh raw	1 (3 g)	3	tr	0	tr
GRAPEFRUIT					
fresh					
pink	1/2	37	tr	0	0
pink sections	1 cup	69	tr	0	1
red	1/2	37	tr	0	0
red sections	1 cup	69	tr	0	1
white	1/2	39	tr	0	0
white sections	1 cup	76	tr	0	0
Ocean Spray					
Fresh	2 oz	50	0	0	0
GRAPEFRUIT JUICE					
Apple & Eve					
Made In The Shade	8 oz	130	0	0	35
Ruby Red					
Everfresh					
Juice	1 can (8 oz)	90	0	0	0
Ruby Red Cocktail	1 can (8 oz)	130	0	0	0
Fresh Samantha					
Juice	1 cup (8 oz)	90	0	0	0
Mott's					
100% Juice	8 oz	110	0	0	10
Nantucket Nectars					
100% Juice	8 oz	100	0	0	0
100% Ruby Red	8 oz	100	0	0	5
Ocean Spray					
100% Juice	8 oz	100	0	0	35
100% Juice Pink	8 oz	110	0	0	35
Ruby Red Drink	8 oz	130	0	0	35
Tropicana					
Golden	8 oz	90	0	0	0
Ruby Red	8 oz	90	0	0	0
Season's Best	8 oz	90	0	0	15
Twister Pink	1 bottle (10 oz)	140	0	0	20
W/ Double Vitamin C	8 oz	110	0	0	15
Veryfine					
100% Juice	1 bottle (10 oz)	110	0	0	20
Pink	1 bottle (10 oz)	150	0	0	35
Ruby Red	8 oz	120	0	0	25

FOOD	PORTION	CALS	FAT	CHOL	SOD
GRAPES					
fresh	10	36	tr	0	1
thompson seedless in heavy syrup	1/2 cup	94	tr	0	7
thompson seedless water pack	1/2 cup	48	tr	0	7
GRAVY					
(*see also* SAUCE)					
canned					
Campbell					
Beef	1/4 cup	29	1	1	421
Brown	1/4 cup	46	3	tr	350
Chicken	1/4 cup	42	2	3	244
Turkey	1/4 cup	29	1	2	289
mix					
Durkee					
Au Jus as prep	1/4 cup	5	0	0	320
Brown as prep	1/4 cup	10	1	0	250
Brown Mushroom as prep	1/4 cup	15	0	0	300
Brown Onion as prep	1/4 cup	15	0	0	290
Chicken as prep	1/4 cup	20	1	0	350
Country as prep	1/4 cup	35	2	0	370
Homestyle as prep	1/4 cup	15	1	0	240
Pork as prep	1/4 cup	10	0	0	240
Sausage as prep	1/4 cup	35	2	0	570
Swiss Steak as prep	1/4 cup	15	0	0	370
Turkey as prep	1/4 cup	20	0	0	270
French's					
Au Jus as prep	1/4 cup	5	0	0	220
Brown as prep	1/4 cup	10	1	0	250
Chicken as prep	1/4 cup	25	1	0	250
Country as prep	1/4 cup	35	2	0	370
Herb Brown as prep	1/2 cup	15	1	0	350
Homestyle as prep	1/4 cup	10	1	0	230
Mushroom as prep	1/4 cup	10	1	0	250
Onion	1/4 cup	15	1	0	260
Pork as prep	1/4 cup	10	1	0	250
Turkey as prep	1/4 cup	20	0	0	270
Loma Linda					
Quik Gravy Brown	1 tbsp (5 g)	20	0	0	370
Quik Gravy Chicken	1 tbsp (5 g)	20	0	0	410
Quik Gravy Country	1 tbsp (5 g)	25	1	0	250
Quik Gravy Mushroom	1 tbsp (5 g)	15	0	0	300
Quik Gravy Onion	1 tbsp (5 g)	20	0	0	230
McCormick					
Beef & Herb as prep	1/4 cup	30	1	<5	290

FOOD	PORTION	CALS	FAT	CHOL	SOD
GREAT NORTHERN BEANS					
canned					
Green Giant					
Great Northern	1/2 cup (4.4 oz)	100	1	0	290
dried					
cooked	1 cup	210	1	0	4
GREEN BEANS					
canned					
Green Giant					
Cut	1/2 cup (4.2 oz)	20	0	0	400
Cut 50% Less Sodium	1/2 cup (4.2 oz)	20	0	0	200
French Style	1/2 cup (4.1 oz)	20	0	0	390
Kitchen Sliced	1/2 cup (4.2 oz)	20	0	0	400
Whole	1/2 cup (4.1 oz)	25	0	0	330
fresh					
cooked	1/2 cup	22	tr	0	2
raw	1/2 cup	17	tr	0	3
frozen					
Birds Eye					
French w/ Toasted Almonds	3/4 cup (4.1 oz)	80	4	0	500
Green Giant					
Cut	3/4 cup (2.8 oz)	25	0	0	0
Harvest Fresh & Almonds	2/3 cup (2.8 oz)	60	3	0	95
Harvest Fresh Cut	2/3 cup (2.9 oz)	25	0	0	95
Stouffer's					
Green Bean Mushroom Casserole	1 serv (4 oz)	130	8	2	450
GROUPER					
cooked	3 oz	100	1	40	45
cooked	1 fillet (7.1 oz)	238	3	95	107
GUAVA					
fresh	1	45	1	0	2
guava sauce	1/2 cup	43	tr	0	4
GUAVA JUICE					
Nantucket Nectars					
Cocktail	8 oz	130	0	0	5
HADDOCK					
fresh					
cooked	3 oz	95	1	63	74
cooked	1 fillet (5.3 oz)	168	1	110	131
smoked					
smoked	1 oz	33	tr	21	214
take-out					
breaded & fried	1 piece (3.5 oz)	187	9	63	350
HALIBUT					
fresh					
atlantic & pacific cooked	1/2 fillet (5.6 oz)	223	5	65	110
atlantic & pacific cooked	3 oz	119	2	35	59

FOOD	PORTION	CALS	FAT	CHOL	SOD
greenland baked	3 oz	203	15	50	87
greenland baked	5.6 oz	380	28	94	163
HALVA					
(see SESAME)					
HAM					
(see also HAM DISHES, PORK, TURKEY)					
Alpine Lace					
Boneless Cooked 98% Fat Free	2 slices (2 oz)	60	1	25	530
Honey Ham 98% Fat Free	2 slices (2 oz)	60	1	25	530
Smoked Virginia 98% Fat Free	2 slices (2 oz)	60	1	25	400
Armour					
Chopped Ham canned	2 oz	130	11	35	880
Deviled Ham Spread	1 pkg (3 oz)	210	18	60	700
Lean Slices Brown Sugar	1 pkg (2.5 oz)	90	2	35	700
Boar's Head					
Black Forest Smoked	2 oz	60	1	30	580
Cappy	2 oz	60	2	15	530
Deluxe	2 oz	60	1	25	590
Deluxe Lowered Sodium	2 oz	50	1	20	460
Maple Glazed Honey	2 oz	60	1	20	570
Pepper	2 oz	60	1	20	610
Rosemary & Sundried Tomato	2 oz	70	3	10	590
Sweet Slice Smoked	3 oz	100	3	30	780
Virginia	2 oz	60	1	25	590
Virginia Smoked	2 oz	60	1	25	590
Carl Buddig					
Ham Sliced w/ Natural Juices	1 pkg (2.5 oz)	120	7	40	980
Honey Ham Sliced w/ Natural Juice	1 pkg (2.5 oz)	120	7	40	760
Lean Slices Oven Roasted Honey Ham	1 pkg (2.5 oz)	90	2	35	850
Lean Slices Smoked	1 pkg (2.5 oz)	80	2	35	850
Hormel					
Black Label Canned (refrigerated)	3 oz	100	5	40	1020
Black Label Canned (self stable)	3 oz	110	5	45	970
Cure 81 Half Ham	3 oz	100	5	45	890
Curemaster	3 oz	80	3	40	940
Deviled Ham	4 tbsp (2 oz)	150	12	40	430
Ham & Cheese Patties	1 patty (2 oz)	190	17	45	470
Ham Patties	1 (2 oz)	180	17	35	550
Light & Lean 97 Sliced	1 slice (1 oz)	25	1	15	340
Primissimo Proscuitti	2 oz	120	7	50	1080
Spiral Cure 81	3 oz	150	9	50	1090

FOOD	PORTION	CALS	FAT	CHOL	SOD
Jordan's					
Healthy Trim 97% Fat Free Cooked	1 slice (1 oz)	30	1	10	180
Healthy Trim 97% Fat Free EZ Serve	1 slice (1 oz)	30	1	15	180
Healthy Trim 97% Fat Free Virginia	1 slice (1 oz)	30	1	15	180
Louis Rich					
Carving Board Baked	2 slices (1.6 oz)	50	2	25	550
Carving Board Honey Glazed Thin	6 slices (2.1 oz)	70	2	30	750
Carving Board Honey Glazed Traditional	2 slices (1.6 oz)	50	2	25	560
Carving Board Smoked	1 slice (1.6 oz)	45	2	20	570
Dinner Slices Baked	1 slice (3.3 oz)	80	2	40	1150
Oscar Mayer					
Baked	3 slices (2.2 oz)	70	3	30	790
Boiled	3 slices (2.2 oz)	60	3	30	820
Chopped	1 slice (1 oz)	50	3	15	340
Dinner Slice	3 oz	80	3	40	1010
Dinner Steaks	1 (2 oz)	60	2	30	750
Free Baked	3 slices (1.6 oz)	35	0	15	520
Free Honey	3 slices (1.6 oz)	35	0	15	580
Free Smoked	3 slices (1.6 oz)	35	0	15	550
Honey	3 slices (2.2 oz)	70	3	30	760
Lower Sodium	3 slices (2.2 oz)	70	3	30	520
Smoked	3 slices (2.2 oz)	60	3	30	760
Spam					
Spread	4 tbsp (2 oz)	140	12	40	570
Wampler					
Black Forest	2 oz	60	2	25	650

HAM SUBSTITUTES

FOOD	PORTION	CALS	FAT	CHOL	SOD
Yves					
Veggie Ham Deli Slices	1 serv (2.2 oz)	80	0	0	480

HAMBURGER

(*see* BEEF, HAMBURGER SUBSTITUTES, MEAT SUBSTITUTES)

HAMBURGER SUBSTITUTES

(*see also* MEAT SUBSTITUTES)

FOOD	PORTION	CALS	FAT	CHOL	SOD
Amy's Organic					
Veggie Burger California	1 (2.5 oz)	100	3	0	290
Veggie Burger Chicago	1 (2.5 oz)	100	4	5	190
Veggie Burger Texas	1 (2.5 oz)	130	3	0	270
Boca Burgers					
Hint of Garlic	1 patty (2.5 oz)	110	2	3	296
Vegan Original	1 patty (2.5 oz)	84	0	0	269
Franklin Farms					
Veggiburger Portabella	1 (3 oz)	120	2	0	460

FOOD	PORTION	CALS	FAT	CHOL	SOD
GardenVegan					
Fat-Free Patty	1 patty (2.5 oz)	140	0	0	250
Gardenburger					
Classic Greek	1 (2.5 oz)	120	3	10	310
Fire Roasted Vegetable	1 (2.5 oz)	120	3	10	270
Hamburger Style	1 (2.5 oz)	90	0	0	370
Hamburger Style w/ Cheese	1 (2.5 oz)	110	3	5	380
Savory Mushroom	1 (2.5 oz)	120	3	10	270
Green Giant					
Southwestern Style	1 patty (3.2 oz)	140	4	0	370
Lightlife					
Barbecue Grilles	1 patty (2.7 oz)	120	4	0	180
Lemon Grilles	1 patty (2.7 oz)	140	6	0	280
Light Burgers	1 (3 oz)	130	1	0	410
Tamari Grilles	1 patty (2.7 oz)	120	5	0	260
Loma Linda					
Patty Mix not prep	1/3 cup (0.9 oz)	90	1	0	480
Redi-Burger	5/8 in slice (3 oz)	120	3	0	450
Vege-Burger	1/4 cup (1.9 oz)	70	2	0	115
Morningstar Farms					
Better'n Burger	1 (2.7 oz)	80	0	0	360
Garden Grille	1 patty (2.5 oz)	120	3	<5	280
Garden Veggie Patties	1 patty (2.4 oz)	100	3	0	350
Hard Rock Cafe Veggie Burger	1 (3 oz)	170	8	0	340
Harvest Burger Italian Style	1 patty (3.2 oz)	140	5	0	370
Harvest Burger Original	1 (3.2 oz)	140	4	0	370
Harvest Burger Southwestern	1 (3.2 oz)	140	4	0	370
Spicy Black Bean Burger	1 (2.7 oz)	110	1	0	470
Natural Touch					
Garden Veggie Pattie	1 (2.4 oz)	110	3	0	280
Okara Pattie	1 (2.2 oz)	110	5	0	360
Original Veggie Burger Kit not prep	1/4 pkg (0.8 oz)	80	0	0	360
Southwestern Veggie Burger Kit not prep	1/4 pkg (0.9 oz)	90	0	0	360
Spicy Black Bean Burger	1 (2.7 oz)	100	1	0	330
Vegan Burger	1 (2.7 oz)	70	0	0	370
NewMenu					
VegiBurger	1 patty (3 oz)	110	1	0	320
Quorn					
Burger	1 patty (3 oz)	100	4	0	420
Superburgers					
Vegan Organic Original	1 (3 oz)	98	2	0	350
Vegan Organic Smoked	1 (3 oz)	98	2	0	350
Vegan Organic TexMex	1 (3 oz)	110	1	0	195

FOOD	PORTION	CALS	FAT	CHOL	SOD
V'dora					
Vegetable BurgerLites	1 (3.3 oz)	58	0	0	98
Veggie Patch					
Burgeriffics	1 (2.5 oz)	110	3	0	410
Worthington					
Granburger not prep	3 tbsp (0.6 oz)	60	1	0	410
Prosage Patties	1 (1.3 oz)	80	3	0	300
Vegetarian Burger	1/4 cup (1.9 oz)	60	2	0	270
Yves					
Black Bean & Mushroom Burgers	1 (3 oz)	100	0	0	450
Garden Vegetable Patties	1 (3 oz)	90	0	0	470
Veggie Burger	1 (3 oz)	119	2	0	480
HAZELNUTS					
dry roasted	1 oz	188	19	0	1
oil roasted	1 oz	187	18	0	1
HEART					
beef simmered	3 oz	148	5	164	54
chicken simmered	1 cup (5 oz)	268	11	350	69
lamb braised	3 oz	158	7	212	54
pork braised	1	191	7	285	45
pork braised	1 cup	215	7	320	51
turkey simmered	1 cup (5 oz)	257	9	327	79
veal braised	3 oz	158	6	150	50
HEARTS OF PALM					
canned	1 cup (5.1 oz)	41	1	0	622
canned	1 (1.2 oz)	9	tr	0	141
HEMP					
HempNut					
Shelled Hempseed	1 oz	162	13	0	3
Nutiva					
Hempseed	1 1/2 tbsp (0.5 oz)	70	5	0	0
HERBAL TEA					
(*see* TEA/HERBAL TEA)					
HERBS/SPICES					
(*see also individual names*)					
curry powder	1 tsp	6	tr	0	1
poultry seasoning	1 tsp	5	tr	0	tr
pumpkin pie spice	1 tsp	6	tr	0	1
Chi-Chi's					
Seasoning Mix	1 tsp (3 g)	10	0	0	290
Mrs. Dash					
Extra Spicy	1/8 tsp (0.02 oz)	2	0	0	1
Garlic & Herb	1/8 tsp (0.02 oz)	2	tr	tr	tr
Lemon & Herb	1/8 tsp (0.02 oz)	2	0	0	1
Low Pepper No Garlic	1/8 tsp (0.02 oz)	2	0	0	tr
Original Blend	1/8 tsp (0.02 oz)	2	0	0	1
Table Blend	1/8 tsp (0.02 oz)	2	0	0	1

FOOD	PORTION	CALS	FAT	CHOL	SOD
HERRING					
atlantic cooked	3 oz	172	10	65	98
pacific baked	3 oz	213	15	84	81
smoked	3.5 oz	210	14	70	550
take-out					
atlantic kippered	1 fillet (1.4 oz)	87	5	33	367
atlantic pickled	1/2 oz	39	3	2	131
fried	1 serv (3.5 oz)	233	15	69	100
HICKORY NUTS					
dried	1 oz	187	18	0	0
HOMINY					
canned					
Van Camp					
Golden	1/2 cup (4.3 oz)	80	1	0	540
White	1/2 cup (4.3 oz)	80	1	0	530
HONEY					
honey	1 tbsp (0.7 oz)	64	0	0	1
honey	1 cup (11.9 oz)	1031	0	0	12
HONEYDEW					
fresh					
cubed	1 cup	60	tr	0	17
wedge	1/10	46	tr	0	13
HORSE					
roasted	3 oz	149	5	58	47
HORSERADISH					
Boar's Head					
Horseradish	1 tsp (5 g)	5	0	0	30
Kraft					
Cream Style	1 tsp (5 g)	0	0	0	50
Horseradish Sauce	1 tsp (5 g)	20	2	<5	35
Prepared	1 tsp (5 g)	0	0	0	50
HOTCAKES					
(*see* PANCAKES)					
HOT COCOA					
(*see* COCOA)					
HOT DOG					
(*see also* MEAT SUBSTITUTES, SAUSAGE, SAUSAGE SUBSTITUTES)					
Applegate Farms					
Chicken Natural Uncured	1 (1.5 oz)	120	5	40	450
Natural Turkey	1 (1.5 oz)	120	5	40	450
Armour					
Star Jumbo Beef	1	190	18	30	590
Boar's Head					
Beef	1 (2 oz)	160	14	30	440
Beef Lite	1 (1.6 oz)	90	6	25	270
Pork & Beef	1 (2 oz)	150	14	25	460
Health Is Wealth					
Uncured Beef	1 (1.5 oz)	80	6	20	340

FOOD	PORTION	CALS	FAT	CHOL	SOD
Health Is Wealth (cont.)					
Uncured Chicken	1 (1.5 oz)	100	8	30	320
Healthy Choice					
Beef Low Fat	1 (1.8 oz)	70	3	15	440
Low Fat Turkey Pork Beef	1 (1.4 oz)	60	2	10	350
Hormel					
Fat Free	1 (1.8 oz)	45	0	15	580
Fat Free Beef	1 (1.8 oz)	45	0	10	590
Jordan's					
Healthy Trim Low Fat	1 (1.8 oz)	70	3	25	350
Healthy Trim Low Fat Skinless	1 (1.8 oz)	70	3	25	350
Louis Rich					
Bun Length	1 (2 oz)	110	8	55	650
Cheese	1 (1.6 oz)	90	6	40	480
Franks	1 (1.6 oz)	80	6	40	510
Organic Vallely					
All-Natural Beef	1 (1.6 oz)	90	6	25	310
Oscar Mayer					
Beef	1 (1.6 oz)	140	13	30	460
Big & Juicy Franks Deli Style	1 (2.7 oz)	230	22	50	680
Big & Juicy Franks Original	1 (2.7 oz)	240	22	45	700
Big & Juicy Franks Quarter Pound	1 (4 oz)	350	32	65	1050
Big & Juicy Wieners Hot 'N Spicy	1 (2.7 oz)	220	20	45	750
Big & Juicy Wieners Smokie Links	1 (2.7 oz)	220	19	50	770
Big & Juicy Wieners Original	1 (2.7 oz)	240	22	45	690
Bun-Length Beef	1 (2 oz)	180	17	35	580
Cheese	1 (1.6 oz)	140	13	35	510
Fat Free Beef	1 (1.8 oz)	40	0	15	460
Fat Free Turkey & Beef	1 (1.8 oz)	40	0	15	490
Jumbo Beef	1 (2 oz)	180	17	35	580
Light Beef	1 (2 oz)	110	8	30	620
Wieners	1 (1.6 oz)	150	13	35	430
Wieners Bun-Length	1 (2 oz)	190	17	40	550
Wieners Jumbo	1 (2 oz)	180	17	40	550
Wieners Light	1 (2 oz)	110	8	35	590
Wieners Little	6 (2 oz)	180	17	35	570
Wampler					
Chicken	1 (2 oz)	120	11	60	480
take-out					
corndog	1	460	19	79	972
w/ bun chili	1	297	13	51	480
w/ bun plain	1	242	15	44	671

FOOD	PORTION	CALS	FAT	CHOL	SOD
HOT DOG SUBSTITUTES					
Lightlife					
Smart Deli Jumbo's	1 link (2.7 oz)	80	0	0	590
Smart Dogs	1 (1.5 oz)	45	0	0	230
Tofu Pups	1 (1.4 oz)	60	3	0	140
Wonder Dogs	1 (1.5 oz)	60	2	0	320
Loma Linda					
Big Franks	1 (1.8 oz)	110	7	0	240
Big Franks Low Fat	1 (1.8 oz)	80	3	0	220
Corn Dogs	1 (2.5 oz)	150	4	0	500
Morningstar Farms					
America's Original Veggie Dog	1 (2 oz)	80	1	0	580
Meatfree Corn Dog	1 (2.5 oz)	150	4	0	500
Meatfree Mini Corn Dog	4 (2.7 oz)	170	5	0	580
Natural Touch					
Vege Frank	1 (1.6 oz)	100	6	0	470
NewMenu					
VegiDogs	1 (1.5 oz)	45	0	0	170
Veggie Patch					
Perfectly Franks	1 (1.7 oz)	70	2	0	340
Worthington					
Veja Links Low Fat	1 (1.1 oz)	40	2	0	190
Yves					
Good Dog	1 (1.8 oz)	70	2	0	460
Tofu Dogs	1 (1.3 oz)	45	1	0	240
Veggie Dogs	1 (1.6 oz)	60	0	0	400
Veggie Dogs Chili	1 (1.6 oz)	50	0	0	360
Veggie Dogs Jumbo	1 (2.7 oz)	100	2	0	480
Veggie Dogs Jumbo Hot N' Spicy	1 (2.7 oz)	106	2	0	480
HUMMUS					
Athenos					
Roasted Red Pepper	2 tbsp (1.1 oz)	60	4	0	210
take-out					
hummus	1/3 cup	140	7	0	200
HYACINTH BEANS					
dried cooked	1 cup	228	1	0	13
ICE CREAM AND FROZEN DESSERTS					
(*see also* ICES AND ICE POPS, PUDDING POPS, SHERBET, YOGURT FROZEN)					
dixie cup chocolate	1 (3.5 fl oz)	125	6	20	44
dixie cup strawberry	1 (3.5 fl oz)	112	5	17	35
dixie cup vanilla	1 (3.5 fl oz)	116	6	25	46
freeze dried ice cream chocolate strawberry & vanilla	1 pkg (0.75 oz)	158	5	1	97
Ben & Jerry's					
Bovinity Divinity	1/2 cup	290	18	40	65
Butter Pecan	1/2 cup	330	25	65	140

FOOD	PORTION	CALS	FAT	CHOL	SOD
Ben & Jerry's (cont.)					
Cherry Garcia	1/2 cup	260	16	70	60
Chocolate Chip Cookie Dough	1/2 cup	300	16	65	95
Chocolate Fudge Brownie	1/2 cup	280	15	45	90
Chubby Hubby	1/2 cup	350	21	55	250
Chunky Monkey	1/2 cup	310	19	55	55
Coconut Almond Fudge Chip	1/2 cup	310	22	40	70
Coffee Heath Bar Crunch	1/2 cup	310	18	65	125
Dilbert's World Totally Nuts	1/2 cup	310	21	45	105
Low Fat Blackberry Cobbler	1/2 cup	180	3	20	70
Low Fat Coconut Cream Pie	1/2 cup	160	3	15	75
Low Fat Mocha Latte	1/2 cup	150	2	10	70
Low Fat S'mores	1/2 cup	190	2	15	85
Mint Chocolate Cookie	1/2 cup	280	17	70	130
New York Super Fudge Chunk	1/2 cup	320	21	50	65
No Fat Chocolate Comfort	1/2 cup	150	2	10	85
Orange & Cream	1/2 cup	230	14	40	50
Peanut Butter Cup	1/2 cup	380	25	65	130
Phish Food	1/2 cup	300	14	35	80
Phish Stick	1	330	20	25	85
Pistachio Pistachio	1/2 cup	240	15	50	20
Pop Cookie Dough	1	420	25	55	130
Pop Totally Nuts	1	370	29	30	115
Pop Vanilla	1	330	23	75	55
Pop Vanilla Heath Bar Crunch	1	330	22	65	105
S'mores Bar	1	350	18	25	130
Vanilla World's Best	1/2 cup	250	16	75	60
Vanilla Caramel Fudge	1/2 cup	300	17	70	115
Vanilla Heath Bar Crunch	1/2 cup	310	19	70	135
Wavy Gravy	1/2 cup	340	20	60	120
Bon Bons					
Dark Chocolate	5 pieces	190	13	15	35
Milk Chocolate	5 pieces	200	14	10	35
Breyers					
Butter Pecan	1/2 cup (2.4 oz)	180	12	35	115
Caramel Praline Crunch	1/2 cup (2.6 oz)	180	9	30	30
Cherry Vanilla	1/2 cup (2.4 oz)	150	8	30	30
Chocolate	1/2 cup (2.4 oz)	160	9	30	20
Chocolate Chip	1/2 cup (2.4 oz)	170	10	35	35
Chocolate Chip Cookie Dough	1/2 cup (2.5 oz)	180	10	35	50
Chocolate Rainbow	1/2 cup (2.4 oz)	120	10	25	40
Coffee	1/2 cup (2.4 oz)	150	9	35	35
Cookies N Cream	1/2 cup (2.4 oz)	170	9	30	45
Creamsicle	1/2 cup (2.8 oz)	130	4	15	30
Double Chocolate Fudge	1/2 cup (2.6 oz)	150	9	40	50
Fat Free Caramel Praline	1/2 cup (2.5 oz)	120	0	<5	90
Fat Free Chocolate	1/2 cup (2.4 oz)	90	0	0	55

FOOD	PORTION	CALS	FAT	CHOL	SOD
Fat Free Mint Cookies N Cream	1/2 cup (2.4 oz)	100	0	<5	75
Fat Free Strawberry	1/2 cup (2.4 oz)	90	0	0	50
Fat Free Take Two Vanilla Strawberry	1/2 cup (2.4 oz)	80	0	<5	55
Fat Free Vanilla	1/2 cup (2.4 oz)	90	0	0	65
Fat Free Vanilla Chocolate Strawberry	1/2 cup (2.4 oz)	90	0	0	55
Fat Free Vanilla Fudge Twirl	1/2 cup (2.5 oz)	100	0	0	65
French Vanilla	1/2 cup (2.4 oz)	160	10	105	40
Fruit Rainbow	1/2 cup (2.4 oz)	140	8	30	35
Hershey w/ Almonds	1/2 cup (2.7 oz)	190	8	25	20
Light Butter Pecan	1/2 cup (2.3 oz)	120	4	<5	130
Light Caramel Praline Pecan	1/2 cup (3 oz)	180	5	15	90
Light French Chocolate	1/2 cup (2.4 oz)	150	5	30	55
Light Mint Chocolate Chip	1/2 cup (2.4 oz)	140	5	10	50
Light Vanilla	1/2 cup (2.4 oz)	130	5	35	45
Light Vanilla Chocolate Strawberry	1/2 cup (2.4 oz)	120	3	10	50
Light Low Fat Brown Marble Fudge	1/2 cup (2.6 oz)	130	2	5	65
Light Low Fat French Vanilla	1/2 cup (2.3 oz)	110	2	30	45
Light Low Fat Swiss Almond Fudge	1/2 cup (2.5 oz)	130	3	5	60
Low Fat Butter Pecan	1/2 cup (2.6 oz)	150	7	15	125
Low Fat Vanilla	1/2 cup (2.6 oz)	120	3	15	40
Low Fat Vanilla Chocolate Strawberry	1/2 cup (2.6 oz)	120	3	10	40
Mint Chocolate Chip	1/2 cup (2.4 oz)	170	10	35	35
No Sugar Added Fudge Twirl	1/2 cup (2.6 oz)	100	5	25	55
No Sugar Added Mint Chocolate Chip	1/2 cup (2.4 oz)	100	5	25	50
No Sugar Added Vanilla	1/2 cup (2.4 oz)	90	5	25	50
No Sugar Added Vanilla Chocolate Strawberry	1/2 cup (2.4 oz)	90	5	25	45
Peach	1/2 cup (2.4 oz)	130	6	25	25
Peanut Butter Cup	1/2 cup (2.7 oz)	210	12	30	90
Rocky Road	1/2 cup (2.5 oz)	180	9	25	25
Soft'N Creamy Vanilla	1/2 cup (2.3 oz)	150	7	30	35
Soft'N Creamy Vanilla Chocolate Strawberry	1/2 cup (2.3 oz)	150	7	30	35
Strawberry	1/2 cup (2.4 oz)	130	7	30	30
Take Two Vanilla Chocolate	1/2 cup (2.5 oz)	160	9	35	35
Take Two Vanilla Orange Sherbet	1/2 cup (2.7 oz)	130	5	20	30
Vanilla	1/2 cup (2.4 oz)	150	9	35	35
Vanilla Chocolate Strawberry	1/2 cup (2.4 oz)	150	8	30	30

FOOD	PORTION	CALS	FAT	CHOL	SOD
Breyer's (cont.)					
Vanilla Fudge Twirl	1/2 cup (2.6 oz)	160	8	35	35
Viennetta Cappuccino	1/2 cup (2.4 oz)	190	11	35	35
Viennetta Chocolate	1/2 cup (2.4 oz)	190	12	25	40
Viennetta Vanilla	1/2 cup (2.4 oz)	190	11	40	40
Butterfinger					
Bar	1 (2.5 oz)	190	13	15	35
California Joe					
Soft Serve Chocolate	1/2 cup (2.5 oz)	72	0	0	60
Soft Serve Vanilla	1/2 cup (2.5 oz)	70	0	0	60
Carnation					
Cup Chocolate	1 (3 oz)	140	8	25	40
Cup Chocolate Malt	1 (12 oz)	270	6	20	130
Cup Strawberry	1 (3 oz)	100	5	20	25
Cup Vanilla	1 (3 oz)	100	6	20	30
Cup Vanilla	1 (5 oz)	170	10	35	5
Cup Vanilla Malt	1 (12 oz)	260	6	20	130
Sundae Cup Strawberry	1 (5 oz)	200	8	30	55
Sundae Cup Chocolate	1 (5 oz)	210	9	30	55
Cool Creations					
Cookies & Cream Sandwich	1 (3.5 oz)	240	11	15	250
Mickey Mouse Bar	1 (2.5 oz)	120	8	15	25
Mini Sandwich	1 (2.3 oz)	110	5	10	70
Dippin' Dots					
Dipping Dots Chocolate	5/8 cup (3 oz)	190	9	40	70
Drumstick					
Cone Chocolate	1 (4.6 oz)	320	17	25	90
Cone Chocolate Dipped	1 (4.6 oz)	320	16	25	90
Cone Vanilla	1 (4.6 oz)	340	19	20	90
Cone Vanilla Caramel	1 (4.6 oz)	360	20	25	100
Cone Vanilla Fudge	1 (4.6 oz)	360	20	20	100
Flintstones					
Cool Cream	1 (2.75 oz)	90	2	5	30
Push-Up Pebbles Treats	1 (2.75 oz)	120	6	20	25
Klondike					
Oreo Ice Cream Cookie Sandwich	1 (2.6 oz)	240	10	15	310
Original	1 (3.3 oz)	290	19	30	85
Nestle Crunch					
Chocolate	1 bar (3 oz)	200	14	15	40
Crunch King	1 (4 oz)	270	19	20	45
Nuggets	8 pieces	310	21	20	60
Reduced Fat	1 (2.5 oz)	130	7	5	40
Vanilla	1 bar (3 oz)	200	14	15	40
NutraShake					
High Calorie High Protein All Flavors	1 serv (4 oz)	200	10	60	217

FOOD	PORTION	CALS	FAT	CHOL	SOD
Perry's					
No Fat No Sugar Added Caramel	1/2 cup (2.8 oz)	90	0	0	90
No Fat No Sugar Added Chocolate	1/2 cup (2.6 oz)	80	0	0	80
No Fat No Sugar Added Peach	1/2 cup (2.9 oz)	90	0	0	70
No Fat No Sugar Added Strawberry	1/2 cup (2.8 oz)	90	0	0	75
No Fat No Sugar Added Vanilla	1/2 cup (2.6 oz)	80	0	0	80
Rice Dream					
Cappuccino	1/2 cup (3.2 oz)	150	6	0	100
Carob	1/2 cup (3.2 oz)	150	6	0	100
Carob Almong	1/2 cup (3.2 oz)	170	8	0	95
Cherry Vanilla	1/2 cup (3.2 oz)	150	6	0	90
Cocoa Marble Fudge	1/2 cup (3.2 oz)	150	6	0	100
Cookies N' Dream	1/2 cup (3.2 oz)	170	7	0	100
Mint Chocolate Chip	1/2 cup (3.2 oz)	170	8	0	95
Neapolitan	1/2 cup (3.2 oz)	150	6	0	100
Orange Vanilla Swirl	1/2 cup (3.2 oz)	250	6	0	100
Strawberry	1/2 cup (3.2 oz)	140	5	0	85
Vanilla Swiss Almond	1/2 cup (3.2 oz)	180	8	0	95
Rice Dream Supreme					
Cappuccino Almond Fudge	1/2 cup (3.2 oz)	170	8	0	95
Cherry Chocolate Chunk	1/2 cup (3.2 oz)	170	7	0	85
Chocolate Almond Chunk	1/2 cup (3.2 oz)	170	8	0	95
Chocolate Fudge Brownie	1/2 cup (3.2 oz)	170	7	0	95
Double Espresso Bean	1/2 cup (3.2 oz)	160	7	0	100
Mint Chocolate Cookie	1/2 cup (3.2 oz)	170	8	0	100
Peanut Butter Cup	1/2 cup (3.2 oz)	180	8	0	105
Pralines N' Dream	1/2 cup (3.2 oz)	180	9	0	95
Starbucks					
Biscotti Bliss	1/2 cup	240	12	55	70
Caffe Almond Fudge	1/2 cup	260	13	55	80
Caffe Almond Roast	1 bar	280	18	3	45
Dark Roast Expresso Swirl	1/2 cup	220	10	55	60
Frappuccino	1 bar (2.8 oz)	110	2	10	45
Italian Roast Coffee	1/2 cup	230	12	65	50
Javachip	1/2 cup	250	13	60	55
Low Fat Latte	1/2 cup	170	3	10	65
Low Fat Mocha Mambo	1/2 cup	170	3	10	75
Vanilla Mochachip	1/2 cup	270	16	75	60
Tofutti					
Cuties Chocolate	1 (1.4 oz)	130	5	0	110
Cuties Vanilla	1 (1.4 oz)	121	5	0	121
Monkey Bars Peanut Butter	1 bar (2.5 oz)	220	13	0	105

FOOD	PORTION	CALS	FAT	CHOL	SOD
Weight Watchers					
Chocolate Chip Cookie Dough Sundae	1 (2.64 oz)	190	5	5	120
Chocolate Mousse	1 bar	40	1	5	20
Chocolate Treat	1 bar	100	1	0	25
English Toffee Crunch	1 bar	110	6	5	30
Orange Vanilla Treat	1 bar	40	1	5	15
Vanilla Sandwich	1 bar	150	3	5	150
take-out					
cone vanilla light soft serve	1 (4.6 oz)	164	6	28	92
gelato chocolate hazelnut	1/2 cup (5.3 oz)	370	29	92	49
gelato vanilla	1/2 cup (3 oz)	211	15	151	78
ICE CREAM CONES AND CUPS					
sugar cone	1	40	tr	0	32
wafer cone	1	17	tr	0	6
Frookie					
Chocolate Crunch	1 (0.4 oz)	50	1	0	10
Honey Crunch	1 (0.4 oz)	45	1	0	20
Keebler					
Chocolatey Cone	1 (0.4 oz)	50	1	0	40
Fudge Dipped Cup	1 (0.3 oz)	35	2	0	20
Ice Creme Cup	1 (0.2 oz)	15	0	0	20
Sugar Cone	1 (0.4 oz)	50	1	0	15
Waffle Bowl	1 (0.4 oz)	50	1	0	25
Waffle Cone	1 (0.4 oz)	50	1	0	25
ICE CREAM TOPPINGS					
(*see also* SYRUP)					
marshmallow cream	1 oz	88	tr	0	13
marshmallow cream	1 jar (7 oz)	615	tr	0	90
pineapple	2 tbsp (1.5 oz)	106	0	0	26
strawberry	2 tbsp (1.5 oz)	107	tr	0	9
Ben & Jerry's					
Hot Fudge	(1.3 oz)	140	7	10	25
Hershey					
Chocolate Shoppe Double Chocolate	1 tbsp (0.7 oz)	50	0	0	15
Chocolate Shoppe Apple Pie A La Mode	2 tbsp (1.3 oz)	100	0	0	90
Chocolate Shoppe Butterscotch Caramel	1 tbsp (0.7 oz)	70	1	<5	75
Chocolate Shoppe Caramel	2 tbsp (1.3 oz)	100	0	0	95
Chocolate Shoppe Chocolate Mini	1 tbsp (0.7 oz)	50	0	0	15
Chocolate Shoppe Double Chocolate	1 tbsp (0.6 oz)	60	1	0	30
Chocolate Shoppe Hot Fudge	1 tbsp (0.7 oz)	70	3	<5	80
Chocolate Shoppe Hot Fudge Fat Free	2 tbsp (1.4 oz)	100	0	0	135

FOOD	PORTION	CALS	FAT	CHOL	SOD
Chocolate Shoppe Sprinkles Milk Chocolate	1 tbsp (0.5 oz)	70	3	<5	10
Chocolate Shoppe Sprinkles Reeses	1 tbsp (0.5 oz)	70	4	0	25
Chocolate Shoppe Sprinkles York	1 tbsp (0.6 oz)	80	4	0	0
Kraft					
Butterscotch	2 tbsp (1.4 oz)	130	2	<5	150
Caramel	2 tbsp (1.4 oz)	120	0	0	90
Chocolate	2 tbsp (1.4 oz)	110	0	0	30
Hot Fudge	2 tbsp (1.4 oz)	140	5	0	100
Pineapple	2 tbsp (1.4 oz)	110	0	0	15
Strawberry	2 tbsp (1.4 oz)	110	0	0	15

ICED TEA

(*see also* ENERGY DRINKS, TEA/HERBAL TEA)

mix

FOOD	PORTION	CALS	FAT	CHOL	SOD
Crystal Light					
Decaffeinated as prep	1 serv (8 oz)	5	0	0	0
Iced Tea as prep	1 serv (8 oz)	5	0	0	0
Peach Tea as prep	1 serv (8 oz)	5	0	0	0
Raspberry Tea as prep	1 serv (8 oz)	5	0	0	0
Lipton					
100% Tea Decaffeinated as prep	1 serv	0	0	0	0
100% Tea Unsweetened as prep	1 serv	0	0	0	0
100% Tea as prep	1 serv	0	0	0	0
Calorie Free as prep	1 serv	0	0	0	0
Decaffeinated Ice Tea Brew as prep	1 serv (8 oz)	0	0	0	0
Decaffeinated Lemon as prep	1 serv	90	0	0	0
Diet Decaffeinated Lemon as prep	1 serv	5	0	0	0
Diet Lemon as prep	1 serv	5	0	0	0
Diet Peach as prep	1 serv	5	0	0	0
Diet Raspberry as prep	1 serv	5	0	0	0
Diet Tea & Lemonade as prep	1 serv	10	0	0	5
Herbal Iced Collection	1 tea bag	0	0	0	0
Ice Tea Brew as prep	1 serv (8 oz)	0	0	0	0
Lemon as prep	1 serv	90	0	0	0
Lemon as prep	1 pkg (0.5 oz)	50	0	0	0
Natural Brew 100% Tea Decaffeinated as prep	1 serv	0	0	0	0
Natural Brew 100% Tea as prep	1 serv	0	0	0	0
Natural Brew Diet Lemon as prep	1 serv	5	0	0	0

FOOD	PORTION	CALS	FAT	CHOL	SOD
Lipton (cont.)					
Natural Brew Diet Peach as prep	1 serv	5	0	0	0
Natural Brew Diet Tropical as prep	1 serv	5	0	0	0
Natural Brew Tropical as prep	1 serv	90	0	0	0
Natural Brew Unsweetened Lemon as prep	1 serv	0	0	0	0
Peach as prep	1 serv	90	0	0	0
Rasberry as prep	1 serv	90	0	0	0
Tea & Lemonade as prep	1 serv	90	0	0	0
Nestea					
100% Tea	2 tsp (1 g)	0	0	0	0
100% Tea Decafe	2 tsp (1 g)	0	0	0	0
Ice Teasers Lemon	1 serv (0.5 oz)	5	0	0	0
Ice Teasers Orange	1 serv (0.5 oz)	5	0	0	0
Ice Teasers Wild Cherry	1 serv (0.5 oz)	5	0	0	0
Lemon	2 tsp (1 g)	5	0	0	0
Lemon & Sugar	2 tbsp (0.7 oz)	80	0	0	0
Lemonade Tea	2 tbsp (0.7 oz)	80	0	0	0
Sugar Free	2 tbsp (0.7 oz)	5	0	0	0
Sugar Free Decafe	1 tbsp (0.7 oz)	5	0	0	0
Sun Tea	1 tsp (1 g)	0	0	0	0
ready-to-drink					
Arizona					
Lemon	1 bottle (16 oz)	180	0	0	40
Crystal Light					
Lemon	1 serv (8 oz)	5	0	0	40
Peach Tea	1 serv (8 oz)	5	0	0	40
Raspberry Tea	1 serv (8 oz)	5	0	0	40
Lipton					
Carribean Cooler	1 can (12 oz)	130	0	0	75
Diet Lemon	8 oz	0	0	0	10
Diet Lemon	1 bottle (16 oz)	10	0	0	10
Green Tea & Passion Fruit	1 bottle (16 oz)	160	0	0	10
Lemon	1 can (12 oz)	120	0	0	75
Lemon	8 oz	80	0	0	15
Lemon	1 bottle (16 oz)	180	0	0	10
Natural Lemon	1 box (8 oz)	100	0	0	10
Peach	8 oz	80	0	0	15
Peach	1 bottle (16 oz)	220	0	0	10
Raspberry	8 oz	80	0	0	15
Raspberry	1 bottle (16 oz)	220	0	0	10
Raspberry Blast	1 can (12 oz)	130	0	0	75
Southern Style Extra Sweet No Lemon	1 bottle (16 oz)	240	0	0	10
Southern Style Lemon	1 bottle (16 oz)	200	0	0	10

FOOD	PORTION	CALS	FAT	CHOL	SOD
Southern Style Sweetened No Lemon	1 bottle (16 oz)	200	0	0	10
Sweet	8 oz	80	0	0	15
Sweetened No Lemon	1 bottle (16 oz)	140	0	0	10
Sweetened Lemon	8 oz	80	0	0	15
Tangerine Twist	1 can (12 oz)	120	0	0	75
Tea & Lemonade	1 bottle (16 oz)	220	0	0	10
Unsweetened No Lemon	1 bottle (16 oz)	0	0	0	10
Mad River					
Red Tea w/ Guarana	8 oz	90	0	0	10
Nantucket Nectars					
Diet	8 oz	5	0	0	25
Diet Green Tea	8 oz	5	0	0	5
Half & Half	8 oz	90	0	0	0
Iced Tea	8 oz	80	0	0	0
Matt Fee	8 oz	80	0	0	0
Raspberry	8 oz	90	0	0	20
Savannah	8 oz	80	0	0	0
Snapple					
Diet Lemon	8 oz	0	0	0	10
Diet Peach	8 oz	0	0	0	10
Diet Raspberry	8 oz	0	0	0	10
Ginseng Tea	8 oz	80	0	0	10
Green Tea w/ Lemon	8 oz	100	0	0	10
Lemon	8 oz	100	0	0	10
Lemonade Ice Tea	8 oz	110	0	0	10
Peach	8 oz	100	0	0	10
Raspberry	8 oz	100	0	0	10
ICES AND ICE POPS					
(*see also* ICE CREAM AND FROZEN DESSERTS, PUDDING POPS, SHERBET, YOGURT FROZEN)					
Ben & Jerry's					
Sorbet Devil's Food Chocolate	1/2 cup	170	3	0	60
Sorbet Doonesberry	1/2 cup	140	0	0	15
Sorbet Lemon Swirl	1/2 cup	120	0	0	15
Sorbet Purple Passion Fruit	1/2 cup	140	0	0	25
Carnation					
Cup Orange Sherbet	1 (5 oz)	150	2	5	30
Cup Orange Sherbet	1 (3 oz)	90	1	5	20
Cold Fusion					
Protein Juice Bar All Flavors	1 bar (3.8 oz)	130	0	0	0
Cool Creations					
Ice Pop	1 pop (2 oz)	50	0	0	5
Mickey Mouse Bar	1 (4 oz)	170	11	15	40
Surprise Pops	1 (2 oz)	60	0	0	5
Dole					
Fruit'n Juice Coconut	1 bar (4 oz)	210	7	10	50
Fruit'n Juice Lemonade	1 bar (4 oz)	120	0	0	55

FOOD	PORTION	CALS	FAT	CHOL	SOD
Dole (cont.)					
Fruit'n Juice Lime	1 bar (4 oz)	110	0	0	55
Fruit'n Juice Peach Passion	1 bar (2.5 oz)	70	0	0	5
Fruit'n Juice Pineapple Coconut	1 bar (4 oz)	150	4	0	5
Fruit'n Juice Pineapple Orange Banana	1 bar (2.5 oz)	70	0	0	5
Fruit'n Juice Pineapple Orange Banana	1 bar (4 oz)	110	0	0	5
Fruit'n Juice Raspberry	1 bar (2.5 oz)	70	0	0	5
Fruit'n Juice Strawberry	1 bar (4 oz)	110	0	0	5
Fruit'n Juice Strawberry	1 bar (2.5 oz)	70	0	0	5
Grape No Sugar Added	1 bar (1.75 oz)	25	0	0	5
Raspberry	1 bar (1.75 oz)	45	0	0	5
Raspberry No Sugar Added	1 bar (1.75 oz)	25	0	0	5
Strawberry	1 bar (1.75 oz)	45	0	0	5
Strawberry No Sugar Added	1 bar (1.75 oz)	25	0	0	5
Flintstones					
Push-Up Sherbet Treats	1 (2.75 oz)	100	2	5	25
Frozfruit					
Banana Cream	1 bar (4 oz)	150	7	25	20
Cantaloupe	1 bar (4 oz)	60	0	0	5
Cappuccino Cream	1 bar (3 oz)	140	6	25	20
Cherry	1 bar (4 oz)	70	0	0	0
Coconut Cream	1 bar (4 oz)	170	11	20	25
Kiwi Strawberry	1 bar (4 oz)	90	0	0	0
Lemon	1 bar (4 oz)	90	0	0	10
Lemon Iced Tea	1 bar (4 oz)	80	0	0	10
Lime	1 bar (4 oz)	90	0	0	10
Orange	1 bar (4 oz)	90	0	0	15
Pina Colada Cream	1 bar (4 oz)	170	8	20	20
Pineapple	1 bar (4 oz)	80	0	0	0
Raspberry	1 bar (4 oz)	80	0	0	5
Strawberry	1 bar (4 oz)	80	0	0	20
Strawberry Banana Cream	1 bar (4 oz)	140	6	20	20
Strawberry Cream	1 bar (4 oz)	130	5	20	20
Tropical	1 bar (4 oz)	90	0	0	0
Watermelon	1 bar (4 oz)	50	0	0	0
Mr. Freeze					
Assorted	2 bars (3 oz)	45	0	0	20
Tropical	2 bars (3 oz)	45	0	0	20
Natural Choice					
Organic Banana	1/2 cup (3.6 oz)	110	0	0	0
Organic Blueberry	1/2 cup (3.6 oz)	100	0	0	0
Organic Kiwi	1/2 cup (3.6 oz)	110	0	0	10
Organic Lemon	1/2 cup (3.6 oz)	110	0	0	10
Organic Mango	1/2 cup (3.6 oz)	110	0	0	10

FOOD	PORTION	CALS	FAT	CHOL	SOD
Organic Strawberry	1/2 cup (3.6 oz)	110	0	0	10
Organic Strawberry Kiwi	1/2 cup (3.6 oz)	110	0	0	10
ICING					
(see CAKE ICING)					
INSTANT BREAKFAST					
(see BREAKFAST DRINKS)					
JACKFRUIT					
fresh	3 1/2 oz	70	tr	0	2
JALAPENO					
(see PEPPERS)					
JAM/JELLY/PRESERVES					
apple butter	1 tbsp (0.6 oz)	33	0	0	0
apple jelly	1 tbsp (0.7 oz)	52	0	0	7
orange marmalade	1 tbsp (0.7 oz)	49	0	0	11
strawberry jam	1 tbsp (0.7 oz)	48	0	0	8
Estee					
Fruit Spread Apple Spice	1 tbsp	16	0	0	20
Fruit Spread Apricot	1 tbsp	16	0	0	20
Fruit Spread Grape	1 tbsp	16	0	0	20
Fruit Spread Peach	1 tbsp	16	0	0	20
Fruit Spread Red Raspberry	1 tbsp	16	0	0	25
Tabasco					
Spicy Pepper Jelly	1 tbsp (0.6 oz)	50	0	0	40
White House					
Apple Butter	1 tbsp (0.6 oz)	35	0	0	5
JAPANESE FOOD					
(see ASIAN FOOD, SUSHI)					
JELLY					
(see JAM/JELLY/PRESERVE)					
JERUSALEM ARTICHOKE					
(see ARTICHOKE)					
JAVA PLUM					
fresh	3	5	tr	0	1
fresh	1 cup	82	tr	0	18
JUJUBE					
fresh	3 1/2 oz	105	tr	0	3
KALE					
fresh					
chopped cooked	1/2 cup	21	tr	0	15
raw chopped	1/2 cup	21	tr	0	15
scotch chopped cooked	1/2 cup	18	tr	0	29
KETCHUP					
ketchup	1 tbsp	16	tr	0	178
ketchup	1 pkg (0.2 oz)	6	tr	0	71
low sodium	1 tbsp	16	tr	0	3

FOOD	PORTION	CALS	FAT	CHOL	SOD
Estee					
Ketchup	1 tbsp	15	0	0	190
Healthy Choice					
Ketchup	1 tbsp (0.5 oz)	9	tr	0	97
Heinz					
Ketchup	1 tbsp (0.6 oz)	15	0	0	190
Hunt's					
Ketchup	1 tbsp (0.6 oz)	16	tr	0	198
No Salt Added	1 tbsp (0.6 oz)	16	tr	0	6
McIlhenny					
Spicy	1 tbsp (0.6 oz)	20	0	0	160
KIDNEY					
beef simmered	3 oz	122	3	329	114
lamb braised	3 oz	117	3	481	128
pork cooked	3 oz	128	4	408	68
pork cooked	1 cup	211	7	672	112
veal braised	3 oz	139	5	672	93
KIDNEY BEANS					
canned					
Eden					
Organic	1/2 cup (4.6 oz)	100	0	0	15
Green Giant					
Dark Red	1/2 cup (4.5 oz)	110	0	0	400
Light Red	1/2 cup (4.5 oz)	110	0	0	340
Hunt's					
Kidney	1/2 cup (4.5 oz)	94	1	0	484
Progresso					
Dark Red	1/2 cup (4.5 oz)	110	0	0	340
S&W					
Dark Red Premium	1/2 cup (4.6 oz)	100	1	0	460
Van Camp					
Dark Red	1/2 cup (4.6 oz)	90	0	0	760
Light Red	1/2 cup (4.6 oz)	90	0	0	390
dried					
california red cooked	1 cup	219	tr	0	7
cooked	1 cup	225	1	0	4
red cooked	1 cup	225	1	0	4
KIWIS					
fresh	1 med	46	tr	0	4
KNISH					
take-out					
potato	1 lg (7 oz)	332	12	72	470
potato	1 med (3.5 oz)	166	6	36	235
KOHLRABI					
raw sliced	1/2 cup	19	tr	0	14
sliced cooked	1/2 cup	24	tr	0	17
KUMQUATS					
fresh	1	12	tr	0	1

FOOD	PORTION	CALS	FAT	CHOL	SOD
LAMB					
(*see also* LAMB DISHES)					
cubed lean only braised	3 oz	190	7	92	60
cubed lean only broiled	3 oz	158	6	77	65
ground broiled	3 oz	240	17	82	69
leg lean & fat Choice roasted	3 oz	219	14	79	56
loin chop w/ bone lean only Choice broiled	1 chop (1.6 oz)	100	5	44	39
rib chop lean & fat Choice broiled	3 oz	307	25	84	64
shank lean & fat Choice braised	3 oz	206	11	90	61
shoulder chop w/ bone lean & fat Choice braised	1 chop (2.5 oz)	244	17	84	51
sirloin lean & fat Choice roasted	3 oz	248	21	82	58
LAMB DISHES					
take-out					
curry	3/4 cup	345	17	89	258
stew	3/4 cup	124	5	29	140
LECITHIN					
(*see* SOY)					
LEEKS					
chopped cooked	1/4 cup	8	tr	0	3
cooked	1 (4.4 oz)	38	tr	0	13
freeze dried	1 tbsp	1	0	0	0
raw	1 (4.4 oz)	76	tr	0	25
raw chopped	1/4 cup	16	tr	0	5
LEMON					
fresh	1 med	22	tr	0	3
peel	1 tbsp	0	tr	0	0
wedge	1	5	tr	0	1
LEMON GRASS					
fresh	1 tbsp (5 g)	5	tr	0	tr
fresh	1 cup (2.4 oz)	66	tr	0	4
LEMON JUICE					
bottled	1 tbsp	3	tr	0	3
fresh	1 tbsp	4	0	0	0
frozen	1 tbsp	3	tr	0	0
Canarino					
Italian Hot Lemon Beverage	1 cup	0	0	0	0
Realemon					
Juice	1 tsp (5 ml)	0	0	0	0
LEMONADE					
mix					
Country Time					
Lem'n Berry Sippers Cranberry Raspberry Lemonade as prep	1 serv (8 oz)	90	0	0	0

FOOD	PORTION	CALS	FAT	CHOL	SOD
Country Time (cont.)					
Lem'n Berry Sippers Raspberry Lemonade as prep	1 serv (8 oz)	90	0	0	0
Lem'n Berry Sippers Strawberry Lemonade as prep	1 serv (8 oz)	90	0	0	0
Lem'n Berry Sippers Wildberry Lemonade as prep	1 serv (8 oz)	90	0	0	0
Lem'n Berry Sippers Sugar Free Strawberry Lemonade as prep	1 serv (8 oz)	5	0	0	0
Lemonade as prep	1 serv (8 oz)	70	0	0	15
Pink as prep	1 serv (8 oz)	70	0	0	15
Sugar Free Pink as prep	1 serv (8 oz)	5	0	0	0
Sugar Free as prep	1 serv (8 oz)	5	0	0	0
Crystal Light					
Lemonade as prep	1 serv (8 oz)	5	0	0	0
Pink as prep	1 serv (8 oz)	5	0	0	0
Kool-Aid					
Lemonade as prep	1 serv (8 oz)	70	0	0	0
Mix as prep w/ sugar	1 serv (8 oz)	100	0	0	10
Pink as prep w/ sugar	1 serv (8 oz)	100	0	0	10
Soarin' Strawberry Lemonade as prep	1 serv (8 oz)	70	0	0	15
Soarin' Strawberry Lemonade as prep w/ sugar	1 serv (8 oz)	100	0	0	0
Sugar Free Soarin' Strawberry Lemonade as prep	1 serv (8 oz)	5	0	0	0
Sugar Free Mix as prep	1 serv (8 oz)	5	0	0	0
ready-to-drink					
Crystal Light					
Lemonade	1 serv (8 oz)	5	0	0	20
Pink	1 serv (8 oz)	5	0	0	20
Everfresh					
Lemonade	1 can (8 oz)	120	0	0	0
Ruby Red	1 can (8 oz)	110	0	0	0
Nantucket Nectars					
Authentic	8 oz	120	0	0	0
Pink	8 oz	120	0	0	0
Newman's Own					
Lemonade	1 bottle (10 oz)	140	0	0	45
Roadside Virginia	8 oz	110	0	0	40
Santa Cruz					
Organic	8 oz	100	0	0	0
Shasta Plus					
Lemonade	1 can (11.5 oz)	160	0	0	45

FOOD	PORTION	CALS	FAT	CHOL	SOD
Snapple					
Diet Pink	8 oz	20	0	0	10
Lemonade	8 oz	120	0	0	10
Pink	8 oz	120	0	0	10
Veryfine					
Chillers	1 can (11.5 oz)	190	0	0	15
Chillers Cherry	8 oz	120	0	0	15
Chillers Peach	8 oz	120	0	0	15
Chillers Pink	1 can (11.5 oz)	180	0	0	15
Chillers Strawberry	1 can (11.5 oz)	170	0	0	20
LENTILS					
dried cooked	1 cup	231	1	0	4
Eden					
Organic w/ Sweet Onion & Bay Leaf	1/2 cup (4.6 oz)	90	0	0	210
Natural Touch					
Lentil Rice Loaf	1 in slice (3.2 oz)	170	9	0	370
take-out					
indian sambar	1 serv	236	5	10	189
yemiser selatta ethiopian lentil salad	1 serv (3 oz)	115	7	0	536
LETTUCE					
(*see also* SALAD)					
bibb	1 head (6 oz)	21	tr	0	8
boston	1 head (6 oz)	21	tr	0	8
boston	2 leaves	2	tr	0	1
iceberg	1 leaf	3	tr	0	2
iceberg	1 head (19 oz)	70	1	0	48
looseleaf shredded	1/2 cup	5	tr	0	3
romaine shredded	1/2 cup	4	tr	0	2
Dole					
Iceberg	1 cup (3 oz)	15	0	0	10
Romaine	1 1/2 cups (3 oz)	15	0	0	5
Shredded	1 1/2 cup (3 oz)	15	0	0	10
Earthbound Farm					
Romaine Salad Organic	1 1/2 cups (2.9 oz)	15	0	0	5
LIMA BEANS					
dried					
cooked	1/2 cup	104	tr	0	14
Hurst					
HamBeens Baby Limas w/ Ham	1 serv	120	1	0	63
HamBeens Large Limas w/ Ham	1 serv	120	1	0	63
frozen					
Birds Eye					
Baby	1/2 cup (3.3 oz)	130	0	0	115
Fordhook	1/2 cup (3.3 oz)	100	0	0	10

FOOD	PORTION	CALS	FAT	CHOL	SOD
Green Giant					
Butter Sauce	2/3 cup (3.6 oz)	120	3	<5	330
Harvest Fresh Baby	1/2 cup (2.7 oz)	80	0	0	130
LIME					
fresh	1	20	tr	0	1
LIME JUICE					
bottled	1 tbsp	3	tr	0	2
fresh	1 tbsp	4	tr	0	0
Realime					
Juice	1 tsp (5 ml)	0	0	0	0
LINGCOD					
baked	3 oz	93	1	57	64
fillet baked	5.3 oz	164	2	101	114
LIQUOR/LIQUEUR					
(*see also* BEER AND ALE, DRINK MIXERS, WINE)					
bloody mary	5 oz	116	tr	0	332
bourbon & soda	4 oz	105	0	0	16
coffee liqueur	1.5 oz	174	tr	0	4
creme de menthe	1.5 oz	186	tr	0	3
daiquiri	2 oz	111	0	0	1
gin	1.5 oz	110	0	0	1
gin & tonic	7.5 oz	171	0	0	10
long island ice tea	1 serv (7.5 oz)	159	0	0	12
manhattan	2 oz	128	0	0	2
martini	2.5 oz	156	0	0	2
pina colada	4.5 oz	262	3	0	9
rum	1.5 oz	97	0	0	0
screwdriver	7 oz	174	tr	0	2
sloe gin fizz	2.5 oz	132	0	0	1
tequila sunrise	5.5 oz	189	tr	0	7
tom collins	7.5 oz	121	0	0	39
vodka	1.5 oz	97	0	0	0
whiskey	1.5 oz	105	0	0	0
whiskey sour	3 oz	123	tr	0	10
LIVER					
(*see also* PATÉ)					
beef braised	3 oz	137	4	331	59
beef pan-fried	3 oz	184	7	410	90
chicken stewed	1 cup (5 oz)	219	8	883	71
lamb braised	3 oz	187	7	426	48
lamb fried	3 oz	202	11	419	105
pork braised	3 oz	140	4	302	42
turkey simmered	1 cup (5 oz)	237	8	876	89
veal braised	3 oz	140	6	477	45
veal fried	3 oz	208	10	280	112
Shady Brook					
Turkey	4 oz	160	5	530	110

FOOD	PORTION	CALS	FAT	CHOL	SOD
LOBSTER					
canned					
(*see also* CRAYFISH)					
Progresso					
Lobster Sauce	1/2 cup (4.3 oz)	100	7	5	430
fresh					
northern cooked	1 cup	142	1	104	551
northern cooked	3 oz	83	1	61	323
spiny steamed	1 (5.7 oz)	233	3	146	370
spiny steamed	3 oz	122	2	76	193
LOGANBERRIES					
frozen	1 cup	80	tr	0	1
LONGANS					
fresh	1	2	0	0	0
LOQUATS					
fresh	1	5	tr	0	0
LOTUS					
root raw sliced	10 slices	45	tr	0	33
root sliced cooked	10 slices	59	tr	0	40
seeds dried	1 oz	94	1	0	1
LOX					
(*see* SALMON)					
LUPINES					
dried cooked	1 cup	197	5	0	7
LYCHEES					
fresh	1	6	tr	0	0
MACADAMIA NUTS					
Hawaiian Host					
Chocolate Covered	1 piece (0.5 oz)	53	6	2	15
MacFarms of Hawaii					
Chocolate Covered	1/4 cup (1.3 oz)	210	16	5	25
Dry Roasted Salted	1/4 cup (1.3 oz)	220	23	0	65
Kona Coffee Dark Chocolate	1/4 cup (1.3 oz)	210	16	5	25
Covered					
MACARONI					
(*see* PASTA)					
MACE					
ground	1 tsp	8	1	0	1
MACKEREL					
canned					
jack	1 cup	296	12	150	720
fresh					
atlantic cooked	3 oz	223	15	64	71
jack baked	3 oz	171	9	51	94
king baked	3 oz	114	2	58	172
pacific baked	3 oz	171	9	51	94
spanish cooked	3 oz	134	5	62	56

FOOD	PORTION	CALS	FAT	CHOL	SOD
smoked					
atlantic	3.5 oz	296	24	93	384
MALTED MILK					
Carnation					
Chocolate	3 tbsp (0.7 oz)	90	1	0	40
Original	3 tbsp (0.7 oz)	90	2	5	40
MAMMY-APPLE					
fresh	1	431	4	0	127
MANGO					
fresh	1	135	1	0	4
dried					
Rainforest Farms					
Slices	6 slices (1.3 oz)	140	1	0	108
MANGO JUICE					
Fresh Samantha					
Mango Mama	1 cup (8 oz)	120	0	0	0
Guzzler					
Mango Passion	8 oz	140	0	0	30
Ocean Spray					
Mango Mango	8 oz	130	0	0	35
Snapple					
Mango Madness	8 oz	110	0	0	10
Tang					
Drink Mix as prep	1 serv (8 oz)	100	0	0	0
MARGARINE					
(*see also* BUTTER BLENDS, BUTTER SUBSTITUTES)					
stick corn	1 tsp	34	4	0	44
tub corn	1 tsp	34	4	0	51
tub diet	1 tsp	17	2	0	46
Benecol					
Single Serve Light	1 pkg (0.3 oz)	30	3	0	65
Tub Light	1 tbsp (0.5 oz)	45	5	0	110
Tub Regular	1 tbsp (0.5 oz)	80	9	0	110
Smart Balance					
No Trans Fat	1 tbsp (0.5 oz)	120	14	0	0
No Trans Fat Light	1 tbsp (0.5 oz)	45	5	0	100
No Trans Fat Spread	1 tbsp (0.5 oz)	80	9	0	90
Smart Beat					
Light Unsalted	1 tbsp (0.5 oz)	25	3	0	0
Squeeze Fat Free	1 tbsp (0.5 oz)	5	0	0	100
Super Light Trans Fat Free	1 tbsp (0.5 oz)	20	2	0	105
Take Control					
Spread	1 tbsp (0.5 oz)	50	6	<5	110
Weight Watchers					
Light	1 tbsp	45	4	0	70
Light Sodium Free	1 tbsp	45	4	0	0
MARINADE					
(*see* SAUCE)					

FOOD	PORTION	CALS	FAT	CHOL	SOD
MARJORAM					
dried	1 tsp	2	tr	0	tr
MARSHMALLOW					
marshmallow	1 reg (0.3 oz)	23	0	0	3
marshmallow	1 cup (1.6 oz)	146	tr	0	22
Just Born					
Peeps	5 (1.5 oz)	160	0	0	15
MATZO					
plain	1 (1 oz)	112	tr	0	0
whole wheat	1 (1 oz)	99	tr	0	1
MAYONNAISE					
(*see also* MAYONNAISE TYPE SALAD DRESSING, SAUCE)					
mayonnaise	1 cup	1577	175	130	1250
mayonnaise	1 tbsp	99	11	8	78
reduced calorie	1 cup	556	46	58	1193
reduced calorie	1 tbsp	34	3	4	75
Kraft					
Fat Free	1 tbsp (0.6 oz)	10	0	0	120
Light	1 tbsp (0.5 oz)	50	5	5	90
Real	1 tbsp (0.5 oz)	100	11	5	75
Smart Beat					
Fat Free	1 tbsp	10	0	0	135
Weight Watchers					
Fat Free	1 tbsp	10	0	0	105
Light	1 tbsp	25	2	5	130
Light Low Sodium	1 tbsp	25	2	5	40
MAYONNAISE TYPE SALAD DRESSING					
(*see also* RELISH)					
Miracle Whip					
Free	1 tbsp (0.5 oz)	15	0	0	125
Light	1 tbsp (0.5 oz)	35	3	<5	130
Salad Dressing	1 tbsp (0.6 oz)	70	7	5	95
Nayonaise					
Cholesterol Free	1 tbsp (0.5 oz)	35	3	0	104
Fat Free	1 tbsp (0.5 oz)	11	tr	0	107
Weight Watchers					
Fat Free Whipped Dressing	1 tbsp	15	0	0	95
MEAT STICKS					
(*see also* BEEF DRIED)					
jerky beef	1 oz	96	4	32	815
smoked	1 oz	156	14	38	420
Big Ones					
BBQ	1 (1 oz)	130	12	35	680
Hot n'Spicy	1 (1 oz)	130	12	35	580
Original	1 (1 oz)	130	12	35	620
Teriyaki	1 (1 oz)	130	12	35	440
Jack Link's					
Kippered Beefsteak Teriyaki	1 oz	80	1	25	440

FOOD	PORTION	CALS	FAT	CHOL	SOD
Lance					
Beef & Cheese	1 pkg (1.5 oz)	150	11	45	630
Beef Jerky	1 piece (0.25 oz)	30	2	<5	160
Beef Snack	1 piece (0.63 oz)	100	8	10	290
Hot Sausage	1 piece (0.9 oz)	60	5	15	540
Lowrey's					
Smokehouse Tender Hickory Smoked	1 pkg (1 oz)	80	2	25	710
Smokehouse Tender Original	1 pkg (1 oz)	60	1	25	750
Smokehouse Tender Peppered	1 pkg (1 oz)	60	1	25	720
Oberto					
Beef Jerky	1 pkg (1.3 oz)	100	1	25	780
Pemmican					
Original Tender Kippered Beef Steak	1	110	5	35	1100
Peppered Tender Kippered Beef Steak	1	110	5	35	1170
Rough Cut					
Beef Steak Hot	1 pkg (1 oz)	70	1	25	710
Beef Steak Original	1 pkg (1 oz)	60	1	25	730
Beef Steak Peppered	1 pkg (1 oz)	60	1	25	740
Rustlers Roundup					
Beef Jerky	1 serv (5 g)	20	2	5	115
Flamin' Hot	1 serv (8 g)	40	3	10	140
Smoky Steak	1 serv (0.8 oz)	60	2	20	580
Spicy	1 serv (0.5 oz)	70	6	20	250
Slim Jim					
Spicy	1 (4 1/2 in) (0.3 oz)	50	4	5	125
Spicy Big	1 (.44 oz)	70	6	10	190
Spicy Giant	1 (0.97 oz)	150	14	15	410
Spicy Super	1 (0.64 oz)	100	9	10	260
MEAT SUBSTITUTES					
(*see also* BACON SUBSTITUTES, CANADIAN BACON SUBSTITUTES, CHICKEN SUBSTITUTES, HAMBURGER SUBSTITUTES, SAUSAGE SUBSTITUTES, TURKEY SUBSTITUTES)					
Amy's Organic					
Whole Meals Veggie Loaf	1 pkg (10 oz)	260	5	0	690
Boca Burgers					
Chef Max's Original	1 patty (2.5 oz)	110	2	3	296
Frieda's					
SoyTaco	1 oz	50	3	0	180
Soyrizo	4 tbsp (1.9 oz)	120	9	0	440
Ken & Robert's					
Veggie Pockets	1 (4.5 oz)	250	8	0	490
Veggie Pockets Bar B Que	1 (4.5 oz)	290	8	0	450
Veggie Pockets Broccoli & Cheddar	1 (4.5 oz)	250	8	0	490

FOOD	PORTION	CALS	FAT	CHOL	SOD
Veggie Pockets Greek	1 (4.5 oz)	250	8	0	450
Veggie Pockets Indian	1 (4.5 oz)	260	8	0	490
Veggie Pockets Pizza	1 (4.5 oz)	270	8	0	490
Veggie Pockets Pot Pie	1 (4.5 oz)	250	9	0	410
Veggie Pockets Potato & Cheddar	1 (4.5 oz)	260	8	0	370
Veggie Pockets Santa Fe	1 (4.5 oz)	250	8	0	550
Veggie Pockets Tex Mex	1 (4.5 oz)	260	8	0	490
Lightlife					
Foney Baloney	3 slices (1.5 oz)	60	3	0	240
Gimme Lean Beef	2 oz	70	0	0	240
Smart Deli Bologna	3 slices (1.5 oz)	50	0	0	300
Smart Deli Ham	3 slices (1.5 oz)	50	0	0	300
Smart Deli Peppercorn	3 slices (1.5 oz)	45	0	0	300
Smart Deli Sticks Soylami	1 oz	40	0	0	280
Smart Deli Sticks Pepperoni	1 oz	45	0	0	300
Smart Ground Original	1/3 cup (1.9 oz)	70	0	0	180
Smart Ground Taco	1/3 cup (2 oz)	60	0	0	170
Loma Linda					
Dinner Cuts	2 slices (3.2 oz)	90	2	0	500
Nuteena	3/8 in slice (1.9 oz)	160	13	0	120
Sandwich Spread	1/4 cup (1.9 oz)	80	5	0	260
Savory Dinner Loaf Mix not prep	1/3 cup (0.9 oz)	90	2	0	560
Swiss Stake	1 piece (3.2 oz)	120	6	0	430
Tender Bits	6 pieces (3 oz)	110	5	0	440
Tender Rounds	6 pieces (2.8 oz)	120	5	0	330
Vita Burger Chunks not prep	1/4 cup (0.7 oz)	70	1	0	350
Vita Burger Granules	3 tbsp (0.7 oz)	70	1	0	350
Morningstar Farms					
Burger Style Recipe Crumbles	2/3 cup (1.9 oz)	80	3	0	210
Ground Meatless	1/2 cup (1.9 oz)	60	0	0	260
Harvest Burger Recipe Crumbles	1/2 cup (2 oz)	70	0	0	200
Quarter Prime	1 patty (3.4 oz)	140	2	0	370
Natural Touch					
Dinner Entree	1 patty (3 oz)	220	15	0	380
Loaf Mix not prep	4 tbsp (1 oz)	100	1	0	700
Stroganoff Mix not prep	4 tbsp (0.8 oz)	90	4	10	610
Taco Mix not prep	3 tbsp (0.6 oz)	60	1	0	590
Vegan Burger Crumbles	1/2 cup (1.9 oz)	60	0	0	260
Soy Is Us					
Beef Not!	1/2 cup (1.75 oz)	140	2	0	5
Veggie Patch					
Veggie Rounds	1 (2.5 oz)	120	3	0	250
Veggitinos Meatballs	5 (2.8 oz)	120	4	0	470

FOOD	PORTION	CALS	FAT	CHOL	SOD
Worthington					
Beef Style Meatless	3/8 in slice (1.9 oz)	110	7	0	620
Bolono	3 slices (2 oz)	80	4	0	720
Choplets	2 slices (3.2 oz)	90	2	0	500
Corned Beef Meatless	4 slices (2 oz)	140	9	0	520
Country Stew	1 cup (8.4 oz)	210	9	0	830
Dinner Roast	3/4 in slice (3 oz)	180	12	<5	580
FriPats	1 patty (2.2 oz)	130	6	0	320
Multigrain Cutlets	2 slices (3.2 oz)	100	2	0	390
Numete	3/8 in slice (1.9 oz)	130	10	0	270
Prime Stakes	1 piece (3.2 oz)	120	7	0	440
Prosage Roll	5/8 in slice (1.9 oz)	140	10	0	390
Protose	3/8 in slice (1.9 oz)	130	7	0	280
Salami Meatless	3 slices (2 oz)	130	8	0	930
Savory Slices	3 slices (2.9 oz)	150	9	0	540
Smoked Beef Meatless	6 slices (2 oz)	120	6	0	730
Stakelets	1 piece (2.5 oz)	140	8	0	480
Veelets	1 patty (2.5 oz)	180	9	0	390
Vegetable Skallops	1/2 cup (3 oz)	90	2	0	410
Vegetable Steaks	2 pieces (2.5 oz)	80	2	0	300
Wham	2 slices (1.6 oz)	80	5	0	430
Yves					
Veggie Bologna	4 slices (2.2 oz)	70	0	0	460
Veggie Ground Italian	1/3 cup (2 oz)	60	0	0	270
Veggie Ground Round Italian	1/3 cup (1.9 oz)	60	0	0	270
Veggie Ground Round Original	2 oz	60	0	0	270
Veggie Pizza Pepperoni Slices	1 serv (1.7 oz)	70	0	0	480
Veggie Salami Deli Slices	1 serv (2.2 oz)	90	0	0	390
MELON					
(see also individual names)					
melon balls frozen	1 cup	55	tr	0	53
MELON JUICE					
Ocean Spray					
Mega Melon	8 oz	130	0	0	35
MEXICAN FOOD					
(see SALSA, SAUCE, SPANISH FOOD, TORTILLA)					
MILK					
(see also CHOCOLATE, COCOA, MILK DRINKS, MILKSHAKE)					
canned					
Carnation					
Evaporated	1/2 cup	150	8	10	30
Evaporated Fat Free	1/2 cup (4 fl oz)	100	0	0	40
Evaporated Lowfat	1/2 cup	110	2	5	35
Sweetened Condensed	1/3 cup	330	8	10	45
dried					
buttermilk	1 tbsp	25	tr	5	34
Carnation					
Nonfat	1/3 cup	80	0	<5	125

FOOD	PORTION	CALS	FAT	CHOL	SOD
Saco					
Cultured Buttermilk	4 tbsp (0.8 oz)	80	tr	4	166
Sanalac					
Powder	1/4 cup (0.8 oz)	85	tr	6	117
refrigerated					
1%	1 cup	102	3	10	123
1%	1 qt	409	10	39	493
2%	1 cup	121	5	18	122
2%	1 qt	485	19	73	487
buttermilk	1 cup	99	2	9	257
buttermilk	1 qt	396	9	34	1028
goat	1 cup	168	10	28	122
human	1 cup	171	11	34	42
nonfat	1 cup	86	tr	4	125
nonfat	1 qt	342	2	18	505
whole	1 cup	150	8	33	120
Cool Cow					
Low Fat	1 cup (8 oz)	110	3	<5	125
Farmland					
Skim Plus	1 cup (8 oz)	110	0	<5	170
Horizon Organic					
Fat Free	1 cup (8 oz)	80	0	4	125
Land O'Lakes					
1% Lowfat	1 carton (10 oz)	120	3	15	135
Fat Free	1 carton (10 oz)	100	5	5	140
Whole	1 carton (10 oz)	180	10	45	135
NutraBalance					
LactaCare	1 pkg (8 oz)	500	18	0	240
Organic Valley					
Low Fat	1 cup	100	3	10	120
Nonfat	1 cup	80	0	5	125
Reduced Fat	1 cup	130	5	20	120
Whole	1 cup	150	8	30	120
Stonyfield Farm					
Organic Whole Milk	1 cup (8 oz)	180	10	40	125
Organic Whole Milk Vanilla	1 cup (8 oz)	230	8	30	130
MILK DRINKS					
(*see also* BREAKFAST DRINKS, CHOCOLATE, COCOA, MILKSHAKES)					
chocolate milk 1%	1 cup	158	3	7	152
chocolate milk 2%	1 cup	179	5	17	150
Horizon Organic					
Lowfat Chocolate Milk	1 cup (8 oz)	160	3	10	200
Land O'Lakes					
Chocolate	1 cup (8.4 oz)	200	7	30	180
Organic Valley					
Chocolate Milk Reduced Fat	1 cup	180	5	10	190

FOOD	PORTION	CALS	FAT	CHOL	SOD
Quik					
Banana Lowfat	1 cup (8.4 oz)	200	5	20	95
Banana Powder	2 tbsp (0.8 oz)	90	0	0	0
Chocolate	1 cup (8.4 oz)	230	8	30	130
Chocolate Lowfat	1 carton (8.4 oz)	200	5	20	130
Cookies n Cream Powder	2 tbsp (0.8 oz)	100	1	0	190
Strawberry	1 cup (8.4 oz)	230	8	30	100
Strawberry Lowfat	1 carton (8.4 oz)	210	5	20	100
Strawberry Powder	2 tbsp (0.8 oz)	90	0	0	0
MILK SUBSTITUTES					
(*see also* COFFEE WHITENERS)					
Blue Diamond					
Almond Breeze Original	8 oz	60	2	0	150
Almond Breeze Vanilla	8 oz	90	3	0	150
Edensoy					
Extra Original	8 oz	130	4	0	105
Extra Vanilla	8 oz	150	3	0	90
Original	8 oz	130	4	0	105
Vanilla	8 oz	150	3	0	90
Galaxy					
Veggi Milk Chocolate	1 cup (8 oz)	150	2	0	130
Veggie Milk Original	1 cup (8 oz)	110	3	0	130
Harmony Farms					
Original Rice Beverage	1 cup (8 oz)	90	0	0	100
Harmony House					
Enriched Rice Beverage	1 cup (8 oz)	90	0	0	100
Enriched Soy Beverage	1 cup (8 oz)	90	0	0	100
Original Soy Beverage	1 cup (8 oz)	90	0	0	100
Health Valley					
Soo Moo	1 cup	110	0	0	60
NutraBalance					
NuTaste	1 pkg (8 oz)	80	2	0	210
Rice Dream					
Carob	1 box (8 oz)	150	3	0	100
Chocolate	1 box (8 oz)	170	3	0	115
Chocolate Enriched	1 box (8 oz)	170	3	0	115
Organic Original	1 box (8 oz)	120	2	0	90
Organic Original Enriched	1 box (8 oz)	120	2	0	90
Vanilla	1 box (8 oz)	130	2	0	90
Vanilla Enriched	1 box (8 oz)	130	2	0	90
Vitamite					
Non-Dairy 2% Fat	1 cup (8 oz)	110	5	0	120
Non-Diary Nonfat	1 cup (8 oz)	90	0	0	70
Vitasoy					
Carob Supreme	8 oz	210	6	0	160
Cocoa Light	8 oz	130	2	0	130
Original Creamy	8 oz	160	7	0	180
Original Light	8 oz	90	2	0	95

FOOD	PORTION	CALS	FAT	CHOL	SOD
Rich Cocoa	8 oz	210	6	0	180
Vanilla Light	8 oz	110	2	0	95
Vanilla Delite	8 oz	190	6	0	130
White Wave					
Silk Chocolate Organic	1 cup (8.3 oz)	108	3	0	95
MILKSHAKE					
chocolate	10 oz	360	11	37	273
strawberry	10 oz	319	8	31	234
vanilla	10 oz	314	8	32	232
D'Frosta Shake					
Vanilla	1 serv (13.5 oz)	340	9	40	200
Freeze Flip					
Fruit Shake No Fat Lactose Free Black Raspberry	1 serv (6 oz)	150	0	0	25
MILLET					
cooked	1 cup (6.1 oz)	207	2	0	3
MINERAL WATER					
(*see* WATER)					
MISO					
miso	1/2 cup	284	8	0	5036
MOLASSES					
blackstrap	1 tbsp (0.7 oz)	47	0	0	11
molasses	1 tbsp (0.7 oz)	53	0	0	7
Mott's					
Sulphured	1 tbsp	50	0	0	10
Unsulphured	1 tbsp	50	0	0	0
MONKFISH					
baked	3 oz	82	2	27	20
MOOSE					
roasted	3 oz	114	1	66	58
MOTH BEANS					
dried cooked	1 cup	207	1	0	17
MOUSSE					
frozen					
Sara Lee					
Chocolate Mint Mousse	1/5 pkg (4.3 oz)	440	28	30	100
Weight Watchers					
Chocolate Mousse	1 (2.75 oz)	190	5	5	150
take-out					
chocolate	1/2 cup (7.1 oz)	447	33	299	87
MUFFIN					
frozen					
Pepperidge Farm					
Blueberry	1 (2 oz)	180	7	30	260
Bran w/ Raisins	1 (2 oz)	180	6	25	310
Corn	1 (2 oz)	190	7	30	270
Orange Cranberry	1 (2 oz)	180	6	36	190

FOOD	PORTION	CALS	FAT	CHOL	SOD
Sara Lee					
Blueberry	1 (2.2 oz)	220	11	15	170
Corn	1 (2.2 oz)	260	14	25	220
Weight Watchers					
Chocolate Chocolate Chip	1 (2.5 oz)	190	2	0	350
Fat Free Banana	1 (2.5 oz)	170	0	0	310
Fat Free Blueberry	1 (2.5 oz)	160	0	0	290
mix					
Betty Crocker					
Apple Cinnamon Low Fat Recipe	1	120	1	20	190
Banana Nut	1	150	5	20	200
Banana Nut No Cholesterol Recipe	1	140	4	0	200
Blueberry Low Fat Recipe	1	120	1	20	200
Cinnamon Streusel	1	170	7	20	180
Fat Free Apple Cinnamon	1	120	0	0	200
Fat Free Blueberry	1	120	0	0	200
Lemon Poppyseed	1	190	7	20	220
Lemon Poppyseed No Cholesterol Recipe	1	190	7	0	220
Twice The Blueberry	1	140	4	20	180
Twice The Blueberry No Cholesterol Recipe	1	130	3	0	180
Gold Medal					
Banana Nut	1	170	8	35	190
Caramel Nut	1	170	7	35	230
Corn	1	160	6	35	270
Robin Hood					
Apple Cinnamon	1	170	8	35	220
Banana Nut	1	170	8	35	190
Blueberry	1	160	6	35	220
Caramel Nut	1	170	7	35	230
Sweet Rewards					
Fat Free Apple Cinnamon	1	120	0	0	200
Fat Free Wild Blueberry	1	120	0	0	200
Low Fat Recipe Apple Cinnamon	1	130	1	6	200
Low Fat Recipe Wild Blueberry	1	120	1	20	200
ready-to-eat					
blueberry	1 (2 oz)	158	4	17	255
oat bran wheat free	1 (2 oz)	154	4	0	224
Dolly Madison					
Blueberry	1 (1.75 oz)	170	7	0	280
Mega Banana Nut	1 (5.9 oz)	620	31	75	540
Mega Blueberry	1 (5.9 oz)	590	28	80	590
Mega Chocolate Chip	1 (5.9 oz)	620	29	80	580

FOOD	PORTION	CALS	FAT	CHOL	SOD
Mega Cranberry Orange	1 (5.9 oz)	590	28	90	580
Mega Cream Cheese	1 (5.9 oz)	620	33	90	630
Dutch Mill					
Apple Oat Bran	1 (2 oz)	180	5	0	210
Banana Walnut	1 (2 oz)	220	6	5	210
Carrot	1 (2 oz)	190	7	30	230
Corn	1 (2 oz)	190	6	40	280
Cranberry Orange	1 (2 oz)	170	6	55	290
Raisin Bran	1 (2 oz)	230	5	30	330
Hostess					
Banana Bran Low Fat	1 (2.7 oz)	240	3	0	270
Blueberry Low Fat	1 (2.7 oz)	230	3	0	350
Hearty Banana Nut	1 (5.9 oz)	620	31	75	540
Hearty Blueberry	1 (5.9 oz)	590	28	80	590
Hearty Chocolate Chip	1 (5.9 oz)	620	29	80	580
Hearty Cranberry Orange	1 (5.9 oz)	590	28	90	580
Hearty Cream Cheese	1 (5.9 oz)	620	33	90	630
Mini Banana Walnut	3 (1.2 oz)	160	9	25	100
Mini Blueberry	3 (1.2 oz)	150	8	25	110
Mini Chocolate Chip	3 (1.2 oz)	160	9	20	100
Mini Cinnamon Apple	3 (1.2 oz)	160	9	25	110
Mini Cinnamon Bites	3 (1.1 oz)	130	6	15	110
Mini Rocky Road	3 (1.2 oz)	160	9	20	140
Muffin Loaf Apple Spice	1 (3.7 oz)	430	18	80	350
Muffin Loaf Banana Nut	1 (3.8 oz)	460	20	60	300
Muffin Loaf Blueberry	1 (3.8 oz)	440	19	80	460
Muffin Loaf Chocolate Chocolate Chip	1 (3.8 oz)	400	17	45	330
Muffin Loaf Raspberry	1 (3.8 oz)	440	19	80	460
Oat Bran	1 (1.5 oz)	160	8	0	150
Otis Spunkmeyer					
Mayport Almond Poppy Seed	1/2 muffin (2 oz)	210	12	40	230
Mayport Apple Cinnamon	1 (2.25 oz)	240	13	40	240
Mayport Banana Nut	1 (2.25 oz)	270	14	30	210
Mayport Cheese Streusel	1/2 muffin (2 oz)	220	10	25	170
Mayport Chocolate Chocolate Chip	1 (2.25 oz)	260	13	40	190
Mayport Chocolate Chip	1/2 muffin (2 oz)	240	13	35	210
Mayport Cinnamon Spice	1/2 muffin (2 oz)	230	13	40	250
Mayport Corn	1/2 muffin (2 oz)	230	13	50	240
Mayport Harvest Bran	1 (2.25 oz)	240	10	35	240
Mayport Lemon	1/2 muffin (2 oz)	230	13	40	280
Mayport Orange	1/2 muffin (2 oz)	230	13	40	230
Mayport Pineapple	1/2 muffin (2 oz)	210	12	40	270
Mayport Wild Blueberry	1 (2.25 oz)	230	13	45	230
Mayport Low Fat Apple Cinnamon	1 (4 oz)	380	6	65	300

FOOD	PORTION	CALS	FAT	CHOL	SOD
Otis Spunkmeyer (cont.)					
Mayport Low Fat Banana Nut	1 (4 oz)	350	6	65	400
Mayport Low Fat Chocolate Chocolate Chip	1 (4 oz)	370	6	65	290
Mayport Low Fat Wild Blueberry	1 (4 oz)	350	6	60	280
Sara Lee					
Bran	1 (4 oz)	430	20	50	550
Uncle Wally's					
Fat Free Apple Cinnamon Delight	1 (1.9 oz)	110	0	0	280
Weight Watchers					
Fat Free Apple Crisp	1 (2.5 oz)	160	0	0	290
Fat Free Cranberry Orange	1 (2.5 oz)	160	0	0	290
Fat Free Double Chocolate	1 (2.5 oz)	180	0	0	300
Fat Free Wild Blueberry	1 (2.5 oz)	160	0	0	280
Low Fat Apple Cinnamon	1 (2.5 oz)	170	3	0	200
Low Fat Blueberry	1 (2.5 oz)	180	3	0	200
Low Fat Carrot	1 (2.5 oz)	160	3	0	200
Low Fat Chocolate Chip	1 (2.5 oz)	180	3	0	200
Low Fat Cranberry Orange	1 (2.5 oz)	180	3	0	190
Low Fat Lemon Poppy	1 (2.5 oz)	190	3	0	200
MULBERRIES					
fresh	1 cup	61	1	0	14
MULLET					
striped cooked	3 oz	127	4	54	61
MUNG BEANS					
dried					
cooked	1 cup	213	1	0	4
MUNGO BEANS					
dried cooked	1 cup	190	1	1	13
MUSHROOMS					
canned					
chanterelle	3 1/2 oz	12	1	0	165
straw	1 cup (6.4 oz)	58	1	0	699
BinB					
Pieces & Stems	1 can (4.2 oz)	30	0	0	460
Sliced	1 can (4.2 oz)	30	0	0	460
Sliced With Garlic	1 can (4.2 oz)	35	1	0	410
Whole	1 can (4.2 oz)	30	0	0	460
Green Giant					
Pieces & Stems	1/2 cup (4.2 oz)	30	0	0	440
Sliced	1/2 cup (4.2 oz)	30	0	0	440
Whole	1/2 cup (4.2 oz)	30	0	0	440
dried					
chanterelle	3 1/2 oz	89	2	0	32
cloud ear	1 (5 g)	13	tr	0	2

FOOD	PORTION	CALS	FAT	CHOL	SOD
cloud ear	1 cup (1 oz)	80	tr	0	10
shiitake	4 (1/2 oz)	44	tr	0	2
straw	1 piece (6 g)	2	tr	0	21
fresh					
chanterelle	3 1/2 oz	11	tr	0	3
enoki raw	1 (4 in)	2	tr	0	0
morel	3 1/2 oz	9	tr	0	2
oyster raw	1 lg (5.2 oz)	55	1	0	46
oyster raw	1 sm (0.5 oz)	6	tr	0	5
portabello sliced	1 serv (2 oz)	4	0	0	0
raw	1 (1/2 oz)	5	tr	0	1
raw sliced	1/2 cup	9	tr	0	1
shitake cooked	4 (2.5 oz)	40	tr	0	3
sliced cooked	1/2 cup	21	tr	0	2
whole cooked	1 (0.4 oz)	3	tr	0	0
Mother Earth					
Organic	4 oz	35	1	0	0
MUSSELS					
blue raw	3 oz	73	2	24	243
blue raw	1 cup	129	3	42	429
fresh blue cooked	3 oz	147	4	48	313
MUSTARD					
dry mustard	1 tsp	15	1	0	tr
ready-to-use					
Boar's Head					
Delicatessen Style	1 tsp (5 g)	0	0	0	40
Honey	1 tsp (5 g)	10	0	0	25
Hunt's					
Mustard	1 tsp (5 g)	3	tr	0	64
Kraft					
Horseradish Mustard	1 tsp (5 g)	0	0	0	55
Mustard	1 tsp (5 g)	0	0	0	60
MUSTARD GREENS					
fresh chopped cooked	1/2 cup	11	tr	0	11
Birds Eye					
Chopped	1 cup (3 oz)	30	0	0	20
NATTO					
natto	1/2 cup	187	10	0	6
NAVY BEANS					
canned					
navy	1 cup	296	1	0	1173
Eden					
Organic	1/2 cup (4.6 oz)	110	1	0	15
dried					
cooked	1 cup	259	1	0	2
Hurst					
HamBeens w/ Ham	3 tbsp (1.2 oz)	120	1	0	63

FOOD	PORTION	CALS	FAT	CHOL	SOD
NECTARINE					
fresh	1	67	1	0	0
NEUFCHATEL					
neufchatel	1 oz	74	7	22	113
neufchatel	1 pkg (3 oz)	221	20	65	339
Horizon Organic					
Neufchatel	2 tbsp	70	6	20	120
Organic Valley					
Neufchatel	1 oz	70	6	20	115
Philadelphia					
Neufchatel	1 oz	70	6	20	120
NON-DAIRY CREAMERS					
(*see* COFFEE WHITENERS)					
NON-DAIRY WHIPPED TOPPINGS					
(*see* WHIPPED TOPPINGS)					
NOODLE DISHES					
(*see also* NOODLES, PASTA DINNERS)					
mix					
Kraft					
Noodle Classics Cheddar Cheese as prep	1 cup (7.4 oz)	400	19	70	760
Noodle Classics Savory Chicken as prep	1 cup (8.5 oz)	340	13	55	1370
Lipton					
Noodles & Sauce Alfredo Broccoli as prep	1 cup (2.2 oz)	340	14	80	970
Noodles & Sauce Alfredo as prep	1 cup (2.2 oz)	330	14	80	1040
Noodles & Sauce Beef as prep	1 cup (2.1 oz)	280	10	60	910
Noodles & Sauce Butter as prep	1 cup (2.2 oz)	310	14	70	870
Noodles & Sauce Butter & Herb as prep	1 cup (2.2 oz)	300	13	65	780
Noodles & Sauce Chicken Broccoli as prep	1 cup (2.1 oz)	310	11	70	840
Noodles & Sauce Chicken Tetrazzini as prep	1 cup (2 oz)	300	12	70	950
Noodles & Sauce Chicken as prep	1 cup (2.1 oz)	290	11	65	830
Noodles & Sauce Creamy Chicken as prep	1 cup (2.1 oz)	320	13	75	810
Noodles & Sauce Parmesan as prep	1 cup (2.1 oz)	330	15	75	850
Noodles & Sauce Sour Cream & Chives as prep	1 cup (2.2 oz)	310	14	70	870
Noodles & Sauce Stroganoff as prep	1 cup (2 oz)	300	11	70	950

FOOD	PORTION	CALS	FAT	CHOL	SOD
shelf-stable					
Hormel					
Microcup Meals Noodles & Chicken	1 cup (7.5 oz)	200	9	40	1140
take-out					
noodle pudding	1/2 cup	132	7	27	222
NOODLES					
cellophane	1 cup	492	tr	0	14
chow mein	1 cup (1.6 oz)	237	14	0	189
egg cooked	1 cup (5.6 oz)	213	2	53	11
japanese soba cooked	1 cup (4 oz)	113	tr	0	68
japanese somen cooked	1 cup (6.2 oz)	231	tr	0	283
rice cooked	1 cup (6.2 oz)	192	tr	0	33
spinach/egg cooked	1 cup (5.6 oz)	211	3	53	19
Chun King					
Chow Mein	1/2 cup (1 oz)	137	6	0	217
La Choy					
Chow Mein	1/2 cup (1 oz)	137	6	0	217
Chow Mein Crispy Wide	1/2 cup (1 oz)	148	8	0	289
Rice	1/2 cup (1 oz)	121	3	0	378
NOPALES					
cooked	1 cup (5.2 oz)	23	tr	0	30
raw sliced	1 cup (3 oz)	14	tr	0	19
raw sliced	1/2 cup (1.5 oz)	7	tr	0	9
NUTMEG					
ground	1 tsp	12	1	0	tr
NUTRITION SUPPLEMENTS					
(*see also* BREAKFAST DRINKS, CEREAL BARS, ENERGY BARS, ENERGY DRINKS, SPORTS DRINKS)					
Ensure					
Supplement All Flavors	1 can (8 fl oz)	250	6	<5	200
Essential					
Protein Powder	1 serv (0.6 oz)	70	tr	0	5
GeniSoy					
Soy Protein Powder	1 scoop (0.6 oz)	60	0	0	180
NutraBalance					
EggPro	1 tbsp (7.5 g)	30	0	0	96
Pounds Off					
All Flavors	1 bar (2.1 oz)	210	5	0	25
NUTS MIXED					
(*see also individual names*)					
dry roasted w/ peanuts salted	1 oz	169	15	0	223
oil roasted w/ peanuts salted	1 oz	175	16	0	217
Estee					
Fruit & Nut Mix	1/4 cup	210	12	<5	45
OHELOBERRIES					
fresh	1 cup	39	tr	0	2

FOOD	PORTION	CALS	FAT	CHOL	SOD
OIL					
(see also FAT)					
olive	1 tbsp	119	14	0	0
olive	1 cup	1909	216	0	tr
peanut	1 tbsp	119	14	0	tr
peanut	1 cup	1909	216	0	tr
soybean	1 cup	1927	218	0	tr
soybean	1 tbsp	120	14	0	0
Crisco					
Oil	1 tbsp (0.5 oz)	120	14	0	0
Eden					
Safflower	1 tbsp (0.5 oz)	120	14	0	0
Sesame	1 tbsp (0.5 oz)	140	15	0	0
House Of Tsang					
Hot Chili Sesame	1 tsp (5 g)	45	5	0	0
Mongolian Fire	1 tsp (5 g)	45	5	0	0
Pure Sesame	1 tsp (5 g)	45	5	0	0
Singapore Curry	1 tsp (5 g)	45	5	0	0
Wok Oil	1 tbsp (0.5 oz)	130	14	0	0
Orville Redenbacher's					
Popping	1 tbsp (0.5 oz)	120	14	0	0
Pam					
Butter	1/3 sec spray (0.3 g)	0	0	0	0
Cooking Spray	1/3 sec spray (0.3 g)	0	0	0	0
Olive Oil	1/3 sec spray (0.3 g)	0	0	0	0
Progresso					
Olive Extra Mild	1 tbsp (0.5 oz)	120	14	0	0
Olive Extra Virgin	1 tbsp (0.5 oz)	120	14	0	0
Olive Riviera Blend	1 tbsp (0.5 oz)	120	14	0	0
Smart Beat					
Canola	1 tbsp	120	14	0	0
Weight Watchers					
Butter Spray	1/3 sec spray	0	0	0	0
Cooking Spray	1/3 sec spray	0	0	0	0
OKRA					
fresh					
sliced cooked	1/2 cup	25	tr	0	4
sliced cooked	8 pods	27	tr	0	5
frozen					
sliced cooked	1/2 cup	34	tr	0	3
sliced cooked	1 pkg (10 oz)	94	1	0	8
Birds Eye					
Cut	3/4 cup (2.9 oz)	25	0	0	35
Whole	9 pods (3 oz)	25	0	0	35
OLIVES					
green	4 med	15	2	0	312
green	3 extra lg	15	2	0	312
ripe	1 sm	4	tr	0	28

FOOD	PORTION	CALS	FAT	CHOL	SOD
ripe	1 lg	5	tr	0	38
ripe	1 jumbo	7	1	0	75
ripe	1 colossal	12	1	0	136
spanish stuffed	5 (0.5 oz)	15	1	0	320
Italia In Tavola					
Black Olives Paste	1 tbsp (0.5 oz)	20	2	0	470
Progresso					
Olive Salad (drained)	2 tbsp (0.8 oz)	25	3	0	360
Vlasic					
Ripe Colossal Pitted	2 (0.6 oz)	20	2	0	110
Ripe Jumbo Pitted	3 (0.6 oz)	25	2	0	135
Ripe Large Pitted	4 (0.5 oz)	25	3	0	115
Ripe Medium Pitted	5 (0.5 oz)	25	3	0	115
Ripe Sliced	1/4 cup (0.5 oz)	25	3	0	115
Ripe Small Pitted	6 (0.5 oz)	25	3	0	115
ONION					
canned					
chopped	1/2 cup	21	tr	0	416
whole	1 (2.2 oz)	12	tr	0	234
Boar's Head					
Sweet Vidalia In Sauce	1 tbsp	10	0	0	15
dried					
flakes	1 tbsp	16	tr	0	1
powder	1 tsp	7	tr	0	1
fresh					
chopped cooked	1/2 cup	47	tr	0	3
raw chopped	1/2 cup	30	tr	0	2
scallions raw chopped	1 tbsp	2	tr	0	1
Antioch Farms					
Vidalia	1 med	60	0	0	10
frozen					
chopped cooked	1/2 cup	30	tr	0	12
Birds Eye					
Diced	2/3 cup (3 oz)	30	0	0	30
Pearl Onions In Cream Sauce	1/2 cup (4.4 oz)	60	2	10	280
take-out					
rings breaded & fried	8 to 9	275	16	14	430
ORANGE					
canned					
Dole					
FruitBowls Mandarin Oranges	1 pkg (4 oz)	70	0	0	10
fresh					
california navel	1	65	tr	0	1
california valencia	1	59	tr	0	0
florida	1	69	tr	0	1
peel	1 tbsp	6	tr	0	0
sections	1 cup	85	tr	0	0

FOOD	PORTION	CALS	FAT	CHOL	SOD
ORANGE JUICE					
canned	1 cup	104	tr	0	6
chilled	1 cup	110	1	0	2
fresh	1 cup	111	tr	0	2
frozen as prep	1 cup	112	tr	0	2
frozen not prep	6 oz	339	tr	0	7
orange drink	6 oz	94	0	0	31
Big Juicy					
Drink	8 oz	110	0	0	55
Capri Sun					
Drink	1 pkg (7 oz)	100	0	0	20
Everfresh					
Juice	1 can (8 oz)	100	0	0	0
Ruby Red Orange Drink	1 can (8 oz)	130	0	0	0
Fresh Samantha					
Juice	1 cup (8 oz)	100	0	0	0
Horizon Organic					
Juice Pulp Free	8 oz	110	0	0	0
Juicy Juice					
Punch	1 box (4.23 oz)	60	0	0	5
Kool-Aid					
Drink Mix Orange as prep	1 serv (8 oz)	60	0	0	5
Orange Drink as prep w/ sugar	1 serv (8 oz)	100	0	0	10
Minute Maid					
Simply Orange 100%	8 oz	110	0	0	0
Simply Orange Calcium Fortified	8 oz	110	0	0	0
Simply Orange Grove Made	8 oz	110	0	0	0
Mott's					
100% Juice	1 box (8 oz)	130	0	0	10
100% Juice	8 oz	130	0	0	10
Nantucket Nectars					
100% Juice	8 oz	120	0	0	0
NutraShake					
Fourtified	1 pkg (4 oz)	50	0	0	0
Ocean Spray					
100% Juice	8 oz	120	0	0	35
Shasta Plus					
Orange Drink	1 can (11.5 oz)	160	0	0	45
Snapple					
Orangeade	8 oz	120	0	0	10
Tang					
Orange Drink as prep	1 serv (8 oz)	90	0	0	0
Sugar Free Orange as prep	1 serv (8 oz)	5	0	0	0
Tropicana					
Double Vitamin C	8 oz	110	0	0	0
Juice	8 oz	110	0	0	0
Ruby Red	8 oz	110	0	0	0

FOOD	PORTION	CALS	FAT	CHOL	SOD
Season's Best	8 oz	110	0	0	15
Season's Best Homestyle	8 oz	110	0	0	15
Tropical	8 oz	110	0	0	0
With Calcium	8 oz	110	0	0	0
Veryfine					
100% Juice	1 bottle (10 oz)	150	0	0	45
Chillers Arctic Orange	8 oz	130	0	0	10
Juice Blend	1 can (11.5 oz)	160	0	0	10
Orange Drink	1 bottle (10 oz)	160	0	0	90
OREGANO					
ground	1 tsp	5	tr	0	tr
ORGAN MEATS					
(*see* BRAINS, GIBLETS, GIZZARD, HEART, KIDNEY, LIVER, SWEETBREADS)					
ORIENTAL FOOD					
(*see* ASIAN FOOD, EGG ROLLS, DINNER, NOODLES, RICE, SUSHI)					
OYSTERS					
canned					
eastern	1 cup	170	6	136	277
fresh					
eastern cooked	6 med	58	2	46	94
eastern raw	6 med	58	2	46	94
take-out					
battered & fried	6 (4.9 oz)	368	18	109	677
breaded & fried	6 (4.9 oz)	368	18	109	677
oysters rockefeller	3 oysters	66	2	38	80
stew	1 cup	278	18	100	928
PANCAKE/WAFFLE SYRUP					
(*see also* SYRUP)					
maple	1 tbsp (0.8 oz)	52	0	0	2
pancake syrup	1 tbsp (0.7 oz)	57	0	0	17
Estee					
Maple	1/4 cup	80	0	0	125
Mrs. Butterworth's					
Original	1/4 cup (2 oz)	230	0	0	95
PANCAKES					
frozen					
buttermilk	1 (4 in diam) 1.3 oz	83	1	3	183
plain	1 (4 in diam) 1.3 oz	83	1	3	183
Eggo					
Buttermilk	3 (4.1 oz)	270	8	15	610
mix					
buckwheat	1 (4 in diam)	62	2	20	160
sugar free low sodium	1 (3 in diam)	44	tr	0	58
whole wheat	1 (4 in diam)	92	3	27	252
Betty Crocker					
Buttermilk as prep	3	200	3	10	540
Original as prep	3	200	3	10	540

FOOD	PORTION	CALS	FAT	CHOL	SOD
Bisquick					
Shake 'N Pour Blueberry as prep	3	210	4	0	640
Shake 'N Pour as prep	3	200	5	0	680
Bruce					
Sweet Potato Pancakes	2	210	3	0	670
Estee					
Pancake Mix as prep	4 (4 in diam)	180	0	0	255
Hungry Jack					
Potato as prep	3 (3 in diam)	90	2	50	380
Robin Hood					
Buttermilk as prep	3	230	6	60	560
take-out					
blueberry	1 (4 in diam)	84	4	21	157
buckwheat	1 (4 in diam)	55	2	20	125
potato	1 (4 in diam)	78	6	60	238
w/ butter & syrup	2 (8.1 oz)	520	14	58	1104
PANCREAS					
(*see* SWEETBREADS)					
PAPAYA					
fresh	1	117	tr	0	8
fresh cubed	1 cup	54	tr	0	4
PAPAYA JUICE					
nectar	1 cup	142	tr	0	14
Everfresh					
Premium Drink	1 can (8 oz)	140	0	0	0
Nantucket Nectars					
Cocktail	8 oz	120	0	0	0
PAPRIKA					
paprika	1 tsp	6	tr	0	1
PARSLEY					
dry	1 tsp	1	tr	0	1
dry	1 tbsp	1	tr	0	2
fresh chopped	1/2 cup	11	tr	0	17
PARSNIPS					
fresh sliced cooked	1/2 cup	63	tr	0	8
PASSION FRUIT					
purple fresh	1	18	tr	0	5
PASSION FRUIT JUICE					
yellow	1 cup	149	tr	0	15
PASTA					
(*see also* NOODLES, PASTA DINNERS, PASTA SALAD)					
dry					
corn cooked	1 cup (4.9 oz)	176	1	0	0
elbows cooked	1 cup (4.9 oz)	197	1	0	1
shells small cooked	1 cup (4 oz)	162	1	0	1
spinach spaghetti cooked	1 cup (4.9 oz)	182	1	0	20

FOOD	PORTION	CALS	FAT	CHOL	SOD
Annie Chun's					
Soba Noodles	2 oz	200	1	0	390
Barilla					
Conchiglie Rigate	1 cup (2 oz)	200	1	0	0
Gemelli	1 cup (2 oz)	200	1	0	0
Pennette Rigate	1 1/3 cups (2 oz)	200	1	0	0
Cuore					
Capellini cooked	1 1/3 cup (2 oz)	190	1	0	0
Fusilli cooked	1 1/3 cup (2 oz)	190	1	0	0
Tortiglioni cooked	1 1/3 cup (2 oz)	190	1	0	0
DeCecco					
Whole Wheat Linguine cooked	2 oz	180	2	<5	0
Eden					
Organic Endless Tubes	1/2 cup (1.9 oz)	210	1	0	0
Soba	2 oz	200	2	0	70
Somen	2 oz	200	2	0	80
Udon	2 oz	200	2	0	80
Udon Brown Rice	2 oz	200	2	0	80
Goya					
Coditos not prep	1/2 cup	230	1	0	0
Lundberg					
Spaghetti Organic Brown Rice	2 oz	210	2	0	5
fresh					
cooked	2 oz	75	1	33	3
spinach cooked	2 oz	74	1	19	3
Di Giorno					
Angel's Hair	1 cup	160	2	0	115
Beef & Roasted Garlic Tortellini	1 cup	340	11	50	390
Fettuccine	1 cup	200	2	0	140
Four Cheese Ravioli	1 cup	350	15	70	390
Herb Linguine	1 cup	200	2	0	140
Italian Sausage Ravioli In Green Bell Pepper Pasta	1 1/4 cup	350	12	55	570
Lemon Chicken Tortellini In Cracked Black Pepper Pasta	1 cup	270	5	40	290
Light Cheese Ravioli	1 cup	280	7	40	400
Linguine	1 cup	200	2	0	140
Mozzarella Garlic Tortelloni	1 cup	300	8	45	400
Pesto Tortelloni	1 cup	320	8	45	430
Portabello Mushroom Tortelloni	1 cup	310	7	40	490
Red Bell Pepper Fettuccine	1 cup	200	2	0	140
Spinach Fettuccine	1 cup	190	2	0	160

FOOD	PORTION	CALS	FAT	CHOL	SOD
Di Giorno (cont.)					
Sun-Dried Tomato Ravioli	1 1/3 cup	380	14	55	600
Three Cheese Tortellini	3/4 cup	250	7	35	300
PASTA DINNERS					
(*see also* DINNER, PASTA SALAD)					
canned					
Chef Boyardee					
Beef Ravioli 99% Fat Free	1 cup (8.6 oz)	210	1	15	1150
Franco-American					
Beef Raviolios	1 can (7.7 oz)	250	5	12	911
Beefy Mac	1 can (7.5 oz)	228	8	10	1144
Elbow Macaroni & Cheese	1 can (7.5 oz)	187	6	7	875
Spaghetti 'N Beef	1 can (7.5 oz)	226	8	14	1063
Spaghetti w/ Meatballs	1 can (7.2 oz)	249	9	14	917
Kid's Kitchen					
Microwave Meals Cheezy Mac & Beef	1 cup (7.5 oz)	260	7	30	910
Microwave Meals Noodle Rings & Chicken	1 cup (7.5 oz)	150	4	30	1110
Microwave Meals Spaghetti Rings & Franks	1 cup (7.5 oz)	240	9	30	810
Progresso					
Beef Ravioli	1 cup (9.1 oz)	260	5	5	940
Cheese Ravioli	1 cup (9.1 oz)	220	2	<5	930
frozen					
Amy's Organic					
Macaroni & Cheese	1 pkg (9 oz)	390	14	40	550
Macaroni & Soy Cheese	1 pkg (9 oz)	360	14	0	500
Pasta Primavera	1 pkg (9.5 oz)	320	12	65	680
Ravioli w/ Sauce	1 pkg (9.5 oz)	340	12	20	580
Tofu Vegetable Lasagna	1 pkg (9.5 oz)	300	10	0	630
Vegetable Lasagna	1 pkg (9.5 oz)	300	10	15	680
Whole Meals Cannelloni	1 pkg (9 oz)	260	11	20	560
Birds Eye					
Easy Recipe Meal Starter Cheesy Cheese	1 serv	280	8	69	336
Easy Recipe Meal Starter Chicken Primavera as prep	1 serv	280	8	69	336
Easy Recipe Meal Starter Chicken Alfredo as prep	1 serv	280	8	69	336
Pasta Secrets Creamy Peppercorn	2 1/3 cups (6.6 oz)	300	15	25	460
Pasta Secrets Italian Pesto	2 1/3 cups (6.4 oz)	240	9	5	700
Pasta Secrets Primavera	2 1/3 cups (6.6 oz)	230	10	10	430
Pasta Secrets Three Cheese	2 cups (6.1 oz)	230	8	5	590
Pasta Secrets White Cheddar	2 cups (6.3 oz)	240	10	10	560
Pasta Secrets Zesty Garlic	2 cups (5.9 oz)	240	10	5	310

FOOD	PORTION	CALS	FAT	CHOL	SOD
Green Giant					
Create A Meal Creamy Alfredo as prep	1 1/4 cups (10 oz)	380	12	75	990
Create A Meal Creamy Cheddar as prep	1 1/2 cups (10 oz)	290	10	45	1470
Create A Meal Creamy Chicken Noodle as prep	1 1/4 cups (10 oz)	350	11	65	970
Pasta Accents Alfredo	2 cups (5.6 oz)	210	5	15	480
Pasta Accents Creamy Cheddar	2 1/3 cups (6.7 oz)	250	8	15	700
Pasta Accents Florentine	2 cups (7.3 oz)	310	9	20	910
Pasta Accents Garden Herb Seasoning	2 cups (6.8 oz)	230	7	15	750
Pasta Accents Garlic Seasoning	2 cups (6.6 oz)	260	10	15	640
Pasta Accents Primavera	2 1/4 cups (7 oz)	320	12	20	500
Pasta Accents White Cheddar Sauce	1 3/4 cups (5.6 oz)	300	12	20	570
Lean Cuisine					
Cafe Classics Bow Tie Pasta & Chicken	1 pkg (9.5 oz)	220	4	40	690
Cafe Classics Cheese Lasagna w/ Chicken Scaloppini	1 pkg (10 oz)	270	8	35	690
Cafe Classics Shrimp & Angel Hair Pasta	1 pkg (10 oz)	240	5	45	670
Everyday Favorites	1 pkg (10 oz)	270	6	10	590
Everyday Favorites Alfredo Pasta Primavera	1 pkg (10 oz)	290	7	10	570
Everyday Favorites Angel Hair Pasta	1 pkg (10 oz)	240	4	5	500
Everyday Favorites Cheese Cannelloni	1 pkg (9.1 oz)	230	4	15	590
Everyday Favorites Cheese Ravioli	1 pkg (8.5 oz)	260	7	35	590
Everyday Favorites Chicken Lasagna	1 pkg (10 oz)	280	7	40	590
Everyday Favorites Classic Cheese Lasagna	1 pkg (11.5 oz)	290	6	25	590
Everyday Favorites Fettucini Alfredo	1 pkg (9.25 oz)	280	7	15	540
Everyday Favorites Fettucini Primavera	1 pkg (10 oz)	270	7	15	580
Everyday Favorites Lasagna w/ Meat Sauce	1 pkg (10.5 oz)	300	8	30	570
Everyday Favorites Macaroni & Cheese	1 pkg (10 oz)	290	7	20	630

FOOD	PORTION	CALS	FAT	CHOL	SOD
Lean Cuisine (cont.)					
Everyday Favorites Macaroni & Beef	1 pkg (10 oz)	270	4	25	590
Everyday Favorites Penne Pasta	1 pkg (10 oz)	260	4	0	390
Everyday Favorites Spaghetti w/ Meat Sauce	1 pkg (11.5 oz)	290	5	20	570
Everyday Favorites Spaghetti w/ Meatballs	1 pkg (9.5 oz)	270	6	20	590
Family Style Favorites Five Cheese Lasagna	1 serv (8 oz)	210	5	20	690
Skillet Sensations Chicken Alfredo	1 serv	280	6	30	590
Stouffer's					
Cheddar Pasta w/ Beef & Tomatoes	1 pkg (11 oz)	450	19	51	1130
Cheese Manicotti	1 pkg (9 oz)	380	17	45	880
Cheese Ravioli	1 pkg (10.6 oz)	380	13	100	700
Chicken Lasagna	1 serv (7.8 oz)	320	17	30	750
Fettucini Alfredo	1 pkg (10 oz)	520	28	100	1060
Fettucini Primavera	1 pkg (10 oz)	430	20	50	1100
Five Cheese Lasagna	1 pkg (10.75 oz)	360	13	35	960
Grilled Chicken & Angel Hair Pasta	1 pkg (10.9 oz)	380	13	40	750
Homestyle Chicken Fettucini	1 pkg (10.5 oz)	390	15	65	1250
Homestyle Chicken Parmigiana w/ Spaghetti	1 pkg (12 oz)	460	16	45	1060
Homestyle Veal Parmigiana w/ Spaghetti	1 pkg (11.9 oz)	430	17	80	1120
Lasagna Bake	1 pkg (10.25 oz)	370	12	30	900
Lasagna w/ Meat Sauce	1 pkg (10.5 oz)	370	14	45	1050
Macaroni & Cheese	1 cup (6 oz)	320	16	30	990
Macaroni & Cheese w/ Broccoli	1 pkg (10.5 oz)	360	17	25	1050
Macaroni & Beef	1 pkg (11.5 oz)	420	20	50	1530
Noodles Romanoff	1 pkg (12 oz)	490	25	60	1400
Pasta Shells w/ American Cheese	1 cup (6 oz)	260	10	20	1190
Salisbury Steak w/ Macaroni & Cheese	1 serv (11.3 oz)	410	19	70	1230
Spaghetti w/ Meat Sauce	1 pkg (10 oz)	350	12	35	570
Spaghetti w/ Meatballs	1 pkg (12.6 oz)	440	15	50	830
Tuna Noodle Casserole	1 pkg (10 oz)	320	10	40	1130
Turkey Tettrazini	1 pkg (10 oz)	360	17	55	1060
Vegetable Lasagna	1 pkg (10.5 oz)	440	20	35	1110
Weight Watchers					
Garden Lasagna	1 pkg (11 oz)	270	7	30	610
Homestyle Macaroni & Cheese	1 pkg (9 oz)	290	7	10	630
Smart Ones Angel Hair Pasta	1 pkg (9 oz)	180	2	0	600

FOOD	PORTION	CALS	FAT	CHOL	SOD
Smart Ones Bowtie Pasta & Mushrooms Marsala	1 pkg (9.65 oz)	270	7	40	520
Smart Ones Chicken Fettucini	1 pkg (10 oz)	300	7	70	590
Smart Ones Creamy Rigatoni w/ Broccoli & Chicken	1 pkg (9 oz)	230	2	20	670
Smart Ones Fettucini Alfredo w/ Broccoli	1 pkg (8.5 oz)	230	6	20	540
Smart Ones Lasagna Florentine	1 pkg (10 oz)	200	2	10	640
Smart Ones Lasagna Alfredo	1 pkg (9 oz)	300	7	25	680
Smart Ones Lasagna w/ Meat Sauce	1 pkg (10.25 oz)	270	6	55	570
Smart Ones Lasagna w/ Meat Sauce	1 pkg (9 oz)	240	2	10	520
Smart Ones Macaroni & Cheese	1 pkg (9 oz)	220	2	5	640
Smart Ones Pasta & Spinach Romano	1 pkg (10.4 oz)	260	8	15	510
Smart Ones Pasta w/ Tomato Basil Sauce	1 pkg (9.6 oz)	260	7	10	360
Smart Ones Penne Pasta w/ Sun-Dried Tomatoes	1 pkg (10 oz)	280	8	15	560
Smart Ones Penne Pollo	1 pkg (10 oz)	290	6	55	590
Smart Ones Ravioli Florentine	1 pkg (8.5 oz)	220	2	5	490
Smart Ones Spaghetti Marinara	1 pkg (9 oz)	280	7	5	690
Smart Ones Spaghetti w/ Meat Sauce	1 pkg (10 oz)	280	6	15	560
Smart Ones Spicy Penne & Ricotta	1 pkg (10.2 oz)	280	6	5	400
Smart Ones Tuna Noodle Casserole	1 pkg (9.5 oz)	270	7	45	670
Smart Ones Ziti Mozzarella	1 pkg (9 oz)	290	7	5	600
Yves					
Veggie Lasagna	1 pkg (10.5 oz)	300	3	0	650
Veggie Macaroni	1 pkg (10.5 oz)	230	2	0	580
Veggie Penne	1 pkg (10.5 oz)	220	2	0	730
mix					
Hamburger Helper					
Ravioli as prep	1 cup	280	10	50	840
Ravioli w/ White Cheese Topping as prep	1 cup	310	10	50	960
Kraft					
Deluxe Macaroni & Cheese Four Cheese Blend as prep	1 cup (6.2 oz)	320	10	25	910
Deluxe Macaroni & Cheese Original as prep	1 cup (6.1 oz)	320	10	25	730

FOOD	PORTION	CALS	FAT	CHOL	SOD
Kraft (cont.)					
Light Deluxe Macaroni & Cheese as prep	1 cup (6.5 oz)	290	5	15	810
Macaroni & Cheese All Shapes as prep	1 cup (6.9 oz)	410	18	10	750
Macaroni & Cheese Original as prep	1 cup (6.9 oz)	410	18	10	750
Macaroni & Cheese Original as prep light recipe	1 cup (6.4 oz)	290	6	10	580
Premium Macaroni & Cheese Cheesy Alfredo as prep	1 cup (6.9 oz)	410	19	10	810
Premium Macaroni & Cheese Mild White Cheddar as prep	1 cup (6.8 oz)	410	19	10	740
Premium Macaroni & Cheese Thick 'N Creamy as prep	1 cup (7.6 oz)	420	19	15	760
Premium Macaroni & Cheese Three Cheese as prep	1 cup (6.9 oz)	410	18	10	790
Spaghetti Classics Mild Italian as prep	1 cup (9.1 oz)	240	3	<5	850
Spaghetti Classics Tangy Italian as prep	1 cup (8.9 oz)	240	2	0	830
Spaghetti Classics Zesty Cheese as prep	1 cup (8.6 oz)	240	2	5	800
Spaghetti Classics w/ Meat Sauce as prep	1 cup (8.2 oz)	330	10	15	810
Lipton					
Pasta & Sauce Angel Hair Chicken Broccoli as prep	1 cup	260	8	0	810
Pasta & Sauce Angel Hair Parmesan as prep	1 cup	280	11	10	960
Pasta & Sauce Bow Tie Chicken Primavera as prep	1 cup	290	10	10	820
Pasta & Sauce Bow Tie Italian Cheese as prep	1 cup	300	12	15	900
Pasta & Sauce Butter & Herbs as prep	1 cup	270	10	5	830
Pasta & Sauce Cheddar Broccoli as prep	1 cup	340	11	15	970
Pasta & Sauce Chicken Herb Parmesan as prep	1 cup	80	9	5	910
Pasta & Sauce Chicken Stir-Fry as prep	1 cup	270	8	0	900
Pasta & Sauce Creamy Garlic as prep	1 cup	350	13	15	980
Pasta & Sauce Creamy Mushroom as prep	1 cup	320	11	15	870

FOOD	PORTION	CALS	FAT	CHOL	SOD
Pasta & Sauce Garlic & Butter Linguine as prep	1 cup	260	9	5	850
Pasta & Sauce Mild Cheddar Cheese as prep	1 cup	290	10	10	930
Pasta & Sauce Roasted Garlic Chicken as prep	1 cup	290	10	10	880
Pasta & Sauce Roasted Garlic & Olive Oil w/ Tomato as prep	1 cup	270	9	0	880
Pasta & Sauce Rotini Primavera as prep	1 cup	320	12	15	980
Pasta & Sauce Savory Herb w/ Garlic as prep	1 cup	280	9	5	890
Pasta & Sauce Three Cheese Rotini as prep	1 cup	320	12	15	970
Melting Pot					
Terrazza Black Beans & Penne	1 cup	180	1	0	480
Terrazza Florentine Red Beans & Fusilli	1 cup	220	1	<5	350
Terrazza Red Lentils & Bow Ties	1 cup	240	2	40	390
Terrazza Tuscan White Beans & Gemelli	1 cup	220	1	<5	450
Velveeta					
Rotini & Cheese w/ Broccoli as prep	1 cup (7.2 oz)	400	16	50	1230
Shells & Cheese Bacon as prep	1 cup (6.8 oz)	360	14	40	1140
Shells & Cheese Original as prep	1 cup (6.6 oz)	360	13	40	1030
Shells & Cheese Salsa as prep	1 cup (7.5 oz)	380	14	40	1180
ready-to-eat					
Tyson					
Rosemary Penne	1 pkg (12.5 oz)	330	5	45	860
shelf-stable					
Hormel					
Microcup Meals Lasagna	1 cup (7.5 oz)	250	14	25	950
Microcup Meals Macaroni & Cheese	1 cup (7.5 oz)	260	11	35	690
Microcup Meals Ravioli w/ Tomato Sauce	1 cup (7.5 oz)	220	6	15	840
Microcup Meals Spaghetti & Meatballs	1 cup (7.5 oz)	220	7	25	930
Kid's Kitchen					
Microwave Meals Beefy Macaroni	1 cup (7.5 oz)	190	6	30	790
Microwave Meals Macaroni & Cheese	1 cup (7.5 oz)	260	11	35	690

FOOD	PORTION	CALS	FAT	CHOL	SOD
Kid's Kitchen (cont.)					
Microwave Meals Mini Ravioli	1 cup (7.5 oz)	240	7	20	950
Microwave Meals Spaghetti & Meatballs	1 cup (7.5 oz)	220	7	25	950
Microwave Meals Spaghetti Rings & Meatballs	1 cup (7.5 oz)	250	7	20	1200
Lunch Bucket					
Beef Ravioli In Tomato Sauce	1 pkg (7.5 oz)	180	4	5	740
Italian Pasta w/ Chicken	1 pkg (7.5 oz)	130	2	10	610
Lasagna 'n Meatsauce	1 pkg (7.5 oz)	160	3	5	850
Macaroni 'n Beef in Meatsauce	1 pkg (7.5 oz)	180	5	10	820
Macaroni 'n Cheese	1 pkg (7.5 oz)	190	7	20	930
Pasta 'n Chicken	1 pkg (7.5 oz)	150	5	20	810
Spaghetti 'n Meatsauce	1 pkg (7.5 oz)	160	3	5	850
take-out					
macaroni & cheese	1 cup	230	10	24	730
manicotti	3/4 cup (6.4 oz)	273	12	77	414
rigatoni w/ sausage sauce	3/4 cup	260	12	59	106
spaghetti w/ meatballs & cheese	1 cup	407	19	104	696
PASTA SALAD					
mix					
Kraft					
Herb & Garlic as prep	3/4 cup (4.9 oz)	280	14	0	670
Pasta Salad Classic Ranch w/ Bacon as prep	3/4 cup (4.7 oz)	350	22	10	480
Pasta Salad Creamy Ceasar as prep	3/4 cup (4.8 oz)	340	21	15	630
Pasta Salad Garden Primavera as prep	3/4 cup (5 oz)	240	8	<5	710
Pasta Salad Italian 97% Fat Free as prep	3/4 cup (4.9 oz)	190	2	<5	740
Pasta Salad Parmesan Peppercorn as prep	3/4 cup (4.9 oz)	360	23	15	570
Suddenly Salad					
Classic Pasta	3/4 cup	250	8	0	910
Classic Pasta Reduced Fat Recipe	3/4 cup	210	4	0	910
Garden Italian 98% Fat Free	3/4 cup	140	1	0	520
take-out					
elbow macaroni salad	3.5 oz	160	5	0	590
italian style pasta salad	3.5 oz	140	7	0	480
mustard macaroni salad	3.5 oz	190	10	0	560
pasta salad w/ vegetables	3.5 oz	140	4	0	210

PASTRY

(*see* BROWNIE, CAKE, DANISH PASTRY)

FOOD	PORTION	CALS	FAT	CHOL	SOD
PATÉ					
antipasto paté	1 can (2.25 oz)	110	9	5	530
mushroom anchovy paté	1 can (2.25 oz)	130	11	5	400
paté foie gras	1 oz	127	13	109	211
pork paté	1 oz	107	10	51	189
pork paté en croute	1 oz	91	7	32	214
rabbit paté	1 oz	66	5	21	97
salmon paté	1 can (2.25 oz)	140	10	10	420
shrimp	1 can (2.25 oz)	140	10	25	450
smoked turkey	1 can (2.25 oz)	170	13	15	480
PEACH					
canned					
halves in heavy syrup	1 half	60	tr	0	5
halves in light syrup	1 half	44	tr	0	4
halves juice pack	1 half	34	tr	0	3
halves water pack	1 half	18	tr	0	3
spiced in heavy syrup	1 fruit	66	tr	0	3
spiced in heavy syrup	1 cup	180	tr	0	9
Del Monte					
Fruit Pleasures Raspberry Flavored Peaches	1/2 cup (4.5 oz)	80	0	0	10
Sliced Cling Fruit Naturals	1/2 cup (4.4 oz)	60	0	0	10
dried					
halves	10	311	1	0	9
halves cooked w/o sugar	1/2 cup	99	tr	0	3
fresh					
peach	1	37	tr	0	0
sliced	1 cup	73	tr	0	1
frozen					
slices sweetened	1 cup	235	tr	0	16
PEACH JUICE					
nectar	1 cup	134	tr	0	17
Nantucket Nectars					
The Original	8 oz	120	0	0	15
PEANUT BUTTER					
chunky	2 tbsp	188	16	0	156
chunky w/o salt	2 tbsp	188	16	0	5
smooth	2 tbsp	188	16	0	153
smooth w/o salt	2 tbsp	188	16	0	5
Estee					
Creamy Low Sodium	2 tbsp (1 oz)	190	15	0	0
Jif					
Creamy	2 tbsp (1.1 oz)	190	16	0	150
Extra Crunchy	2 tbsp (1.1 oz)	190	16	0	130
Reese's					
Peanut Butter Chips	1 tbsp (0.5 oz)	80	4	0	35
Tree Of Life					
Peanut Wonder	2 tbsp (1.1 oz)	100	3	0	220

FOOD	PORTION	CALS	FAT	CHOL	SOD
PEANUTS					
chocolate coated	10 (1.4 oz)	208	13	4	16
cooked	1/2 cup	102	7	0	240
dry roasted w/ salt	30 nuts (1 oz)	170	14	0	230
Estee					
Candy Coated	1/4 cup	200	9	<5	45
Frito Lay					
Honey Roasted	1 serv (1.5 oz)	270	21	0	80
Hot	1 serv (1.1 oz)	190	16	0	250
Salted	1 oz	200	16	0	180
Lance					
Honey Toasted	1 pkg (1 3/8 oz)	220	15	0	170
Roasted	1 pkg (1 3/4 oz)	190	14	0	0
Salted	1 pkg (1 1/8 oz)	200	15	0	150
Salted Long Tube	1/4 cup (1 oz)	180	14	0	135
Little Debbie					
Salted	1/4 cup (1 oz)	160	14	0	130
Pennant					
Oil Roasted	1 oz	170	14	0	115
Tom's					
Double Coated	1 pkg (1.35 oz)	220	15	0	60
Toasted	1 pkg (1.4 oz)	240	19	0	160
Weight Watchers					
Honey Roasted	1 pkg (0.7 oz)	100	5	0	100
PEAR					
canned					
halves in heavy syrup	1 half	68	tr	0	4
halves in light syrup	1 half	45	tr	0	4
halves water pack	1 half	22	tr	0	41
dried					
halves	10	459	1	0	10
halves cooked w/o sugar	1/2 cup	163	tr	0	4
fresh					
asian	1 (4.3 oz)	51	tr	0	0
pear	1	98	1	0	1
sliced w/ skin	1 cup	97	1	0	1
PEAR JUICE					
nectar	1 cup	149	tr	0	9
PEAS					
canned					
Green Giant					
Sweet	1/2 cup (4.3 oz)	60	0	0	390
Sweet 50% Less Sodium	1/2 cup (4.3 oz)	60	0	0	195
LeSueur					
Early Peas	1/2 cup (4.2 oz)	60	0	0	380
Early Peas 50% Less Sodium	1/2 cup (4.2 oz)	60	0	0	190
Sweet	1/2 cup (4.2 oz)	60	0	0	380
Sweet 50% Less Sodium	1/2 cup (4.2 oz)	60	0	0	190

FOOD	PORTION	CALS	FAT	CHOL	SOD
dried					
split cooked	1 cup	231	1	0	4
Bascom's					
Yellow Split as prep	1/2 cup	110	0	0	0
Hurst					
HamBeens Green Split Peas w/ Ham	1 serv	120	1	0	63
fresh					
green cooked	1/2 cup	67	tr	0	2
green raw	1/2 cup	58	tr	0	3
snap peas cooked	1/2 cup	34	tr	0	3
snap peas raw	1/2 cup	30	tr	0	3
frozen					
green cooked	1/2 cup	63	tr	0	70
snap peas cooked	1/2 cup	42	tr	0	4
snap peas cooked	1 pkg (10 oz)	132	1	0	12
Birds Eye					
Baby Pea Blend	3/4 cup (2.6 oz)	40	0	0	40
Baby Sweet	2/3 cup (3.1 oz)	70	1	0	105
Field Peas w/ Snaps	2/3 cup (3.4 oz)	130	1	0	15
Purple Hull Peas	1/2 cup (2.8 oz)	110	1	0	10
Green Giant					
Butter Sauce	3/4 cup (4 oz)	100	2	<5	400
Butter Sauce LeSueur Baby Baby Peas	3/4 cup (4 oz)	100	2	<5	370
Harvest Fresh LeSueur Baby Peas	2/3 cup (3.2 oz)	70	0	0	220
Harvest Fresh Sugar Snap	2/3 cup (3.2 oz)	50	0	0	95
Harvest Fresh Sweet	2/3 cup (3.3 oz)	60	0	0	200
LaSueur Baby Sweet	2/3 cup (2.8 oz)	60	0	0	150
LaSueur Early June	2/3 cup (2.8 oz)	80	0	0	150
LaSueur Early June w/ Mushrooms	3/4 cup (3 oz)	60	0	0	105
Select Sugar Snap	3/4 cup (2.8 oz)	35	0	0	0
Sweet	2/3 cup (3.1 oz)	70	0	0	135
PECANS					
halves dry roasted w/ salt	20 (1 oz)	200	21	0	110
PECTIN					
Slim Set					
Powder	1 tbsp	3	0	0	1
Sure Jell					
For Lower Sugar Recipes	1/4 tsp (0.7 g)	5	0	0	10
Pectin	1/4 tsp (0.9 g)	5	0	0	0
PEPEAO					
dried	1/2 cup	36	tr	0	8
raw sliced	1 cup	25	tr	0	9

FOOD	PORTION	CALS	FAT	CHOL	SOD
PEPPER					
black	1 tsp	5	tr	0	1
cayenne	1 tsp	6	tr	0	1
red	1 tsp	6	tr	0	1
white	1 tsp	7	tr	0	tr
PEPPERS					
canned					
Chi-Chi's					
Chilies Diced Green	2 tbsp (1.2 oz)	10	0	0	20
Chilies Green Whole	3/4 pepper (1 oz)	10	0	0	15
Progresso					
Cherry Sliced & So Hot	2 tbsp (1 oz)	25	2	0	30
Hot Cherry	1 (1 oz)	10	0	0	150
Pepper Salad (drained)	2 tbsp (1 oz)	15	1	0	160
Roasted	1 piece (1 oz)	10	0	0	55
Sweet Fried w/ Onions	2 tbsp (0.9 oz)	20	2	0	130
Tuscan	3 (1 oz)	10	0	0	450
Rosarita					
Chilies Diced Green	2 tbsp (1 oz)	6	tr	0	85
Chilies Green Strips	1/4 cup (1.2 oz)	5	tr	0	74
Chilies Whole Green	2 tbsp (1.2 oz)	5	tr	0	74
Jalapeno Whole w/ Escabeche	1/4 cup (1.2 oz)	8	tr	0	430
Jalapenos Diced	2 tbsp (1 oz)	5	tr	0	121
Jalapenos Nacho Sliced	2 tbsp (1 oz)	2	tr	0	224
Vlasic					
Hot Sliced Cherry	1 oz	5	0	0	480
Jalapeno Sliced	1 oz	10	0	0	480
Mild Cherry	1 oz	5	0	0	480
Pepper Rings Hot	1 oz	5	0	0	480
Pepper Rings Mild	1 oz	5	0	0	480
dried					
ancho	1 (0.6 oz)	48	1	0	7
green	1 tbsp	1	tr	0	1
pasilla	1 (7 g)	24	1	0	6
red	1 tbsp	1	tr	0	1
fresh					
banana raw	1 (4 in) (1.2 oz)	9	tr	0	4
chili green hot raw	1	18	tr	0	3
chili red hot raw	1 (1.6 oz)	18	tr	0	3
green raw	1 (2.6 oz)	20	tr	0	1
hungarian raw	1 (0.9 oz)	8	tr	0	tr
jalapeno raw	1 (0.5 oz)	4	tr	0	tr
red raw	1 (2.6 oz)	20	tr	0	1
serrano raw	1 (6 g)	2	tr	0	1
yellow raw	1 (6.5 oz)	50	tr	0	3
frozen					
Birds Eye					
Diced Green	3/4 cup (2.9 oz)	20	0	0	10

FOOD	PORTION	CALS	FAT	CHOL	SOD
PERCH					
fresh					
cooked	3 oz	99	1	98	67
PERSIMMONS					
dried japanese	1	93	tr	0	1
fresh	1	32	tr	0	0
fresh japanese	1	118	tr	0	3
PHEASANT					
roasted	3.5 oz	215	9	120	100
PHYLLO DOUGH					
phyllo dough	1 oz	85	2	0	137
sheet	1	57	1	0	92
PICANTE					
(see SALSA)					
PICKLES					
Claussen					
Bread 'N Butter Chips	4 slices (1 oz)	20	0	0	170
Kosher Dill Spears	1 spear (1.2 oz)	5	0	0	320
Kosher Dills Halves	1 half (1 oz)	5	0	0	330
Kosher Dills Mini	1 (0.8 oz)	5	0	0	300
Sandwich Slices Deli Style Hearty Garlic	2 (1.2 oz)	5	0	0	320
Sandwich Slices Kosher Dills	2 (1.2 oz)	5	0	0	440
Super Slices For Burgers	1 (0.8 oz)	5	0	0	320
Vlasic					
Hamburger Dill Chips	1 oz	5	0	0	400
Kosher Cross Cuts	1 oz	5	0	0	220
Kosher Spears	1 oz	5	0	0	220
Kosher Whole	1 oz	5	0	0	220
Sweet Butter Chips	1 oz	30	0	0	190
Sweet Gerkins	1 oz	35	0	0	260
Whole Dills	1 oz	5	0	0	390
PIE					
(see also PIE CRUST)					
filling					
apple	1 can (21 oz)	599	1	0	259
Comstock					
MoreFruit Light Cherry	1/3 cup (2.9 oz)	60	0	0	30
Libby					
Pumpkin Pie Mix	1/3 cup	90	1	0	115
frozen					
Mrs. Smith's					
Peach Deep Dish	1/12 pie (4.1 oz)	300	14	0	330
Sara Lee					
Chocolate Silk	1/5 pie (4.8 oz)	500	32	<5	440
Coconut Cream	1/5 pie (4.8 oz)	480	31	0	430
Fruit's Of The Forest	1/8 pie (4.6 oz)	340	19	0	420

FOOD	PORTION	CALS	FAT	CHOL	SOD
Sara Lee (cont.)					
Homestyle Apple	1/8 pie (4.6 oz)	340	16	0	310
Homestyle Blueberry	1/8 pie (4.6 oz)	360	15	0	340
Homestyle Cherry	1/8 pie (4.6 oz)	330	15	0	290
Homestyle Dutch Apple	1/8 pie (4.6 oz)	350	15	0	320
Homestyle Mince	1/8 pie (4.6 oz)	390	17	0	450
Homestyle Peach	1/8 pie (4.6 oz)	330	13	0	250
Homestyle Pecan	1/8 pie (4.2 oz)	520	24	45	480
Homestyle Pumpkin	1/8 pie (4.6 oz)	260	11	30	460
Homestyle Raspberry	1/8 pie (4.6 oz)	380	19	5	330
Lemon Meringue	1/6 pie (5 oz)	350	11	0	460
Slice Lemon Icebox	1 (3.5 oz)	260	9	<5	180
Slice Southern Pecan	1 (4 oz)	470	23	25	420
Weight Watchers					
Mississippi Mud	1 piece (2.45 oz)	160	5	5	120
mix					
Jell-O					
No Bake Chocolate Silk as prep	1/6 pie (4.4 oz)	320	16	5	490
snack					
Dolly Madison					
Apple	1 (4.5 oz)	480	22	15	390
Blueberry	1 (4.5 oz)	480	21	20	460
Cherry	1 (4.5 oz)	470	22	20	470
Chocolate Pudding	1 (4.5 oz)	530	25	30	410
Lemon	1 (4.5 oz)	500	24	20	430
Peach	1 (4.5 oz)	480	21	25	460
Pecan	1 (3 oz)	360	19	70	320
Pecan Fried	1 (4.5 oz)	530	21	10	430
Pineapple	1 (4.5 oz)	460	21	15	340
Hostess					
Apple	1 (4.5 oz)	480	22	15	390
Blackberry	1 (4.5 oz)	520	21	15	400
Blueberry	1 (4.5 oz)	480	21	20	460
Cherry	1 (4.5 oz)	470	22	20	470
French Apple	1 (4.5 oz)	480	22	15	390
Lemon	1 (4.5 oz)	500	24	20	430
Peach	1 (4.5 oz)	480	21	25	460
Pineapple	1 (4.5 oz)	460	21	15	430
Strawberry	1 (4.5 oz)	510	23	15	360
Lance					
Pecan	1 (3 oz)	350	17	25	200
Tastykake					
Apple	1 (4 oz)	270	11	0	300
Blueberry	1 (4 oz)	300	11	0	300
Cherry	1 (4 oz)	290	11	0	300
Coconut Creme	1 (4 oz)	370	21	55	420
French Apple	1 (4.2 oz)	310	11	0	290

FOOD	PORTION	CALS	FAT	CHOL	SOD
Lemon	1 (4 oz)	300	13	40	320
Peach	1 (4 oz)	280	11	0	300
Pineapple	1 (4 oz)	290	12	20	310
Pineapple Cheese	1 (4 oz)	320	12	20	410
Pumpkin	1 (4 oz)	340	14	35	530
Strawberry	1 (3.5 oz)	320	12	0	300
Tastyklair	1 (4 oz)	400	20	90	290
Tom's					
Apple	1 pkg (3 oz)	330	17	5	250
Banana Marshmallow	1 pkg (2.75 oz)	320	11	0	190
Cherry	1 pkg (3 oz)	320	18	5	240
Chocolate Marshmallow	1 pkg (2.75 oz)	320	11	0	190
take-out					
apple	1/8 of 9 in pie	411	19	0	327
banana cream	1/8 of 9 in pie	398	20	75	355
blueberry	1/8 of 9 in pie	360	18	0	272
butterscotch	1/8 of 9 in pie	355	18	78	335
cherry	1/8 of 9 in pie	486	22	0	343
coconut creme	1/8 of 9 in pie	396	21	77	356
coconut custard	1/6 of 8 in pie	271	14	36	348
custard	1/8 of 9 in pie	262	11	87	256
lemon meringue	1/8 of 9 in pie	362	16	68	307
mince	1/8 of 9 in pie	477	18	0	419
pecan	1/6 of 8 in pie	452	21	36	480
pumpkin	1/6 of 8 in pie	229	10	22	308
vanilla cream	1/8 of 9 in pie	350	18	78	327
PIE CRUST					
(*see also* PIE)					
frozen					
Pepperidge Farm					
Puff Pastry Sheets	1/6 sheet (1.4 oz)	170	11	0	200
Puff Pastry Shell	1 (1.6 oz)	190	13	0	230
Puff Pastry Squares	1 sq (2 oz)	240	16	0	250
Pet-Ritz					
Deep Dish	1/8 pie (0.7 oz)	90	5	<5	75
Regular	1/8 pie (0.6 oz)	80	5	<5	60
Tart Shells	1 (1 oz)	130	8	0	170
mix					
as prep	9 in crust (5.6 oz)	801	49	0	1167
Betty Crocker					
Pie Crust	1/8 crust	110	8	0	150
ready-to-eat					
chocolate cookie crumb baked	1/8 of 9 in pie (1 oz)	139	9	0	185
graham cracker baked	1/8 of 9 in pie (1 oz)	148	8	0	171
vanilla wafer cracker crumbs baked	1/8 of 9 in pie (0.8 oz)	119	8	9	116
Keebler					
Graham Single Serve	1 (0.8 oz)	120	6	0	150

FOOD	PORTION	CALS	FAT	CHOL	SOD
refrigerated					
All Ready					
Crust	1/8 pie (0.9 oz)	120	7	5	100
PIEROGI					
Health Is Wealth					
Potato & Cheddar	2 (2.8 oz)	140	2	0	360
Potato & Onion	2 (2.8 oz)	140	2	0	300
Mrs. T's					
Jalapeno & Cheddar	3 (4.2 oz)	190	3	10	490
Potato & Cheddar	3 (4.2 oz)	180	3	10	430
Potato & Onion	3 (4.2 oz)	180	2	<5	340
Sweet Potato	3 (4.2 oz)	300	0	<5	250
PIG'S EARS AND FEET					
ear simmered	1	184	12	100	185
Hormel					
Pickled Feet	2 oz	80	6	45	530
Pickled Hocks	2 oz	110	8	45	530
PIGEON					
w/ skin & bone	3.5 oz	169	10	110	90
PIGEON PEAS					
dried cooked	1/2 cup	102	tr	0	5
PIGNOLIA					
(*see* PINE NUTS)					
PIKE					
northern cooked	3 oz	96	1	43	42
walleye baked	3 oz	101	1	94	56
PILLNUTS					
canarytree dried	1 oz	204	23	0	1
PIMIENTOS					
canned	1 slice	0	0	0	0
canned	1 tbsp	3	tr	0	2
Dromedary					
Peeled	1/2 tsp (4 g)	0	0	0	0
Unpeeled	1/2 tsp (4 g)	0	0	0	0
PINE NUTS					
pignolia dried	1 oz	146	14	0	1
pignolia dried	1 tbsp	51	5	0	0
pinyon dried	1 oz	161	17	0	20
Progresso					
Pignoli	1 jar (1 oz)	170	13	0	0
PINEAPPLE					
canned					
chunks in heavy syrup	1 cup	199	tr	0	3
chunks juice pack	1 cup	150	tr	0	4
crushed in heavy syrup	1 cup	199	tr	0	3
slices in heavy syrup	1 slice	45	tr	0	1
slices in light syrup	1 slice	30	tr	0	1

FOOD	PORTION	CALS	FAT	CHOL	SOD
slices juice pack	1 slice	35	tr	0	1
slices water pack	1 slice	19	tr	0	1
tidbits in heavy syrup	1 cup	199	tr	0	3
tidbits in juice	1 cup	150	tr	0	4
tidbits in water	1 cup	79	tr	0	3
fresh					
diced	1 cup	77	tr	0	1
slice	1 slice	42	tr	0	1
Bonita Hill					
Golden Extra Sweet	2 slices (3.9 oz)	60	0	0	10
frozen					
chunks sweetened	1/2 cup	104	tr	0	2
PINEAPPLE JUICE					
canned	1 cup	139	tr	0	2
frozen as prep	1 cup	129	tr	0	3
frozen not prep	6 oz	387	tr	0	6
Dole					
Chilled	8 oz	130	0	0	10
PINK BEANS					
dried					
cooked	1 cup	252	1	0	3
PINTO BEANS					
canned					
Chi-Chi's					
Pinto Beans	1/2 cup (4.3 oz)	100	1	0	540
Eden					
Organic	1/2 cup (4.6 oz)	100	0	0	15
Organic Spicy w/ Jalapeno & Red Peppers	1/2 cup (4.6 oz)	125	0	0	195
Green Giant					
Pinto Beans	1/2 cup (4.4 oz)	110	1	0	280
Progresso					
Pinto Beans	1/2 cup (4.6 oz)	110	1	0	250
dried					
cooked	1 cup	235	1	0	3
Hurst					
HamBeens w/ Ham	3 tbsp (1.2 oz)	120	1	0	63
PINYON					
(*see* PINE NUTS)					
PISTACHIOS					
dry roasted w/ salt	47 nuts (1 oz)	160	13	0	120
Lance					
Pistachios	1 pkg (1 1/8 oz)	90	7	0	105
PITANGA					
fresh	1 cup	57	1	0	5
fresh	1	2	tr	0	0

FOOD	PORTION	CALS	FAT	CHOL	SOD
PIZZA					
(see also pizza restaurants in Part 2, PIZZA DOUGH, PIZZA SAUCE)					
Amy's Organic					
Cheese	1 (13 oz)	310	11	15	490
Pocket Sandwich Cheese Pizza	1 (4.5 oz)	290	9	20	390
Pocket Sandwich Veggie Pepperoni Pizza	1 (4.5 oz)	220	7	15	490
Roasted Vegetable	1 (12 oz)	270	8	0	470
Spinach	1 (14 oz)	320	11	15	490
Appian Way					
Pizza Mix Thick Crust	1/3 pie (4.2 oz)	290	5	10	830
Pizza Mix Thin Crust	1/3 pie (4.1 oz)	250	3	0	740
Di Giorno					
Rising Crust 12 inch Four Cheese	1/6 pie (4.9 oz)	320	11	25	870
Rising Crust 12 inch Italian Sausage	1/6 pie (5.3 oz)	360	14	35	1000
Rising Crust 12 inch Pepperoni	1/6 pie (5.2 oz)	370	16	35	1080
Rising Crust 12 inch Supreme	1/6 pie (5.8 oz)	380	17	40	1100
Rising Crust 12 inch Three Meat	1/6 pie (5.4 oz)	380	16	40	1100
Rising Crust 12 inch Vegetable	1/6 pie (5.6 oz)	310	10	20	830
Rising Crust 8 inch Chicken Supreme	1/3 pie (4.8 oz)	270	9	30	740
Rising Crust 8 inch Four Cheese	1/3 pie (4 oz)	260	9	20	720
Rising Crust 8 inch Italian Sausage	1/3 pie (4.4 oz)	300	12	25	830
Rising Crust 8 inch Pepperoni	1/3 pie (4.2 oz)	300	13	30	880
Rising Crust 8 inch Spinach	1/3 pie (4.3 oz)	250	8	15	670
Rising Crust 8 inch Supreme	1/3 pie (4.7 oz)	310	14	30	900
Rising Crust 8 inch Three Meat	1/3 pie (4.4 oz)	310	13	30	900
Rising Crust 8 inch Vegetable	1/3 pie (4.6 oz)	250	8	15	680
Health Is Wealth					
Pizza Munchees	6 (3 oz)	190	5	0	560
Jack's					
Great Combinations 12 inch Bacon Cheeseburger	1/4 pie (4.7 oz)	360	18	45	770
Great Combinations 12 inch Double Cheese	1/4 pie (4.9 oz)	380	19	50	670
Great Combinations 12 inch Pepperoni	1/4 pie (5.2 oz)	410	19	40	830
Great Combinations 12 inch Pepperoni & Mushrooms	1/4 pie (4.8 oz)	340	16	35	740

FOOD	PORTION	CALS	FAT	CHOL	SOD
Great Combinations 12 inch Sausage	1/4 pie (5.4 oz)	390	18	40	700
Great Combinations 12 inch Sausage & Mushroom	1/4 pie (4.9 oz)	310	15	30	610
Great Combinations 12 inch Sausage & Pepperoni	1/4 pie (4.8 oz)	350	19	40	770
Great Combinations 12 inch Supreme	1/4 pie (5.2 oz)	350	18	40	750
Great Combinations 9 inch Double Cheese	1/2 pie (5.5 oz)	430	21	55	740
Great Combinations 9 inch Pepperoni & Sausage	1/2 pie (5.1 oz)	380	18	40	790
Naturally Rising 12 inch Bacon Cheeseburger	1/6 pie (5 oz)	350	15	40	680
Naturally Rising 12 inch Canadian Bacon	1/6 pie (4.9 oz)	280	9	30	590
Naturally Rising 12 inch Cheese	1/6 pie (4.5 oz)	290	10	25	500
Naturally Rising 12 inch Combination w/ Sausage & Pepperoni	1/6 pie (5.2 oz)	360	17	40	680
Naturally Rising 12 inch Pepperoni	1/6 pie (4.9 oz)	350	16	40	710
Naturally Rising 12 inch Pepperoni Supreme	1/6 pie (5.1 oz)	340	16	35	670
Naturally Rising 12 inch Sausage	1/6 pie (5.1 oz)	340	15	35	600
Naturally Rising 12 inch Spicy Italian Sausage	1/6 pie (5.1 oz)	330	14	40	680
Naturally Rising 12 inch The Works	1/6 pie (5.3 oz)	330	14	35	580
Naturally Rising 9 inch Cheese	1/3 pie (4.7 oz)	300	10	25	500
Naturally Rising 9 inch Combination w/ Sausage & Pepperoni	1/4 pie (4.2 oz)	300	14	35	560
Naturally Rising 9 inch Pepperoni	1/3 pie (5.2 oz)	360	16	40	720
Naturally Rising 9 inch Sausage	1/3 pie (5.4 oz)	360	16	35	620
Naturally Rising 9 inch The Works	1/4 pie (4.5 oz)	280	12	30	480
Original 12 inch Canadian Bacon	1/4 pie (4.4 oz)	280	10	30	620
Original 12 inch Cheese	1/3 pie (5 oz)	360	13	30	650
Original 12 inch Hamburger	1/4 pie (4.4 oz)	300	14	35	580
Original 12 inch Pepperoni	1/4 pie (4.3 oz)	330	15	35	720
Original 12 inch Sausage	1/4 pie (4.3 oz)	300	14	30	580

FOOD	PORTION	CALS	FAT	CHOL	SOD
Jack's (cont.)					
Original 12 inch Spicy Italian Sausage	1/4 pie (4.3 oz)	290	13	35	650
Original 9 inch Pepperoni	1/2 pie (5 oz)	380	18	40	820
Original 9 inch Sausage	1/2 pie (5.1 oz)	360	16	35	660
Pizza Bursts Combination Sausage & Pepperoni	6 pieces (3 oz)	250	12	20	500
Pizza Bursts Pepperoni	6 pieces (3 oz)	260	14	20	560
Pizza Bursts Sausage	6 pieces (3 oz)	250	12	20	490
Pizza Bursts Supercheese	6 pieces (3 oz)	250	12	20	460
Pizza Bursts Supreme	6 pieces (3 oz)	250	13	20	520
Lean Cuisine					
Everyday Favorites French Bread Cheese	1 pkg (6 oz)	320	7	15	580
Everyday Favorites French Bread Deluxe	1 pkg (6.1 oz)	290	6	25	550
Everyday Favorites French Bread Pepperoni	1 pkg (5.25 oz)	300	8	25	590
Everyday Favorites French Bread Sun Dried Tomatoes	1 serv (6 oz)	340	8	20	580
Pepperidge Farm					
Gourmet Crust Cheese	1 (4.4 oz)	390	20	90	770
Gourmet Crust Pepperoni	1 (4.5 oz)	420	23	90	810
Stouffer's					
French Bread Bacon Cheddar	1 piece (5.7 oz)	430	21	25	880
French Bread Cheese	1 piece (5.2 oz)	370	16	15	880
French Bread Cheeseburger	1 piece (6 oz)	420	20	30	800
French Bread Deluxe	1 piece (6.2 oz)	430	21	20	990
French Bread Double Cheese	1 piece (5.9 oz)	400	16	25	950
French Bread Pepperoni	1 piece (5.6 oz)	430	20	15	990
French Bread Pepperoni & Mushroom	1 piece (6.1 oz)	440	20	30	910
French Bread Sausage	1 piece (6 oz)	420	18	20	1260
French Bread Sausage & Pepperoni	1 piece (6.25 oz)	470	23	25	1340
French Bread Three Meat	1 piece (6.25 oz)	460	21	35	1200
French Bread Vegetable Deluxe	1 piece (6.4 oz)	380	16	20	780
French Bread White Pizza	1 piece (5.1 oz)	460	23	20	700
Tombstone					
Double Top Pepperoni	1/6 pie (4.5 oz)	340	19	45	810
Double Top Sausage	1/6 pie (4.6 oz)	320	17	40	760
Double Top Sausage & Pepperoni	1/6 pie (4.6 oz)	340	19	45	820
Double Top Supreme	1/6 pie (4.7 oz)	330	18	40	780
Double Top Two Cheese	1/6 pie (5.2 oz)	380	19	50	760
For One 1/2 Less Fat Cheese	1 pie (6.5 oz)	460	10	20	940
For One 1/2 Less Fat Vegetable	1 pie (7.2 oz)	360	9	10	860

FOOD	PORTION	CALS	FAT	CHOL	SOD
For One Extra Cheese	1 pie (6.9 oz)	520	28	50	940
For One Pepperoni	1 pie (6.9 oz)	550	32	55	1160
For One Supreme	1 pie (7.5 oz)	550	32	55	1090
Light Supreme	1/5 pie (4.8 oz)	270	9	20	720
Light Vegetable	1/5 pie (4.6 oz)	240	7	10	500
Original 12 inch Canadian Bacon	1/4 pie (5.5 oz)	350	14	35	890
Original 12 inch Deluxe	1/5 pie (4.8 oz)	310	14	30	690
Original 12 inch Extra Cheese	1/4 pie (5.1 oz)	350	15	30	680
Original 12 inch Hamburger	1/5 pie (4.4 oz)	310	15	30	670
Original 12 inch Pepperoni	1/4 pie (5.3 oz)	400	21	40	930
Original 12 inch Sausage	1/5 pie (4.4 oz)	300	14	30	680
Original 12 inch Sausage & Mushroom	1/5 pie (4.6 oz)	300	14	30	680
Original 12 inch Sausage & Pepperoni	1/5 pie (4.4 oz)	320	16	30	740
Original 12 inch Supreme	1/5 pie (5.1 oz)	320	16	30	730
Original 9 inch Deluxe	1/3 pie (4.4 oz)	280	13	25	630
Original 9 inch Extra Cheese	1/2 pie (5.6 oz)	380	19	30	740
Original 9 inch Hamburger	1/3 pie (4.4 oz)	280	13	25	600
Original 9 inch Pepperoni	1/3 pie (4 oz)	300	15	30	680
Original 9 inch Pepperoni & Sausage	1/3 pie (4.1 oz)	300	15	30	710
Original 9 inch Sausage	1/3 pie (4 oz)	280	13	25	610
Original 9 inch Supreme	1/3 pie (4.4 oz)	310	16	30	720
Oven Rising Italian Sausage	1/6 pie (5.1 oz)	320	13	30	700
Oven Rising Pepperoni	1/6 pie (4.9 oz)	340	15	35	750
Oven Rising Supreme	1/6 pie (5.1 oz)	320	14	30	720
Oven Rising Three Cheese	1/6 pie (4.8 oz)	320	13	35	580
Oven Rising Three Meat	1/6 pie (5.1 oz)	340	15	35	750
Thin Crust Four Meat Combo	1/4 pie (5 oz)	380	23	45	890
Thin Crust Italian Sausage	1/4 pie (5 oz)	370	22	45	840
Thin Crust Pepperoni	1/4 pie (4.8 oz)	400	25	50	920
Thin Crust Supreme	1/4 pie (5 oz)	380	22	45	840
Thin Crust Supreme Taco	1/4 pie (5.1 oz)	370	23	50	740
Thin Crust Three Cheese	1/4 pie (4.7 oz)	360	21	45	690
Weight Watchers					
Smart Ones Deluxe Combo	1 (6.57 oz)	380	11	40	550
Smart Ones Pepperoni	1 (5.56 oz)	390	12	45	650
take-out					
cheese	12 in pie	1121	26	74	2680
cheese	1/8 of 12 in pie	140	3	9	336
cheese meat & vegetables	1/8 of 12 in pie	184	5	21	382
cheese meat & vegetables	12 in pie	1472	43	165	3054
pepperoni	12 in pie	1445	56	115	2133
pepperoni	1/8 of 12 in pie	181	7	14	267

FOOD	PORTION	CALS	FAT	CHOL	SOD
PIZZA DOUGH					
crust	1 slice (1.7 oz)	130	2	0	230
Pillsbury					
Crust	1/5 crust (2 oz)	150	2	0	380
Robin Hood					
Crust	1/4 crust	160	2	0	340
PIZZA SAUCE					
Hunt's					
Fully Prepared	1/4 cup (2.2 oz)	21	1	0	251
Pizza Sauce	1/4 cup (2.2 oz)	27	1	0	190
Prima Choice Supper Heavy	1/4 cup (2.2 oz)	28	1	0	36
Progresso					
Pizza Sauce	1/4 cup (2.1 oz)	20	0	0	170
PLANTAINS					
fresh uncooked	1 (6.3 oz)	218	1	0	7
sliced cooked	1/2 cup	89	tr	0	4
Chifles					
Plantain Chips	1 pkg (2 oz)	170	11	0	14
PLUMS					
canned					
purple in heavy syrup	3	119	tr	0	26
purple in light syrup	3	83	tr	0	26
purple juice pack	3	55	tr	0	1
purple water pack	3	39	tr	0	1
fresh					
plum	1	36	tr	0	0
sliced	1 cup	91	1	0	1
POI					
poi	1/2 cup	134	tr	0	14
POLENTA					
(*see also* CORNMEAL)					
Frieda's					
Dried Tomato	4 oz	80	0	0	250
Italian Herb	4 oz	80	0	0	45
Mexicana	4 oz	80	0	0	200
Original	4 oz	80	0	0	198
Wild Mushroom	4 oz	80	0	0	200
Melissa's					
Original	4 oz	80	0	0	198
POLLACK					
atlantic baked	3 oz	100	1	77	94
POMEGRANATE					
fresh	1	104	tr	0	5
Cortas					
Concentrated Juice	1 tbsp (0.6 oz)	40	0	0	0
POMPANO					
florida cooked	3 oz	179	10	54	65

FOOD	PORTION	CALS	FAT	CHOL	SOD
POPCORN					
(*see also* CHIPS, POPCORN CAKES, PRETZELS, SNACKS)					
air-popped	1 cup (0.3 oz)	31	tr	0	0
oil popped	1 cup (0.4 oz)	55	3	0	97
Chester's					
Butter	3 cups	160	12	0	330
Caramel Craze	3/4 cup	130	2	0	220
Cheddar Cheese	3 cups	190	13	<5	300
Microwave Butter	5 cups	200	12	0	300
Cracker Jack					
Fat Free Butter Toffee	3/4 cup	110	0	0	85
Fat Free Caramel	3/4 cup	110	0	0	70
Original	1/2 cup	120	2	0	70
Estee					
Caramel	1 cup	120	2	0	90
Herr's					
Regular	3 cups (1 oz)	140	11	0	250
Jolly Time					
America's Best 94% Fat Free	1 cup	20	0	0	10
Blast O Butter	1 cup	45	3	0	85
Blast O Butter Light	1 cup	30	2	0	75
Butter Licious	1 cup	35	2	0	40
Butter Licious Light	1 cup	30	2	0	25
Crispy & White	1 cup	40	3	0	40
Crispy & White Light	1 cup	25	1	0	25
Healthy Pop 94% Fat Free	1 cup	20	0	0	10
White Air Popped	5 cups	100	1	0	0
Yellow Air Popped	5 cups	100	1	0	0
Lance					
Cheese	1 pkg (0.6 oz)	90	5	0	210
Plain	1 pkg (0.5 oz)	70	3	0	135
White Cheddar	1 pkg (0.6 oz)	100	8	0	170
White Cheddar	1 pkg (0.9 oz)	150	11	0	240
Newman's Own					
Microwave Butter Flavor	3 1/2 cups	170	11	0	180
Microwave Light Butter	3 1/2 cups	110	3	0	90
Microwave Light Natural	3 1/2 cups	110	3	0	90
Microwave Natural	3 1/2 cups	170	11	0	180
Popcorn unpopped	3 tbsp	110	2	0	0
Orville Redenbacher's					
Gourmet Original	3 cups	92	1	0	2
Hot Air	3 cups	92	1	0	2
Microwave Butter	3 cups	168	13	0	388
Microwave Butter No Salt Added	3 cups	176	12	0	2
Microwave Butter Light	3 cups	122	6	0	357
Microwave Caramel	1 serv	179	10	0	47
Microwave Golden Cheddar	1 serv	169	13	0	373

FOOD	PORTION	CALS	FAT	CHOL	SOD
Orville Redenbacher's (cont.)					
Microwave Natural	3 cups	164	11	0	512
Microwave Natural No Salt Added	3 cups	174	12	0	2
Microwave Natural Light	3 cups	118	5	0	382
Microwave Smartpop	1 serv	96	3	0	445
Microwave Smartpop Butter Snack Size	1 bag	155	4	0	477
Microwave Snack Size Butter	1 bag	287	22	0	647
Microwave Snack Size Butter Light	1 bag	183	8	0	539
Microwave White Cheddar	1 serv	169	13	0	373
Redenbudders Microwave Herb & Garlic	1 serv	176	13	0	499
Redenbudders Microwave Zesty Butter	1 serv	177	13	0	429
Redenbudders Movie Theater Butter Light	1 serv	113	5	0	321
Redenbudders Movie Theater Microwave Butter	1 serv	176	13	0	499
Smart Pop Movie Theater Butter	1 serv	92	2	0	307
White	3 cups	92	1	0	2
Planters					
Fiddle Faddle Caramel Fat Free	1 cup (1 oz)	110	0	0	210
Pop Secret					
94% Fat Free Butter	1 cup (5 g)	20	0	0	40
94% Fat Free Natural	1 cup (5 g)	20	0	0	40
Butter	1 cup (7 g)	35	3	0	50
Cheddar Cheese	1 cup (6 g)	30	2	0	45
Jumbo Pop Butter	1 cup (7 g)	40	3	0	55
Jumbo Pop Movie Theater Butter	1 cup (7 g)	40	3	0	55
Light Butter	1 cup (5 g)	20	1	0	45
Light Movie Theater Butter	1 cup (5 g)	25	1	0	45
Light Natural	1 cup (5 g)	25	1	0	45
Movie Theater Butter	1 cup (7 g)	40	3	0	55
Nacho Cheese	1 cup (6 g)	30	2	0	50
Natural	1 cup (7 g)	35	3	0	65
Real Butter	1 cup (7 g)	35	3	0	60
Smartfood					
Butter	3 cups	150	9	5	240
Low Fat Toffee Crunch	3/4 cup	110	1	0	220
Reduced Fat Golden Butter	3 1/3 cups	130	4	0	410
Reduced Fat White Cheddar	3 cups	140	6	<5	280
White Cheddar	2 cups	190	12	5	310
Snyder's Of Hanover					
Butter	5/8 oz	110	10	0	150

FOOD	PORTION	CALS	FAT	CHOL	SOD
Tom's					
Caramel Corn	1 pkg (1.6 oz)	180	3	0	110
Utz					
Au Natural	3 cups (1 oz)	120	1	0	0
Butter	2 cups (1 oz)	170	12	0	210
Cheese	2 cups (1 oz)	150	10	5	250
Hulless Puff'N Corn	2 cups (1 oz)	180	15	0	150
Hulless Puff'N Corn Hot Cheese	1 pkg (1.75 oz)	290	22	0	680
Hulless Puff'N Corn Cheese	2 cups (1 oz)	170	12	<5	210
White Cheddar	2 cups (1 oz)	150	9	<5	270
Weight Watchers					
Butter	1 pkg (0.66 oz)	90	3	0	100
Butter Toffee	1 pkg (0.9 oz)	110	3	0	90
Caramel	1 pkg (0.9 oz)	100	1	0	45
Microwave	1 pkg (1 oz)	100	1	0	0
White Cheddar Cheese	1 pkg (0.66 oz)	90	4	0	125
POPCORN CAKES					
Orville Redenbacher's					
BBQ Mini	8 (0.5 oz)	55	1	0	124
Butter	2 (0.6 oz)	134	1	tr	79
Butter Mini	8 (0.5 oz)	56	1	1	71
Caramel	1 (0.4 oz)	34	tr	0	16
Caramel Mini	7 (0.5 oz)	50	tr	tr	24
Nacho Cheese Mini	8 (0.5 oz)	56	1	1	85
Peanut Crunch Mini	7 (0.5 oz)	55	1	tr	39
White Cheddar	2 (0.6 oz)	63	1	tr	83
White Cheddar Mini	8 (0.5 oz)	56	1	tr	67
POPOVER					
home recipe	1	87	3	46	82
POPPY SEEDS					
poppy seeds	1 tsp	15	1	0	1
PORK					
(*see also* BACON, CANADIAN BACON, DELI MEATS/COLD CUTS, HAM, PORK DISHES, SAUSAGE)					
canned					
Hormel					
Pickled Tidbits	2 oz	100	8	45	530
fresh					
boston blade roast lean & fat cooked	3 oz	229	16	73	57
boston blade steak lean & fat cooked	3 oz	220	14	81	59
center loin roast lean bone in cooked	3 oz	169	8	67	56
center loin chop lean bone in cooked	3 oz	172	7	72	53
center rib chop lean & fat bone in cooked	3 oz	213	13	62	34

FOOD	PORTION	CALS	FAT	CHOL	SOD
center rib roast lean & fat bone in cooked	3 oz	217	13	62	39
fresh ham rump lean roasted	3 oz	175	7	82	55
fresh ham rump lean & fat roasted	3 oz	214	12	82	53
fresh ham shank lean roasted	3 oz	183	9	78	54
fresh ham shank lean & fat roasted	3 oz	246	17	78	50
fresh ham whole lean roasted	3 oz	179	8	80	54
fresh ham whole lean roasted diced	1 cup	285	13	127	86
fresh ham whole lean & fat roasted	3 oz	232	15	80	51
fresh ham whole lean & fat roasted diced	1 cup	369	24	127	81
ground cooked	3 oz	252	18	80	62
loin chop lean bone in braised	3 oz	191	11	71	53
loin chop lean bone in broiled	3 oz	199	12	71	68
loin roast lean bone in roasted	3 oz	210	13	79	25
loin whole lean & fat braised	3 oz	203	12	68	41
loin whole lean & fat broiled	3 oz	206	12	68	53
loin whole lean & fat roasted	3 oz	211	12	70	50
lungs braised	3 oz	84	3	329	69
pancreas cooked	3 oz	186	9	268	36
ribs country style lean & fat braised	3 oz	252	18	74	50
shoulder arm picnic lean & fat roasted	3 oz	269	20	80	60
shoulder whole lean & fat roasted	3 oz	248	18	77	58
shoulder whole lean & fat roasted diced	1 cup	394	29	122	92
shoulder whole lean roasted	3 oz	196	12	77	64
shoulder whole lean roasted diced	1 cup	311	18	122	101
sirloin chop lean & fat bone in braised	3 oz	208	13	70	43
sirloin roast lean & fat bone in cooked	3 oz	222	14	74	51
spareribs braised	3 oz	338	26	103	79
spleen braised	3 oz	127	3	428	91
tail simmered	3 oz	336	30	110	21
tenderloin lean roasted	3 oz	139	4	67	48
top loin chop boneless lean & fat cooked	3 oz	198	11	64	36
top loin roast bonless lean & fat cooked	3 oz	192	10	66	37

FOOD	PORTION	CALS	FAT	CHOL	SOD
Oscar Mayer					
Sweet Morsel Smoked Boneless Pork Shoulder Butt	3 oz	180	15	50	990
ready-to-eat					
Tyson					
Pork Pattie	1 (3.8 oz)	200	11	40	270
POSOLE					
(*see* HOMINY)					
POT PIE					
Amy's Organic					
Broccoli	1 (7.5 oz)	430	22	45	630
Country Vegetable	1 (7.5 oz)	370	16	40	580
Shepard's	1 (8 oz)	160	4	0	490
Vegetable	1 (7.5 oz)	360	18	45	540
Vegetable Non-Dairy	1 (7.5 oz)	320	9	0	590
Lean Cuisine					
Everyday Favorites Chicken Pie	1 pkg (9.5 oz)	300	8	30	580
Everyday Favorites Vegetable Eggroll	1 pkg (9 oz)	300	5	0	610
Mrs. Paterson's					
Aussie Pie Chicken	1 (5.5 oz)	460	25	90	770
Aussie Pie Chicken Low Fat	1 (5.5 oz)	380	17	35	930
Aussie Pie Philly Steak	1 (5.5 oz)	420	24	40	860
Stouffer's					
Beef Pie	1 pkg (10 oz)	450	26	65	1140
Chicken Pie	1 pkg (10 oz)	540	33	25	1080
Turkey	1 pkg (10 oz)	530	33	65	1040
Swanson					
Beef	1 (7 oz)	376	19	22	739
Chicken	1 (7 oz)	416	22	19	814
Turkey	1 (7 oz)	440	24	18	748
take-out					
beef	1/3 of 9 in pie (7.4 oz)	515	30	42	596
chicken	1/3 of 9 in pie (8.1 oz)	545	31	56	594
POTATO					
(*see also* CHIPS, KNISH, PANCAKES)					
canned					
Hormel					
Au Gratin & Bacon	1 can (7.5 oz)	250	14	25	840
fresh					
baked skin only	1 skin (2 oz)	115	tr	0	12
baked w/ skin	1 (6.5 oz)	220	tr	0	16
boiled	1/2 cup	68	tr	0	3
PurelyIdaho					
Oven Roasts	1 serv (3 oz)	70	0	0	0

FOOD	PORTION	CALS	FAT	CHOL	SOD
frozen					
Birds Eye					
Whole	3 (2.6 oz)	50	0	0	25
Lean Cuisine					
Everyday Favorites Deluxe Cheddar Potato	1 pkg (10.4 oz)	250	6	20	590
Everyday Favorites Roasted Potatoes w/ Broccoli	1 pkg (10.25 oz)	260	6	15	590
MicroMagic					
French Fries Low Fat	1 pkg (3 oz)	130	3	0	35
Oh Boy!					
Stuffed With Cheddar Cheese	1 (5 oz)	130	4	<5	270
Stouffer's					
Au Gratin	1/2 cup (5.75 oz)	130	6	15	590
Scalloped	1/2 cup (5.75 oz)	140	6	<5	450
Weight Watchers					
Smart Ones Baked Broccoli & Cheese	1 pkg (10 oz)	250	6	20	570
mix					
instant mashed flakes as prep w/ whole milk & butter	1/2 cup	118	6	15	349
instant mashed flakes not prep	1/2 cup	78	tr	0	24
instant mashed granules as prep w/ whole milk & butter	1/2 cup	114	5	15	270
instant mashed granules not prep	1/2 cup	372	1	0	67
Barbara's					
Mashed not prep	1/3 cup (0.8 oz)	70	0	0	10
Betty Crocker					
Au Gratin Low Fat Recipe	1/2 cup	110	1	<5	560
Au Gratin as prep	1/2 cup	150	6	5	600
Cheddar & Bacon	1/2 cup	150	6	<5	650
Cheddar & Bacon Low Fat Recipe	1/2 cup	120	3	0	620
Cheddar & Sour Cream	1/2 cup	130	3	5	580
Chicken & Vegetable	2/3 cup	140	4	<5	520
Chicken & Vegetable Low Fat Recipe	2/3 cup	120	3	<5	510
Hash Browns	1/2 cup	190	8	0	620
Homestyle Broccoli Au Gratin	1/2 cup	140	6	<5	530
Homestyle Broccoli Au Gratin Low Fat Recipe	1/2 cup	110	3	0	530
Homestyle Cheddar Cheese	1/2 cup	120	3	<5	600
Homestyle Cheddar Cheese Stove Top Recipe	1/2 cup	140	5	5	680

FOOD	PORTION	CALS	FAT	CHOL	SOD
Homestyle Cheesy Scalloped	1/2 cup	140	6	<5	540
Homestyle Cheesy Scalloped Low Fat Recipe	1/2 cup	110	3	<5	540
Julienne	1/2 cup	150	6	<5	630
Mashed Butter & Herb	1/2 cup	160	8	5	470
Mashed Butter & Herb Reduced Fat Recipe	1/2 cup	130	5	<5	450
Mashed Chicken & Herb	1/2 cup	150	7	<5	520
Mashed Chicken & Herb Reduced Fat Recipe	1/2 cup	120	4	0	490
Mashed Four Cheese	1/2 cup	150	7	<5	570
Mashed Four Cheese Reduced Fat Recipe	1/2 cup	120	4	0	540
Mashed Potato Buds	2/3 cup	160	8	<5	460
Mashed Potato Buds Reduced Fat Recipe	2/3 cup	120	4	0	420
Mashed Roasted Garlic	1/2 cup	150	8	<5	400
Mashed Roasted Garlic Reduced Fat Recipe	1/2 cup	130	5	0	380
Mashed Sour Cream & Chives	1/2 cup	150	7	5	440
Mashed Sour Cream & Chives Reduced Fat Recipe	1/2 cup	120	4	<5	420
Potato Shakers Original	2/3 cup	140	4	<5	580
Potato Shakers Original Low Fat Recipe	2/3 cup	120	2	<5	560
Ranch	1/2 cup	160	6	<5	610
Scalloped	1/2 cup	150	6	<5	620
Scalloped Low Fat Recipe	2/3 cup	110	1	0	580
Sour Cream'n Chive	1/2 cup	160	7	5	600
Three Cheese	1/2 cup	150	6	<5	600
Twice Baked Cheddar & Bacon Low Fat Recipe	2/3 cup	130	3	<5	530
Twice Baked Cheddar & Bacon as prep	2/3 cup	210	11	85	580
Hungry Jack					
Au Gratin as prep	1/2 cup	150	5	10	620
Cheddar & Bacon as prep	1/2 cup	150	5	10	540
Cheesy Scalloped as prep	1/2 cup	150	5	10	570
Creamy Scalloped as prep	1/2 cup	150	5	10	460
Mashed Butter Flavored as prep	1/2 cup	150	7	<5	350
Mashed Flakes as prep	1/2 cup	160	7	<5	240
Mashed Garlic Flavored as prep	1/2 cup	150	7	<5	360
Mashed Parsley Butter as prep	1/2 cup	150	7	<5	380
Mashed Sour Cream 'n Chives as prep	1/2 cup	150	7	<5	380
Sour Cream & Chives as prep	1/2 cup	160	6	15	510

FOOD	PORTION	CALS	FAT	CHOL	SOD
Idaho					
Mashed Potato Flakes as prep	1/2 cup	150	6	<5	240
Mashed Potato Granules as prep	1/2 cup	160	7	<5	300
Shake 'N Bake					
Perfect Potatoes Crispy Cheddar	1/6 pkg (7 g)	30	2	5	380
Perfect Potatoes Herb & Garlic	1/6 pkg (7 g)	20	0	0	380
Perfect Potatoes Home Fries	1/6 pkg (7 g)	20	0	0	410
Perfect Potatoes Parmesan Peppercorn	1/6 pkg (7 g)	25	1	<5	300
Perfect Potatoes Savory Onion	1/6 pkg (7 g)	20	0	0	280
shelf-stable					
Lunch Bucket					
Scalloped w/ Ham Chunks	1 pkg (7.5 oz)	170	7	10	660
Micro Cup Meals					
Microcup Meals Scalloped Potatoes w/ Ham	1 cup (7.5 oz)	240	14	35	920
take-out					
au gratin w/ cheese	1/2 cup	178	10	18	548
baked topped w/ cheese sauce	1	475	29	19	381
baked topped w/ cheese sauce & bacon	1	451	26	30	973
baked topped w/ cheese sauce & broccoli	1	402	14	20	484
baked topped w/ cheese sauce & chili	1	481	22	31	701
baked topped w/ sour cream & chives	1	394	22	23	182
french fries	1 lg	355	19	0	187
french fries	1 reg	235	12	0	124
hash brown	1/2 cup (2.5 oz)	151	9	9	290
indian yogurt potatoes	1 serv	315	9	18	216
mashed	1/2 cup	111	4	2	309
mustard potato salad	3.5 oz	120	6	0	393
o'brien	1 cup	157	3	7	421
potato pancakes	1 (1.3 oz)	101	7	35	188
potato salad	1/2 cup	179	10	86	661
potato salad w/ vegetables	3.5 oz	120	3	0	390
scalloped	1/2 cup	127	5	7	435
POTATO STARCH					
potato starch	3 1/2 oz	335	tr	0	8
POUT					
ocean baked	3 oz	86	1	57	66
PRESERVE					
(*see* JAM/JELLY/PRESERVE)					

FOOD	PORTION	CALS	FAT	CHOL	SOD
PRETZELS					
(see also CHIPS, POPCORN, SNACKS)					
Bachman					
Thin'n Right	12 (1 oz)	120	1	0	650
Estee					
Chocolate Covered	7	130	6	0	270
Dutch	2 (1.1 oz)	130	1	0	40
Unsalted	23 (1 oz)	120	1	0	30
Gardetto's					
Mustard	1 pkg (0.5 oz)	50	1	0	110
Herr's					
Hard Sourdough	1 (1 oz)	100	0	0	450
Lance					
Pretzels	1 pkg (1.25 oz)	140	1	0	470
Little Debbie					
Mini Twists	1 pkg (1.2 oz)	140	1	0	470
Nabisco					
Air Crisps Fat Free	23 pieces (1 oz)	110	0	0	550
Nestle					
Flipz Milk Chocolate Covered	9 pieces (1 oz)	130	5	<5	135
Flipz White Fudge Covered	9 pieces (1 oz)	130	6	0	130
Newman's Own					
Salted Rounds Organic	1 pkg (1.4 oz)	150	2	0	530
Rold Gold					
Crispy's Thins	4 (1 oz)	110	2	0	670
Fat Free Cheddar Cheese	17 (1 oz)	110	0	0	440
Fat Free Honey Mustard	17 (1 oz)	110	0	0	380
Fat Free Sticks	48 (1 oz)	110	0	0	530
Fat Free Thins	12 pieces (1 oz)	110	0	0	520
Fat Free Tiny Twists	18 pieces (1 oz)	110	0	0	420
Honey Mustard	16 (1 oz)	110	1	0	370
Rods	3 (1 oz)	110	1	0	610
Sour Dough Nuggets	11 (1 oz)	110	0	0	330
Snyder's Of Hanover					
Dips White Fudge	1 oz	130	6	0	80
Hard Sourdough	1 oz	100	0	0	240
Hard Sourdough Unsalted	1 oz	100	0	0	90
Logs	1 oz	110	1	0	360
Mini	1 oz	120	0	0	250
Mini Unsalted	1 oz	110	0	0	75
Nibblers	1 oz	120	0	0	200
Nibblers Honey Mustard & Onions	1 oz	130	3	0	95
Nibblers Oat Bran	1 oz	130	3	0	170
Nibblers Unsalted	1 oz	120	0	0	50
Oat Bran	1 oz	100	3	0	260
Old Fashioned Dipping Stix	1 oz	100	0	0	330
Old Tyme Unsalted	1 oz	120	1	0	75

FOOD	PORTION	CALS	FAT	CHOL	SOD
Snyder's Of Hanover (cont.)					
Olde Tyme	1 oz	120	1	0	120
Olde Tyme Stix	1 oz	120	1	0	150
Pieces Buttermilk Ranch	1 oz	130	5	0	250
Pieces Cheddar Cheese	1 oz	190	6	0	260
Pieces Honey Mustard & Onions	1 oz	140	7	0	240
Pieces Peppered Pizza	1 oz	150	8	0	340
Rods	1 oz	120	2	0	400
Snaps	24 (1 oz)	120	1	0	390
Thin	1 oz	130	0	0	430
Whole Wheat Honey	1 oz	120	1	0	20
Utz					
Country Store Stix	5 (1 oz)	110	1	0	470
Fat Free Hard	1 (0.8 oz)	90	0	0	470
Fat Free Hard No Salt Added	1 (0.8 oz)	90	0	0	50
Fat Free Sour Dough Nuggets	10 (1 oz)	100	0	0	470
Fat Free Stix	14 (1 oz)	100	0	0	280
Fat Free Thin	10 (1 oz)	100	0	0	480
Honey Mustard & Onion	1/3 cup (1 oz)	130	6	0	270
Rods	3 (1 oz)	120	1	0	400
Specials	5 (1 oz)	110	1	0	470
Specials Extra Dark	5 (1 oz)	110	1	0	470
Specials Unsalted	5 (1 oz)	110	1	0	80
Wheels	20 (1 oz)	100	0	0	480
Weight Watchers					
Oat Bran Nuggets	1 pkg (1.5 oz)	170	3	0	250
PRICKLYPEAR					
fresh	1	42	1	0	6
PRUNE JUICE					
canned	1 cup	181	tr	0	11
PRUNES					
canned					
in heavy syrup	5	90	tr	0	2
dried					
cooked w/o sugar	1/2 cup	113	tr	0	2
dried	10	201	tr	0	3
PUDDING					
(*see also* CUSTARD, PUDDING POPS)					
mix					
Jell-O					
Americana Rice as prep w/ skim milk	1/2 cup (5.2 oz)	140	0	<5	160
Americana Tapioca as prep w/ skim milk	1/2 cup (5.1 oz)	130	0	<5	180
Banana Cream as prep w/ 2% milk	1/2 cup (5.1 oz)	140	3	10	240

FOOD	PORTION	CALS	FAT	CHOL	SOD
Butterscotch as prep w/ 2% milk	1/2 cup (5.2 oz)	160	3	10	190
Chocolate as prep w/ 2% milk	1/2 cup (5.2 oz)	150	3	10	170
Chocolate Fudge as prep w/ 2% milk	1/2 cup (5.2 oz)	150	3	10	170
Coconut Cream as prep w/ 2% milk	1/2 cup (5.1 oz)	150	5	10	210
Fat Free Chocolate as prep w/ skim milk	1/2 cup (5.2 oz)	130	0	<5	170
Fat Free Vanilla as prep w/ skim milk	1/2 cup (5.1 oz)	130	0	<5	200
Instant Banana Cream as prep w/ 2% milk	1/2 cup (5.2 oz)	150	3	10	410
Instant Butterscotch as prep w/ 2% milk	1/2 cup (5.2 oz)	150	3	10	450
Instant Chocolate as prep w/ 2% milk	1/2 cup (5.2 oz)	160	3	10	470
Instant Chocolate Fudge as prep w/ 2% milk	1/2 cup (4.2 oz)	160	3	10	440
Instant Coconut Cream as prep w/ 2% milk	1/2 cup (4.2 oz)	160	5	10	320
Instant French Vanilla as prep w/ 2% milk	1/2 cup (4.2 oz)	150	3	10	410
Instant Lemon as prep w/ 2% milk	1/2 cup (4.2 oz)	150	3	10	370
Instant Pistachio as prep w/ 2% milk	1/2 cup (4.2 oz)	160	3	10	410
Instant Vanilla as prep w/ 2% milk	1/2 cup (4.2 oz)	150	3	10	410
Instant Fat Free Chocolate as prep w/ skim milk	1/2 cup (5.3 oz)	140	0	<5	410
Instant Fat Free Devil's Food as prep w/ skim milk	1/2 cup (5.3 oz)	140	0	<5	420
Instant Fat Free Sugar Free Banana as prep w/ skim milk	1/2 cup (4.6 oz)	70	0	<5	410
Instant Fat Free Sugar Free Butterscotch as prep w/ skim milk	1/2 cup (4.6 oz)	70	0	<5	400
Instant Fat Free Sugar Free Chocolate Fudge as prep w/ skim milk	1/2 cup (4.7 oz)	80	0	<5	390
Instant Fat Free Sugar Free Chocolate as prep w/ skim milk	1/2 cup (4.6 oz)	80	0	<5	390
Instant Fat Free Sugar Free Vanilla as prep w/ skim milk	1/2 cup (4.6 oz)	70	0	<5	400

FOOD	PORTION	CALS	FAT	CHOL	SOD
Jell-O (cont.)					
Instant Fat Free Sugar Free White Chocolate as prep w/ skim milk	1/2 cup (4.6 oz)	70	0	<5	400
Instant Fat Free Vanilla as prep w/ skim milk	1/2 cup (5.2 oz)	140	0	<5	410
Instant Fat Free White Chocolate as prep w/ skim milk	1/2 cup (5.2 oz)	140	0	<5	410
Lemon as prep w/ 2% milk	1/2 cup (4.4 oz)	140	2	75	75
Milk Chocolate as prep w/ 2% milk	1/2 cup (5.2 oz)	150	3	10	170
Sugar Free Chocolate as prep w/ 2% milk	1/2 cup (4.6 oz)	90	3	10	170
Sugar Free Vanilla as prep w/ 2% milk	1/2 cup (4.5 oz)	80	3	10	170
Vanilla as prep w/ 2% milk	1/2 cup (5.1 oz)	140	3	10	200
Louisiana Purchase					
Bread	1 serv (1.3 oz)	150	3	0	220
Lundberg					
Elegant Rice Cinnamon Raisin	1/2 cup (3.9 oz)	70	0	0	0
Elegant Rice Coconut	1/2 cup (3.9 oz)	70	2	0	0
Elegant Rice Honey Almond	1/2 cup (3.9 oz)	70	1	0	0
Uncle Ben's					
Rice Pudding Cinnamon & Raisins as prep	1/2 cup (1.5 oz)	160	1	0	150
ready-to-eat					
Ensure					
All Flavors	1 pkg (4 oz)	170	5	<5	135
Handi-Snacks					
Banana	1 serv (3.5 oz)	120	4	0	150
Butterscotch	1 serv (3.5 oz)	120	4	0	150
Chocolate	1 serv (3.5 oz)	130	4	0	125
Chocolate Fudge	1 serv (3.5 oz)	130	4	0	130
Fat Free Chocolate	1 serv (3.5 oz)	90	0	0	170
Fat Free Vanilla	1 serv (3.5 oz)	90	0	0	180
Tapioca	1 serv (3.5 oz)	120	4	0	120
Vanilla	1 serv (3.5 oz)	120	4	0	150
Healthy Choice					
Low Fat Chocolate Raspberry	1/2 cup (3.5 oz)	102	2	0	111
Low Fat Chocolate Almond	1/2 cup (3.5 oz)	109	2	0	109
Low Fat Double Chocolate Fudge	1/2 cup (3.5 oz)	101	1	0	116
Low Fat French Vanilla	1/2 cup (3.5 oz)	98	1	0	122
Low Fat Tapioca	1/2 cup (3.5 oz)	101	1	1	115

FOOD	PORTION	CALS	FAT	CHOL	SOD
Hunt's					
Snack Pack Banana	1 serv (3.5 oz)	119	4	2	155
Snack Pack Butterscotch	1 serv (3.5 oz)	130	4	2	164
Snack Pack Chocolate	1 serv (3.5 oz)	143	5	1	139
Snack Pack Chocolate Fudge	1 serv (3.5 oz)	147	5	1	153
Snack Pack Chocolate Marshmallow	1 serv (3.5 oz)	134	5	1	212
Snack Pack Fat Free Chocolate	1 serv (3.5 oz)	86	tr	1	134
Snack Pack Fat Free Tapioca	1 serv (3.5 oz)	82	tr	0	141
Snack Pack Fat Free Vanilla	1 serv (3.5 oz)	81	tr	0	146
Snack Pack Lemon	1 serv (3.5 oz)	124	3	0	47
Snack Pack Milk Chocolate Variety	1 serv (3.5 oz)	143	5	2	136
Snack Pack Swirl Chocolate Caramel	1 serv (3.5 oz)	143	5	1	143
Snack Pack Swirl Chocolate Peanut Butter	1 serv (3.5 oz)	146	6	2	156
Snack Pack Swirl Smores	1 serv (3.5 oz)	136	5	1	94
Snack Pack Tapioca	1 serv (3.5 oz)	125	4	1	144
Snack Pack Toppers Chocolate Fudge w/ Rainbow Sprinkles	1 serv (4 oz)	164	6	tr	145
Snack Pack Toppers Chocolate w/ Dinosaurs	1 serv (4 oz)	161	6	tr	164
Snack Pack Toppers Chocolate w/ Fun Chips	1 serv (4 oz)	176	6	1	153
Snack Pack Toppers Vanilla w/ Chocolate Sprinkles	1 serv (4 oz)	164	6	tr	129
Snack Pack Vanilla	1 serv (3.5 oz)	135	5	1	147
Imagine					
Banana	1 pkg (4 oz)	150	3	0	40
Butterscotch	1 pkg (4 oz)	150	3	0	45
Chocolate	1 pkg (4 oz)	170	3	0	65
Lemon	1 pkg (4 oz)	150	3	0	50
Jell-O					
Chocolate	1 serv (4 oz)	160	5	0	190
Chocolate Marshmallow	1 serv (4 oz)	160	5	0	180
Chocolate Vanilla Swirls	1 serv (4 oz)	160	5	0	180
Free Chocolate	1 serv (4 oz)	100	0	0	190
Free Chocolate Vanilla Swirl	1 serv (4 oz)	100	0	0	210
Free Devil's Food	1 serv (4 oz)	100	0	0	210
Free Rocky Road	1 serv (4 oz)	100	0	0	210
Free Vanilla	1 serv (4 oz)	100	0	0	240
Tapioca	1 serv (4 oz)	140	4	0	160
Tapioca	1 serv (4 oz)	100	0	0	240
Vanilla	1 serv (4 oz)	160	5	0	170

FOOD	PORTION	CALS	FAT	CHOL	SOD
Kozy Shack					
Banana	1 pkg (4 oz)	130	3	10	150
Chocolate	1 pkg (4 oz)	140	4	5	150
Light Chocolate	1 pkg (4 oz)	110	1	5	150
Light Vanilla	1 pkg (4 oz)	110	1	10	160
Rice	1 pkg (4 oz)	130	3	17	140
Tapioca	1 pkg (4 oz)	140	3	5	160
Vanilla	1 pkg (4 oz)	130	3	10	150
NutraBalance					
Low Lactose All Flavors	1 serv (4 oz)	225	8	0	220
Swiss Miss					
Butterscotch	1 pkg (4 oz)	156	6	1	182
Chocolate	1 pkg (4 oz)	166	6	1	177
Chocolate Fudge	1 pkg (4 oz)	175	6	1	207
Fat Free Chocolate	1 pkg (4 oz)	98	tr	0	141
Fat Free Chocolate Fudge	1 pkg (4 oz)	101	tr	0	147
Fat Free Tapioca	1 pkg (4 oz)	98	tr	0	184
Fat Free Vanilla	1 pkg (4 oz)	93	tr	0	168
Fat Free Parfait Vanilla Chocolate	1 pkg (4 oz)	96	tr	0	143
Milk Chocolate	1 pkg (4 oz)	166	6	1	165
Parfait Vanilla Chocolate	1 pkg (4 oz)	164	6	1	196
Swirl Chocolate Caramel	1 pkg (4 oz)	169	6	1	178
Swirl Chocolate Vanilla	1 pkg (4 oz)	169	6	1	159
Swirl Chocolate Vanilla Chocolate	1 pkg (4 oz)	169	6	1	159
Tapioca	1 pkg (4 oz)	138	4	1	180
Vanilla	1 pkg (4 oz)	156	6	1	181
take-out					
bread pudding	1/2 cup (4.4 oz)	212	7	83	291
bread w/ raisins	1/2 cup	180	5	77	185
chocolate	1/2 cup (5.5 oz)	206	4	9	157
rice w/ raisins	1/2 cup	246	6	136	270
tapioca	1/2 cup (5.3 oz)	189	7	124	288
vanilla	1/2 cup (4.3 oz)	130	4	17	113
PUDDING POPS					
(*see also* ICE CREAM AND FROZEN DESSERTS, YOGURT FROZEN)					
chocolate	1 (1.6 oz)	72	2	1	77
vanilla	1 (1.6 oz)	75	2	1	50
PUMMELO					
fresh	1	228	tr	0	7
sections	1 cup	71	tr	0	2
PUMPKIN					
canned					
Libby					
Solid Pack	1/2 cup	40	1	0	5
fresh					
cooked mashed	1/2 cup	24	tr	0	2

FOOD	PORTION	CALS	FAT	CHOL	SOD
flowers cooked	1/2 cup	10	tr	0	4
leaves cooked	1/2 cup	7	tr	0	3
seeds					
dried	1 oz	154	13	0	5
roasted	1 oz	148	12	0	5
salted & roasted	1 oz	148	12	0	144
PURSLANE					
cooked	1 cup	21	tr	0	51
raw	1 cup	7	tr	0	20
QUAHOGS					
(see CLAMS)					
QUICHE					
take-out					
lorraine	1/8 of 8 in pie	600	48	285	653
QUINCE					
fresh	1	53	tr	0	4
QUINOA					
quinoa not prep	1 cup (6 oz)	636	10	0	36
RABBIT					
domestic w/o bone roasted	3 oz	167	7	70	40
wild w/o bone stewed	3 oz	147	3	104	38
RADICCHIO					
raw shredded	1/2 cup	5	tr	0	4
RADISHES					
dried					
chinese	1/2 cup	157	tr	0	161
daikon	1/2 cup	157	tr	0	161
fresh					
chinese raw sliced	1/2 cup	8	tr	0	9
daikon raw sliced	1/2 cup	8	tr	0	9
red raw	10	7	tr	0	11
white icicle raw sliced	1/2 cup	7	tr	0	8
take-out					
moo namul saengche korean salad	1 serv (3.7 oz)	34	tr	0	547
RAISINS					
chocolate coated	10 (0.4 oz)	39	2	0	4
Dole					
CinnaRaisins	1 pkg (1 oz)	95	0	0	5
Estee					
Chocolate Covered	1/4 cup	180	6	<5	45
Mariana					
Fruit n Yogurt Milk Chocolate Covered Raisins	32 pieces (1 oz)	130	5	0	40
Nestle					
Chocolate Covered	1 1/3 tbsp	70	3	0	0

FOOD	PORTION	CALS	FAT	CHOL	SOD
RASPBERRIES					
canned					
in heavy syrup	1/2 cup	117	tr	0	4
fresh					
raspberries	1 cup	61	1	0	0
frozen					
Birds Eye					
Red	1/2 cup (4.4 oz)	90	0	0	5
RASPBERRY JUICE					
Crystal Light					
Raspberry Ice Drink	1 serv (8 oz)	5	0	0	20
Raspberry Ice Drink Mix as prep	1 serv (8 oz)	5	0	0	0
Dole					
Country Raspberry	8 oz	140	0	0	35
Kool-Aid					
Drink Mix as prep	1 serv (8 oz)	60	0	0	0
Raspberry Drink as prep w/ sugar	1 serv (8 oz)	100	0	0	30
Splash					
Blue Raspberry Drink	1 serv (8 oz)	120	0	0	35
RED BEANS					
canned					
Green Giant					
Red Beans	1/2 cup (4.5 oz)	100	1	0	350
Hunt's					
Small	1/2 cup (4.5 oz)	89	1	0	713
Van Camp					
Red Beans	1/2 cup (4.6 oz)	90	0	0	560
RELISH					
cranberry orange	1/2 cup	246	tr	0	44
hamburger	1 tbsp	19	tr	0	164
hot dog	1 tbsp	14	tr	0	164
sweet	1 tbsp	19	tr	0	122
Green Giant					
Corn	1 tbsp (0.6 oz)	20	0	0	40
Vlasic					
Fancy Sweet	1 tbsp	15	0	0	140
RHUBARB					
fresh	1/2 cup	13	tr	0	2
frozen	1/2 cup	60	tr	0	1
frozen as prep w/ sugar	1/2 cup	139	tr	0	2
RICE					
(see also BRAN, CEREAL, FLOUR, RICE CAKES, WILD RICE)					
glutinous cooked	1 cup (6.1 oz)	169	tr	0	9
starch	3.5 oz	343	0	0	61

FOOD	PORTION	CALS	FAT	CHOL	SOD
Birds Eye					
Rice & Broccoli In Cheese Sauce	1 pkg (10 oz)	290	9	15	1110
White & Wild	1 cup (6.6 oz)	180	4	10	480
Carolina					
Red Beans & Rice as prep	1/4 pkg	190	1	0	790
Chun King					
Fried Rice Mix	1/2 cup (1.4 oz)	126	tr	0	691
Goya					
Arroz Amarillo	1/4 cup (1.6 oz)	170	0	0	546
Green Giant					
Rice & Broccoli	1 pkg (10 oz)	320	12	15	1000
Rice Medley	1 pkg (10 oz)	240	3	5	880
Rice Pilaf	1 pkg (10 oz)	230	3	5	1020
White & Wild	1 pkg (10 oz)	250	5	0	1000
La Choy					
Fried Rice	1 cup (4.9 oz)	236	1	0	1024
Lipton					
Oriental Stir Fry as prep	1 cup	270	8	0	860
Rice & Sauce Alfredo Broccoli as prep	1 cup	320	12	15	990
Rice & Sauce Beef as prep	1 cup	270	8	0	1010
Rice & Sauce Cajun Style as prep	1 cup	270	7	0	910
Rice & Sauce Cajun Style w/ Beans as prep	1 cup	310	8	0	530
Rice & Sauce Cheddar Broccoli as prep	1 cup	280	9	5	1010
Rice & Sauce Chicken & Parmesan Risotto as prep	1 cup	270	9	0	830
Rice & Sauce Chicken Broccoli as prep	1 cup	280	9	0	910
Rice & Sauce Chicken Flavor as prep	1 cup	280	9	5	960
Rice & Sauce Creamy Chicken as prep	1 cup	290	11	0	830
Rice & Sauce Herb & Butter as prep	1 cup	280	11	10	880
Rice & Sauce Medley as prep	1 cup	270	9	5	870
Rice & Sauce Mushroom as prep	1 cup	270	8	0	960
Rice & Sauce Mushroom & Herb as prep	1 cup	290	8	0	620
Rice & Sauce Oriental as prep	1 cup	280	8	0	940
Rice & Sauce Pilaf as prep	1 cup	260	11	0	930
Rice & Sauce Scampi Style as prep	1 cup	270	9	5	900

FOOD	PORTION	CALS	FAT	CHOL	SOD
Lipton (cont.)					
Rice & Sauce Spanish as prep	1 cup	270	8	0	900
Rice & Sauce Teriyaki as prep	1 cup	270	8	0	910
Roasted Chicken as prep	1 cup	260	8	0	880
Salsa Style as prep	1 cup	220	7	0	540
Southwestern Chicken Flavor as prep	1 cup	260	11	0	840
Lundberg					
One-Step Curry	1 cup (7.4 oz)	160	1	0	400
Risotto Tomato Basil	1 serv	140	1	0	630
Melting Pot					
Risotto Milanese w/ Saffron	1 cup	210	0	0	70
Risotto Primavera	1 cup	200	1	0	85
Risotto Sun-Dried Tomatoes & Peas	1 cup	200	1	0	75
Risotto Three Cheese	1 cup	200	2	5	410
Risotto Wild Mushroom	1 cup	200	1	0	50
Minute					
Boil-In-Bag White as prep	1 cup (5.7 oz)	190	0	0	10
Instant Brown as prep	2/3 cup	170	2	0	10
Instant White as prep	1 cup (5.7 oz)	160	0	0	5
Long Grain & Wild Seasoned w/ Herbs as prep	1 cup (7.8 oz)	230	1	0	950
Success					
Brown & Wild Mix as prep	1/2 cup	120	3	0	432
Van Camp					
Spanish	1/2 cup (4.5 oz)	90	2	0	645
Zatarain's					
Dirty Rice Mix as prep w/o meat and oil	1/2 cup	130	0	0	680
Red Beans & Rice as prep w/o oil	1/2 cup	100	0	0	490
take-out					
nasi goreng indonesian rice & vegetables	1 cup (4.9 oz)	130	0	0	530
paella	1 serv (7 oz)	308	16	92	580
pilaf	1/2 cup	84	3	22	362
spanish	3/4 cup	363	27	35	1339
RICE CAKES					
(*see also* POPCORN CAKES)					
brown rice	1 (0.3 oz)	35	tr	0	29
brown rice unsalted	1 (0.3 oz)	35	tr	0	3
Estee					
Banana Nut	5	60	1	0	30
Cinnamon Spice	5	60	0	0	5
Granny Smith Apple	5	60	0	0	5
Mixed Berry	5	60	0	0	0
Peanut Butter Crunch	5	60	0	0	80

FOOD	PORTION	CALS	FAT	CHOL	SOD
Lundberg					
Nutra Farmed Brown Rice	1 (0.7 oz)	70	0	0	55
Nutra Farmed Sesame Tamari	1 (0.7 oz)	70	1	0	120
Organic Koku Sesame	1 (0.7 oz)	80	0	0	35
Weight Watchers					
Apple Cinnamon	1 oz	110	1	0	0
Butter	1 oz	110	2	0	280
Caramel	1 oz	110	1	0	30
White Cheddar	1 oz	100	1	0	280
ROCKFISH					
pacific cooked	3 oz	103	2	38	65
ROE					
(*see individual fish names*)					
ROLL					
(*see also* BISCUIT, CROISSANT, ENGLISH MUFFIN, MUFFIN, POPOVER, SCONE)					
frozen					
New York					
Garlic	1 (2 oz)	210	10	0	370
Sara Lee					
Deluxe Cinnamon Rolls w/ Icing	1 (2.7 oz)	370	15	40	300
Deluxe Cinnamon Rolls w/o Icing	1 (2.7 oz)	320	15	40	300
ready-to-eat					
Bread Du Jour					
Cracked Wheat	1 (1.2 oz)	100	1	0	200
Italian	1 (1.2 oz)	90	1	0	190
Sourdough	1 (1.2 oz)	90	1	0	190
Freihofer's					
Brown 'N Serve	1 (1 oz)	80	2	0	160
Pepperidge Farm					
Brown & Serve Club	1 (1.6 oz)	120	1	0	240
Dinner Rolls Finger Poppy	1 (0.9 oz)	80	2	<5	125
Parker House	1 (0.9 oz)	80	2	<5	120
Stroehmann					
Hamburger	1 (1.4 oz)	100	2	0	210
Hamburger Potato	1 (1.9 oz)	140	2	0	260
Hot Dog	1 (1.4 oz)	100	2	0	210
Hot Dog Potato	1 (1.9 oz)	140	2	0	260
Wonder					
Brown & Serve	1 (1 oz)	80	2	0	150
Brown & Serve Sourdough	1 (1 oz)	70	2	0	130
Brown & Serve Wheat	1 (1 oz)	80	2	0	140
Bun	1 (3 oz)	220	3	0	430
Club French	1 (1.6 oz)	120	2	0	230
Club Grain	1 (1.6 oz)	120	2	0	210
Club Sourdough	1 (1.6 oz)	120	2	0	230
Dinner	2 (1.6 oz)	130	1	0	240

FOOD	PORTION	CALS	FAT	CHOL	SOD
Wonder (cont.)					
Dinner Honey Rich	1 (1.3 oz)	100	2	0	160
Dinner Wheat	2 (1.6 oz)	140	3	0	240
Hamburger	1 (2.5 oz)	190	3	0	370
Hamburger	1 (1.5 oz)	110	2	0	220
Hamburger	1 (2 oz)	150	2	0	290
Hamburger	1 (2.5 oz)	180	3	0	370
Hamburger Wheat	1 (1.9 oz)	140	2	0	280
Hamburger Wheat	1 (1.5 oz)	120	2	0	210
Hoagie French	1 (3 oz)	220	3	0	410
Hoagie Grain	1 (3 oz)	220	3	0	370
Hoagie Sourdough	1 (3 oz)	220	3	0	410
Hot Dog	1 (2 oz)	160	3	0	300
Kaiser	1 (2.2 oz)	180	3	0	270
Kaiser Hoagie	1 (3 oz)	220	3	0	410
Multigrain	1 (1.8 oz)	140	2	0	210
Potato Bun	1 (1.5 oz)	110	1	0	220
Steak	1 (2.5 oz)	190	3	0	360
refrigerated					
Pillsbury					
Apple Cinnamon	1 (1.5 oz)	150	6	0	320
Caramel	1 (1.7 oz)	170	7	0	330
Cinnamon w/ Icing	1 (1.5 oz)	150	6	0	340
Cinnamon w/ Icing Reduced Fat	1 (1.5 oz)	140	4	0	340
Cinnamon Raisin w/ Icing	1 (1.7 oz)	170	6	0	320
Cornbread Twists	1 (1.4 oz)	140	6	0	330
Crecents Reduced Fat	1 (1 oz)	100	5	0	230
Crescent	1 (1 oz)	110	6	0	220
Dinner	1 (1.4 oz)	110	2	0	270
Dinner Wheat	1 (1.4 oz)	110	2	0	270
Orange Sweet Roll w/ Icing	1 (1.7 oz)	150	7	0	340
ROSE HIP					
fresh	3 1/2 oz	91	0	0	146
ROSELLE					
fresh	1 cup	28	tr	0	3
ROSEMARY					
dried	1 tsp	4	tr	0	1
ROUGHY					
orange baked	3 oz	75	1	22	69
RUTABAGA					
cooked mashed	1/2 cup	41	tr	0	22
SABLEFISH					
baked	3 oz	213	17	53	61
smoked	3 oz	218	17	55	626
SAFFRON					
saffron	1 tsp	2	tr	0	1

FOOD	PORTION	CALS	FAT	CHOL	SOD
SAGE					
ground	1 tsp	2	tr	0	tr
SALAD					
(see also LETTUCE, PASTA SALAD)					
mix					
Dole					
All American Toss	2 cups (3.5 oz)	50	1	<5	160
American Blend	1 1/2 cups (3 oz)	15	0	0	10
Classic	1 1/2 cups (3 oz)	15	0	0	15
Classic Romaine Blend	1 1/2 cups (3 oz)	15	0	0	10
Coleslaw	1 1/2 cups (3 oz)	25	0	0	25
European Special Blend	2 cups (3 oz)	15	0	0	15
Garlic Caesar Complete w/ Dressing	1 1/2 cups (3.5 oz)	180	15	5	420
Greek Marinade	1 1/2 cups (3.5 oz)	100	8	<5	340
Greener Selection	1 1/2 cups (3 oz)	15	0	0	10
Light Caesar Complete w/ Dressing	1 1/2 cups (3.5 oz)	60	1	0	390
Light Herb Ranch Complete w/ Dressing	1 1/2 cups (3.5 oz)	50	1	5	280
Light Roasted Garlic Caesar Complete w/ Dressing	1 1/2 cups (3.5 oz)	60	1	0	400
Light Zesty Italian Complete w/ Dressing	1 1/2 cups (3.5 oz)	50	1	0	290
Mediterranean Marinade	2 cups (3.5 oz)	90	8	0	180
Oriental Complete w/ Dressing	1 1/2 cups (3.5 oz)	120	6	0	240
Romano Complete w/ Dressing	1 1/2 cups (3.5 oz)	150	12	0	570
Sunflower Ranch Complete w/ Dressing	1 1/2 cups (3.5 oz)	160	16	5	220
Tomato & Mozzarella Medley	2 cups (3.5 oz)	60	2	5	80
Triple Cheese Toss	2 cups (3.5 oz)	80	5	15	120
Earthbound Farm					
Baby Caesar Mix	1 pkg (5 oz)	25	0	0	10
Baby Greens w/ Low Fat Honey Dijon Vinaigrette & Tomato Croutons	1 serv (3.5 oz)	90	3	0	380
Caesar w/ Garlic Croutons	1 serv (3.5 oz)	170	15	10	230
Italian Salad Organic	1 2/3 cups (2.9 oz)	15	0	0	10
Mixed Baby Greens Organic	1 pkg (4 oz)	30	0	0	100
Organic Baby Greens w/ Vinaigrette & Garlic Croutons	1 serv (3.5 oz)	230	20	0	290
Organic Baby Spinach w/ Sesame Soy Vinaigrette & Peanuts	1 serv (3.5 oz)	150	11	0	340

FOOD	PORTION	CALS	FAT	CHOL	SOD
Earthbound Farm (cont.)					
Organic Italian Salad w/ Blue Cheese Dressing & Walnuts	1 serv (3.5 oz)	190	17	15	210
Romaine Blend Organic	1 2/3 cups (2.9 oz)	15	0	0	10
Fresh Express					
Fancy Field Greens	1 1/2 cups (3 oz)	15	0	0	15
Original Iceberg Garden w/ Zip	1 1/2 cups (3 oz)	15	0	0	10
Veggie Lover's	1 1/2 cups (3 oz)	20	0	0	15
Suddenly Salad					
Caesar	3/4 cup	220	9	0	580
Caesar Low Fat Recipe	3/4 cup	170	3	0	580
Italian Pepperoni	1 cup	190	4	0	680
Italian Pepperoni Low Fat Recipe	1 cup	180	2	0	680
Ranch & Bacon	3/4 cup	330	20	15	480
Ranch & Bacon Low Fat Recipe	3/4 cup	180	2	<5	530
Weight Watchers					
Caesar Salad	1 serv (3.5 oz)	60	0	0	600
Caesar Salad w/ Cookies	1 pkg (4.3 oz)	160	3	0	670
European Salad	1 serv (3.5 oz)	60	0	0	530
European Salad w/ Cookies	1 pkg (4.3 oz)	160	3	0	620
Garden Salad	1 serv (3.5 oz)	60	0	0	270
Garden Salad w/ Cookies	1 pkg (4 oz)	120	2	0	340
take-out					
caesar	2 cups (5 oz)	235	20	10	440
chef w/o dressing	1 1/2 cups	386	28	244	279
tossed w/o dressing	1 1/2 cups	32	tr	0	53
tossed w/o dressing	3/4 cup	16	0	0	27
tossed w/o dressing w/ cheese & egg	1 1/2 cups	102	6	98	119
tossed w/o dressing w/ chicken	1 1/2 cups	105	2	72	209
tossed w/o dressing w/ pasta & seafood	1 1/2 cups (4.6 oz)	380	21	50	1572
tossed w/o dressing w/ shrimp	1 1/2 cups	107	2	180	487
waldorf	1/2 cup	79	6	8	49
SALAD DRESSING					
mix					
Et Tu					
Caesar Salad Kit	1 serv	140	12	5	115
Good Seasons					
Cheese Garlic as prep	2 tbsp (1 oz)	140	16	0	330
Fat Free Honey Mustard as prep	2 tbsp (1.2 oz)	20	0	0	280
Fat Free Italian as prep	2 tbsp (1.1 oz)	10	0	0	290
Fat Free Ranch as prep	2 tbsp (1.2 oz)	20	0	0	250
Fat Free Zesty Herb as prep	2 tbsp (1.1 oz)	10	0	0	260

FOOD	PORTION	CALS	FAT	CHOL	SOD
Garlic & Herbs as prep	2 tbsp (1 oz)	140	15	0	340
Gourmet Caesar as prep	2 tbsp (1.1 oz)	150	16	0	300
Gourmet Parmesan Italian as prep	2 tbsp (1.1 oz)	150	16	0	330
Honey French as prep	2 tbsp (1.2 oz)	160	15	0	250
Honey Mustard as prep	2 tbsp (1.1 oz)	150	15	0	240
Italian as prep	2 tbsp (1 oz)	140	15	0	320
Mexican Spice as prep	2 tbsp (1.1 oz)	140	15	0	310
Mild Italian as prep	2 tbsp (1.1 oz)	150	15	0	370
Oriental Sesame as prep	2 tbsp (1.1 oz)	150	16	0	360
Reduced Calorie Italian as prep	2 tbsp (1 oz)	50	5	0	280
Reduced Calorie Zesty Italian as prep	2 tbsp (1 oz)	50	5	0	260
Roasted Garlic as prep	2 tbsp (1.1 oz)	150	15	0	340
Zesty Italian as prep	2 tbsp (1 oz)	140	15	0	220
ready-to-eat					
Benecol					
Creamy Italian	2 tbsp	100	10	0	170
French	2 tbsp (0.8 oz)	130	11	0	170
Ranch	2 tbsp	130	13	0	250
Thousand Island	2 tbsp	130	12	0	210
Estee					
Creamy French	2 tbsp (1 oz)	10	0	0	80
Italian	2 tbsp	5	0	0	80
Kraft					
1/3 Less Fat Catalina	2 tbsp (1.2 oz)	80	5	0	400
1/3 Less Fat Cucumber Ranch	2 tbsp (1.1 oz)	60	5	0	480
1/3 Less Fat Italian	2 tbsp (1.1 oz)	70	7	0	240
1/3 Less Fat Ranch	2 tbsp (1.1)	110	11	10	310
1/3 Less Fat Thousand Island	2 tbsp (1.2 oz)	70	5	10	340
Bacon & Tomato	2 tbsp (1.1 oz)	140	14	<5	280
Buttermilk Ranch	2 tbsp (1.1 oz)	150	16	<5	240
Caesar Italian	2 tbsp (1.1 oz)	100	10	0	480
Caesar Ranch	2 tbsp (1.1 oz)	110	11	10	290
Catalina	2 tbsp (1.1 oz)	120	10	0	390
Catalina With Honey	2 tbsp (1.1 oz)	130	11	0	320
Classic Caesar	2 tbsp (1.1 oz)	110	11	10	290
Coleslaw	2 tbsp (1.1 oz)	130	11	15	410
Creamy French	2 tbsp (1.1 oz)	160	15	0	270
Creamy Garlic	2 tbsp (1.1 oz)	110	11	0	360
Creamy Italian	2 tbsp (1.1 oz)	110	11	0	250
Cucumber Ranch	2 tbsp (1.1 oz)	140	15	0	220
Free Blue Cheese	2 tbsp (1.2 oz)	45	0	0	360
Free Caesar Italian	2 tbsp (1.2 oz)	25	0	0	480
Free Catalina	2 tbsp (1.2 oz)	35	0	0	320
Free Classic Caesar	2 tbsp (1.2 oz)	45	0	0	360
Free Creamy Italian	2 tbsp (1.2 oz)	50	0	0	330

FOOD	PORTION	CALS	FAT	CHOL	SOD
Kraft (cont.)					
Free French	2 tbsp (1.2 oz)	45	0	0	300
Free Garlic Ranch	2 tbsp (1.2 oz)	45	0	0	320
Free Honey Dijon	2 tbsp (1.2 oz)	45	0	0	330
Free Italian	2 tbsp (1.2 oz)	20	0	0	430
Free Peppercorn Ranch	2 tbsp (1.2 oz)	45	0	0	330
Free Ranch	1 tbsp (1.2 oz)	50	0	0	350
Free Red Wine Vinegar	2 tbsp (1.1 oz)	15	0	0	410
Free Thousand Island	2 tbsp (1.2 oz)	40	0	0	280
Garlic Ranch	2 tbsp (1.1 oz)	180	19	10	270
Herb Vinaigrette	2 tbsp (1.1 oz)	140	15	0	250
Honey Dijon	2 tbsp (1.1 oz)	110	10	0	210
Honey Mustard	2 tbsp (1.1 oz)	110	10	0	210
House Italian w/ Olive Oil Blend	2 tbsp (1.1 oz)	120	12	<5	240
Peppercorn Ranch	2 tbsp (1 oz)	170	18	10	270
Pesto Italian	2 tbsp (1.1 oz)	90	9	0	310
Ranch	2 tbsp (1 oz)	170	18	10	280
Roka Blue Cheese	2 tbsp (1.1 oz)	130	13	<5	310
Russian	2 tbsp (1.2 oz)	130	10	0	310
Sour Cream & Onion Ranch	2 tbsp (1 oz)	170	18	10	250
Thousand Island	2 tbsp (1.1 oz)	110	10	10	310
Thousand Island With Bacon	2 tbsp (1.1 oz)	130	12	0	200
Tomato & Herb Italian	2 tbsp (1.1 oz)	100	9	0	340
Zesty Italian	2 tbsp (1.1 oz)	110	11	0	540
Nasoya					
Creamy Dill	2 tbsp (1 oz)	63	5	0	145
Creamy Italian	2 tbsp (1 oz)	60	5	0	187
Garden Herb	2 tbsp (1 oz)	61	5	0	148
Sesame Garlic	2 tbsp (1 oz)	63	5	0	137
Thousand Island	2 tbsp (1 oz)	62	4	0	146
Newman's Own					
Balsamic Vinaigrette	2 tbsp (1.1 oz)	90	9	0	350
Caesar	2 tbsp (1.1 oz)	150	16	<5	450
Light Italian	2 tbsp (1.1 oz)	20	1	0	380
Olive Oil & Vinegar	2 tbsp (1 oz)	150	16	0	150
Ranch	2 tbsp (1 oz)	180	19	<5	170
Seven Seas					
1/3 Less Fat Creamy Italian	2 tbsp (1.1 oz)	60	5	0	500
1/3 Less Fat Italian w/ Olive Oil Blend	2 tbsp (1.1 oz)	45	4	0	460
1/3 Less Fat Ranch	2 tbsp (1.1 oz)	100	9	0	320
1/3 Less Fat Red Wine Vinegar & Oil	2 tbsp (1.1 oz)	45	4	0	320
1/3 Less Fat Viva Italian	2 tbsp (1.1 oz)	45	4	0	320
2 Cheese Italian	2 tbsp (1.1 oz)	70	7	0	240
Chunky Blue Cheese	2 tbsp (1.1 oz)	130	13	<5	310
Classic Caesar	2 tbsp (1.1 oz)	100	10	0	480
Creamy Italian	2 tbsp (1.1 oz)	120	12	0	510

FOOD	PORTION	CALS	FAT	CHOL	SOD
Free Ranch	2 tbsp (1.2 oz)	45	0	0	330
Free Red Wine Vinegar	2 tbsp (1.1 oz)	15	0	0	410
Free Sour Cream & Onion Ranch	2 tbsp (1.2 oz)	50	0	0	300
Free Viva Italian	2 tbsp (1.1 oz)	10	0	0	480
Green Goddess	2 tbsp (1.1 oz)	130	13	0	260
Herbs & Spices	2 tbsp (1.1 oz)	90	9	0	290
Ranch	2 tbsp (1.1 oz)	160	17	<5	260
Red Wine Vinegar & Oil	2 tbsp (1.1 oz)	90	9	0	500
Viva Italian	2 tbsp (1.1 oz)	90	9	0	370
Viva Russian	2 tbsp (1.1 oz)	150	16	0	210
Weight Watchers					
Fat Free Caesar	2 tbsp	10	0	0	390
Fat Free Caesar	1 pkg (0.75 oz)	5	0	0	290
Fat Free Creamy Italian	2 tbsp	30	0	0	360
Fat Free French Style	2 tbsp	40	0	0	200
Fat Free Honey Dijon	2 tbsp	45	0	0	150
Fat Free Italian	2 tbsp	10	0	0	360
Fat Free Ranch	1 pkg (0.75 oz)	25	0	0	200
Fat Free Ranch	2 tbsp	35	0	0	270
Wishbone					
Caesar	2 tbsp (1 oz)	90	10	5	300
Chunky Blue Cheese	2 tbsp (1 oz)	150	17	0	290
Classic House Italian	2 tbsp (1 oz)	140	14	5	360
Classic Olive Oil Italian	2 tbsp (1 oz)	60	5	0	350
Creamy Caesar	2 tbsp (1 oz)	180	18	10	290
Creamy Italian	2 tbsp (1 oz)	110	10	0	240
Creamy Roasted Garlic	2 tbsp (1 oz)	110	10	0	240
Deluxe French	2 tbsp (1 oz)	120	11	0	170
Fat Free Chunky Blue Cheese	2 tbsp (1 oz)	35	0	0	290
Fat Free Creamy Italian	2 tbsp (1 oz)	35	0	0	250
Fat Free Creamy Roasted Garlic	2 tbsp (1 oz)	40	0	0	280
Fat Free Deluxe French	2 tbsp (1 oz)	30	0	0	230
Fat Free Honey Dijon	2 tbsp (1 oz)	45	0	0	270
Fat Free Italian	2 tbsp (1 oz)	10	0	0	280
Fat Free Parmesan & Onion	2 tbsp (1 oz)	45	0	0	320
Fat Free Ranch	2 tbsp (1 oz)	40	0	0	280
Fat Free Red Wine Vinaigrette	2 tbsp (1 oz)	35	0	0	230
Fat Free Sweet N' Spicy French	2 tbsp (1 oz)	30	0	0	220
Fat Free Thousand Island	2 tbsp (1 oz)	35	0	0	290
Italian	2 tbsp (1 oz)	80	8	0	490
Lite French	2 tbsp (1 oz)	50	2	5	240
Lite Italian	2 tbsp (1 oz)	15	1	0	500
Lite Ranch	2 tbsp (1 oz)	100	8	5	300
Olive Oil Vinaigrette	2 tbsp (1 oz)	60	5	0	250
Oriental	2 tbsp (1 oz)	70	5	0	440
Parmesan & Onion	2 tbsp (1 oz)	110	10	5	260

FOOD	PORTION	CALS	FAT	CHOL	SOD
Wishbone (cont.)					
Ranch	2 tbsp (1 oz)	160	17	10	200
Red Wine Vinaigrette	2 tbsp (1 oz)	80	5	0	230
Robusto Italian	2 tbsp (1 oz)	90	8	0	550
Russian	2 tbsp (1 oz)	110	6	0	350
Sweet N' Spicy French	2 tbsp (1 oz)	140	12	0	330
Thousand Island	2 tbsp (1 oz)	140	12	10	340
SALMON					
canned					
chum w/ bone	3 oz	120	5	33	414
sockeye w/ bone	3 oz	130	6	37	458
fresh					
atlantic baked	3 oz	155	7	60	48
chinook baked	3 oz	196	11	72	51
chum baked	3 oz	131	4	81	54
coho cooked	3 oz	157	6	42	50
pink baked	3 oz	127	4	57	73
sockeye cooked	3 oz	183	9	74	102
smoked					
chinook	3 oz	99	4	20	666
Lascco					
Nova Sliced	2 oz	60	1	20	960
take-out					
roulette w/ spinach stuffing	1 serv (4 oz)	160	6	45	400
salmon cake	1 (3 oz)	241	15	104	602
SALSA					
(*see also* KETCHUP, SAUCE, SPANISH FOOD)					
Chi-Chi's					
Con Queso	2 tbsp (1.1 oz)	90	7	15	480
Hot	2 tbsp (1 oz)	10	0	0	160
Medium	2 tbsp (1 oz)	10	0	0	140
Mild	2 tbsp (1 oz)	10	0	0	140
Picante Hot	2 tbsp (1 oz)	10	0	0	270
Picante Medium	2 tbsp (1 oz)	10	0	0	200
Picante Mild	2 tbsp (1 oz)	10	0	0	210
Verde Medium	2 tbsp (1.2 oz)	15	0	0	180
Verde Mild	2 tbsp (1.2 oz)	15	0	0	180
Guiltless Gourmet					
Roasted Red Pepper	2 tbsp (1 oz)	10	0	0	120
Southwestern Grill	2 tbsp (1 oz)	10	0	0	150
Hunt's					
Alfresco All Varieties	2 tbsp (1.1 oz)	10	tr	0	161
Hot	2 tbsp (1.1 oz)	27	tr	0	236
Medium	2 tbsp (1.1 oz)	27	tr	0	236
Mild	2 tbsp (1.1 oz)	27	tr	0	236
Picante All Varieties	2 tbsp (1.1 oz)	11	tr	0	256
Squeeze Mild & Medium	2 tbsp (1.1 oz)	27	tr	0	236

FOOD	PORTION	CALS	FAT	CHOL	SOD
Newman's Own					
Bandito Hot	2 tbsp (1.1 oz)	10	0	0	150
Bandito Medium	2 tbsp (1.1 oz)	10	0	0	105
Bandito Mild	2 tbsp (1.1 oz)	10	0	0	105
Peach	2 tbsp (1.1 oz)	25	0	0	90
Pineapple	2 tbsp (1.1 oz)	15	0	0	90
Roasted Garlic	2 tbsp (1.1 oz)	10	0	0	150
Pace					
Picante Mild or Medium	2 tbsp	10	0	0	220
Thick & Chunky Mild or Medium	2 tbsp	10	0	0	220
Rosarita					
Extra Chunky Medium	2 tbsp (1 oz)	7	tr	0	229
Green Tomatillo Medium	2 tbsp (1 oz)	8	tr	0	188
Picante Zesty Jalapeno Hot	2 tbsp (1 oz)	8	tr	0	246
Picante Zesty Jalapeno Medium	2 tbsp (1 oz)	9	tr	0	254
Picante Zesty Jalapeno Mild	2 tbsp (1 oz)	8	tr	0	239
Roasted Mild	2 tbsp (1 oz)	10	tr	0	233
Traditional Medium	2 tbsp (1 oz)	7	tr	0	234
Traditional Mild	2 tbsp (1 oz)	7	tr	0	247
Snyder's Of Hanover					
Mild	2 tbsp	10	0	0	220
Taco Bell					
Smooth 'N Zesty Picante Medium	2 tbsp (1.1 oz)	15	0	0	190
Smooth 'N Zesty Picante Mild	2 tbsp (1.1 oz)	15	0	0	190
Thick 'N Chunky Salsa Hot	2 tbsp (1.1 oz)	15	0	0	240
Thick 'N Chunky Salsa Medium	2 tbsp (1.1 oz)	15	0	0	240
Thick 'N Chunky Salsa Mild	2 tbsp (1.1 oz)	15	0	0	240
Tostitos					
Con Queso	2.3 oz	80	5	<10	560
Hot	2.3 oz	30	0	0	520
Low Fat Con Queso	2.5 oz	80	3	<10	560
Medium	2.3 oz	30	0	0	520
Mild	2.3 oz	30	0	0	520
Restaurant Style	2.2 oz	30	0	0	420
Ultimate Garden	2.4 oz	30	0	0	460
Utz					
Chunky	2 tbsp (1 oz)	60	0	0	190
SALSIFY					
fresh sliced cooked	1/2 cup	46	tr	0	11
raw sliced	1/2 cup	55	tr	0	13
SALT/SEASONED SALT					
(*see also* SALT SUBSTITUTES)					
salt	1 tsp (6 g)	0	0	0	2325

FOOD	PORTION	CALS	FAT	CHOL	SOD
Morton					
Lite	1/4 tsp (1.4 g)	tr	0	0	280
SALT SUBSTITUTES					
Cardia					
Salt Alternative	1 pkg (0.6 g)	0	0	0	135
Estee					
Salt-It	1/4 tsp	0	0	0	560
Morton					
Salt Substitute	1/4 tsp (1.2 g)	tr	0	0	tr
Mrs. Dash					
Onion & Herb	1/8 tsp (0.02 oz)	2	0	0	1
NoSalt					
Salt Alternative	1 pkg (0.75 g)	0	0	0	0
Papa Dash					
Lite Salt	1/2 tsp (1 g)	0	0	0	170
SANDWICHES					
take-out					
chicken fillet plain	1	515	29	60	957
chicken fillet w/ cheese lettuce mayonnaise & tomato	1	632	39	76	1238
croque monsieur	1 (12.4 oz)	765	46	152	1018
fish fillet w/ tartar sauce & cheese	1	524	29	68	939
fried egg w/ cheese	1	340	19	291	804
fried egg w/ cheese & ham	1	348	16	245	1005
ham w/ cheese	1	353	15	58	772
roast beef submarine sandwich w/ tomato lettuce & mayonnaise	1	411	13	73	845
roast beef w/ cheese	1	402	18	77	1634
roast beef plain	1	346	14	52	792
steak w/ tomato lettuce salt & mayonnaise	1	459	14	73	798
submarine w/ salami ham cheese lettuce tomato onion & oil	1	456	19	35	1650
tuna salad submarine sandwich w/ lettuce & oil	1	584	28	47	1294
SAPODILLA					
fresh	1	140	2	0	20
SAPOTES					
fresh	1	301	1	0	21
SARDINES					
canned					
atlantic in oil w/ bone	2	50	3	34	121
pacific in tomato sauce w/ bone	1	68	5	23	157
SAUCE					

(*see also* BARBECUE SAUCE, GRAVY, PIZZA SAUCE, SALSA, SPAGHETTI SAUCE, TOMATO)

FOOD	PORTION	CALS	FAT	CHOL	SOD
jarred					
Armour					
Chili Hot Dog	1/4 cup (2.2 oz)	120	9	20	310
Meatless Sloppy Joe Sauce	1/4 cup (2.2 oz)	30	0	0	430
Boar's Head					
Ham Glaze Brown Sugar & Spice	2 tbsp (1.4 oz)	120	0	0	95
Cheez Whiz					
Cheese	2 tbsp (1.2 oz)	90	7	20	540
Cheese Jalapeno Pepper	2 tbsp (1.2 oz)	90	7	25	510
Cheese Mild Salsa	2 tbsp (1.2 oz)	100	7	25	530
Chi-Chi's					
Enchilada	1/4 cup (2.1 oz)	30	2	0	210
Taco	1 tbsp (0.5 oz)	10	0	0	75
Chun King					
Sweet And Sour	2 tbsp (1.2 oz)	58	tr	0	104
Teriyaki	1 tbsp (0.6 oz)	17	tr	0	917
Teriyaki Hot	1 tbsp (0.6 oz)	17	tr	0	995
Fritos					
Texas-Style Chili Hearty Topping	2.3 oz	50	2	10	330
Utimate Taco Hearty Topping	2.3 oz	50	2	10	330
Gebhardt					
Enchilada Sauce	1/4 cup (2.2 oz)	35	2	0	218
Hot Dog Chili Sauce	1/4 cup (2.2 oz)	60	3	1	274
Hot Sauce	1 tsp (5 g)	1	tr	0	89
Green Giant					
Sloppy Joe	1/4 cup (2.6 oz)	50	0	0	420
Sloppy Joe as prep w/ meat	1 serv (4.4 oz)	200	11	45	470
Hormel					
Not-So-Sloppy-Joe Sauce	1/4 cup (2.2 oz)	70	0	0	720
House Of Tsang					
Bangkok Padang	1 tbsp (0.6 oz)	45	3	0	240
Hoisin	1 tsp (6 g)	15	0	0	120
Mandarin Marinade	1 tbsp (0.6 oz)	25	0	0	680
Saigon Sizzle	1 tbsp (0.6 oz)	40	1	0	350
Spicy Brown Bean	1 tsp (6 g)	15	0	0	130
Stir Fry Classic	1 tbsp (0.6 oz)	25	1	0	570
Stir Fry Sweet & Sour	1 tbsp (0.6 oz)	30	0	0	45
Stir Fry Szechuan Spicy	1 tbsp (0.6 oz)	20	1	0	490
Sweet & Sour Concentrate	1 tsp (6 g)	10	0	0	15
Teriyaki Korean	1 tbsp (0.6 oz)	30	1	0	430
Hunt's					
Light w/ Mushrooms	1/2 cup (4.4 oz)	42	tr	0	438
Steak	1 tbsp (0.6 oz)	10	tr	0	256
Just Rite					
Hot Dog	1/4 cup (2.2 oz)	50	3	2	265

FOOD	PORTION	CALS	FAT	CHOL	SOD
Kraft					
Cocktail	1/4 cup (2.3 oz)	60	1	0	800
Fat Free Tartar Sauce	2 tbsp (1.1 oz)	25	0	0	200
Lemon & Herb Tartar Sauce	2 tbsp (1 oz)	150	16	15	170
Reduced Fat Sandwich Spread	1 tbsp (0.5 oz)	35	3	0	130
Sandwich Spread	1 tbsp (0.5 oz)	50	4	<5	105
Sweet'n Sour	2 tbsp (1.2 oz)	60	0	0	125
Tartar	2 tbsp (1.1 oz)	90	9	10	170
La Choy					
Duck Sauce Sweet & Sour	2 tbsp (1.3 oz)	61	tr	0	128
Sweet & Sour	2 tbsp (1.2 oz)	58	tr	0	104
Teriyaki	1 tbsp (0.6 oz)	17	tr	0	917
Manwich					
BBQ Sloppy Joe	1/4 cup (2.2 oz)	57	tr	0	887
Bold	1/4 cup (2.2 oz)	62	1	0	802
Mexican	1/4 cup (2.2 oz)	27	tr	0	552
Taco Season	1/4 cup (2.2 oz)	27	tr	0	552
Thick & Chunky	1/4 cup (2.3 oz)	44	tr	0	737
Mrs. Dash					
Steak	1 tbsp (0.4 oz)	17	tr	0	10
Newman's Own					
Spicy Simmer Sauce Diavolo	1/2 cup (4.4 oz)	70	3	0	510
Open Range					
Hot Dog Chili	1/4 cup (2.2 oz)	61	3	3	255
Pace					
Enchilada Sauce	1/4 cup	36	0	0	290
Taco Sauce	1/4 cup	32	2	0	150
Progresso					
Alfredo	1/2 cup (4.4 oz)	200	15	50	850
Sauce Arturo					
Original	1/4 cup (2.2 fl oz)	50	1	0	680
Tabasco					
Caribbean Steak Sauce	1 tbsp (0.6 oz)	15	0	0	160
Garlic Basting Sauce	1 tbsp (0.6 oz)	20	0	0	250
Habanero Sauce	1 tsp (0.2 oz)	5	0	0	140
Hot Sauce w/ Garlic	1 tsp (0.2 oz)	0	0	0	95
Jalapeno Pepper Sauce	1 tbsp	15	0	0	320
New Orleans Steak Sauce	1 tbsp (0.6 oz)	15	0	0	270
Pepper Sauce	1 tsp (0.2 oz)	0	0	0	30
Taco Bell					
Taco Sauce Medium	2 tbsp (1.1 oz)	15	0	0	160
Taco Sauce Mild	2 tbsp (1.1 oz)	15	0	0	160
The Restaurant Hot Sauce	1 tsp (5 g)	0	0	0	50
Tostitos					
Beef Fiesta Nacho	2.4 oz	120	8	10	500
Chicken Quesadilla Topping	2.5 oz	90	6	10	600

FOOD	PORTION	CALS	FAT	CHOL	SOD
mix					
bearnaise as prep w/ milk & butter	1 cup	701	68	189	1265
cheese as prep w/ milk	1 cup	307	17	53	1566
curry as prep w/ milk	1 cup	270	15	35	1276
mushroom as prep w/ milk	1 cup	228	10	34	1533
sour cream as prep w/ milk	1 cup	509	30	91	1007
stroganoff as prep	1 cup	271	11	38	1829
sweet & sour as prep	1 cup	294	tr	0	779
teriyaki as prep	1 cup	131	1	0	4791
white as prep w/ milk	1 cup	241	13	34	796
Durkee					
A La King as prep	1 cup	60	4	0	800
Cheese as prep	1/4 cup	25	2	2	260
Hollandaise as prep	2 tbsp	10	0	0	70
White as prep	1/4 cup	20	1	0	330
French's					
Cheese as prep	1/4 cup	25	1	0	250
Hollandaise as prep	2 tbsp	10	0	0	75
Manwich					
Mix	1/4 oz	22	tr	0	355
McCormick					
Chicken Dijon Blend	1 2/3 tbsp (10 g)	40	2	<5	420
Hollandaise Blend	2 tsp (4 g)	15	0	15	110
shelf-stable					
Cheez Whiz					
Cheese Sqeezable	2 tbsp (1.2 oz)	100	8	15	470
take-out					
bearnaise	1 oz	177	19	21	257
SAUERKRAUT					
Boar's Head					
Sauerkraut	2 tbsp (1 oz)	5	0	0	180
Claussen					
Sauerkraut	1/4 cup (1.1 oz)	5	0	0	210
Vlasic					
Fresh	1/4 cup (1 oz)	5	0	0	280
SAUSAGE					
(*see also* HOT DOG, SAUSAGE SUBSTITUTES)					
bratwurst pork cooked	1 link (3 oz)	256	22	51	473
chipolata	3.5 oz	342	32	66	747
chorizo	3.5 oz	499	45	70	2300
kielbasa pork	1 oz	88	8	19	305
vienna canned	1 (1/2 oz)	45	4	8	152
Armour					
Vienna Sausage 25% Less Fat	3 (1.9 oz)	130	11	50	420
Vienna Sausage 50% Less Fat	3 (1.9 oz)	90	7	40	420
Vienna Sausage Chicken & Beef	3 (1.9 oz)	120	10	65	620

FOOD	PORTION	CALS	FAT	CHOL	SOD
Armour (cont.)					
Vienna Sausage Hot'n Spicy	3 (2.1 oz)	150	13	50	660
Vienna Sausage In BBQ Sauce	3 (2.1 oz)	150	13	50	580
Vienna Sausage In Beef Stock	3 (1.9 oz)	150	14	50	430
Vienna Sausage Jalapeno In Beef Stock	3 (1.9 oz)	170	16	50	420
Banner					
Sausage Stomachs	2 oz	90	5	95	430
Sausage Tripe	2 oz	90	5	85	430
Boar's Head					
Bratwurst	1 (4 oz)	300	25	75	650
Hot Smoked	1 (3.2 oz)	280	25	55	740
Kielbasa	2 oz	120	10	50	440
Knockwurst	1 (4 oz)	310	27	50	950
Hormel					
Kielbasa	2 oz	150	13	40	530
Light & Lean 97 Dinner Smoked	2 oz	60	2	20	640
Pickled Hot	6 (2 oz)	140	11	40	380
Pickled Smoked	6 (2 oz)	140	11	40	380
Smoked Summer	2 oz	200	18	55	970
Vienna	2 oz	140	14	45	420
Vienna Chicken	2 oz	110	9	55	400
Little Sizzlers					
Brown & Serve	2 patties (1.8 oz)	190	18	40	560
Brown & Serve	3 links (2.1 oz)	190	22	45	670
Cooked	3 links (1.8 oz)	230	22	45	610
Cooked	2 patties (1.8 oz)	230	22	45	610
Heat & Serve Pork cooked	3 links (1.8 oz)	230	22	45	610
Louis Rich					
Polska Kielbasa	2 oz	90	5	35	490
Turkey Hot	2.5 oz	120	8	55	430
Turkey Original	2.5 oz	120	8	55	430
Turkey Smoked	2 oz	90	5	30	490
Old Smokehouse					
Summer Sausage	2 oz	200	18	55	970
Oscar Mayer					
Pork cooked	2 links (1.7 oz)	170	15	40	410
Smokies Beef	1 (1.5 oz)	120	11	30	420
Smokies Cheese	1 (1.5 oz)	130	12	30	450
Smokies Link	1 (1.5 oz)	130	12	25	430
Smokies Little	6 (2 oz)	170	15	35	570
Smokies Little Cheese	6 (2 oz)	180	16	40	590
Shady Brook					
Turkey Breakfast	2 oz	80	4	35	480
Turkey Hot Italian	2 oz	100	5	40	460
Turkey Old World Style	4 oz	190	11	65	850
Turkey Sweet Italian	2 oz	100	5	40	420

FOOD	PORTION	CALS	FAT	CHOL	SOD
Turkey Store					
Breakfast	2 links (2 oz)	140	11	45	360
Wampler					
Breakfast Turkey	2 (2.4 oz)	110	6	45	440
Italian Turkey	1 (2.7 oz)	120	6	50	480
SAUSAGE SUBSTITUTES					
Boca Burgers					
Breakfast Patties	1 (1.3 oz)	70	3	0	300
GardenSausage					
Patty	1 (2.5 oz)	140	3	5	460
Lightlife					
Gimme Lean	2 oz	70	0	0	290
Lean Links Breakfast	1 (1.2 oz)	60	3	0	130
Lean Links Italian	1 (1.4 oz)	60	2	0	160
Light	2 patties (2.3 oz)	80	0	0	340
Loma Linda					
Linketts	1 (1.2 oz)	70	5	0	160
Little Links	2 (1.6 oz)	90	6	0	230
Morningstar Farms					
Breakfast Links	2 (1.6 oz)	60	2	0	340
Breakfast Patties	1 (1.3 oz)	80	3	0	270
Grillers	1 patty (2.2 oz)	140	7	0	260
Sausage Style Recipe Crumbles	2/3 cup (1.9 oz)	90	3	0	370
Natural Touch					
Vegan Sausage Crumbles	1/2 cup (1.9 oz)	60	0	0	300
Worthington					
Leanies	1 link (1.4 oz)	100	7	0	430
Prosage Links	2 (1.6 oz)	60	3	0	340
Saucettes	1 link (1.3 oz)	90	6	0	200
Super Links	1 (1.7 oz)	110	8	0	350
Veja Links	1 (1.1 oz)	50	3	0	190
Yves					
Veggie Breakfast Links	1 (1.6 oz)	60	0	0	390
Veggie Breakfast Patties	1 (2 oz)	70	2	0	350
SAVORY					
ground	1 tsp	4	tr	0	tr
SCALLOP					
fresh					
raw	3 oz	75	1	28	137
take-out					
breaded & fried	6 (5 oz)	386	19	107	919
SCONE					
Finnegan's					
Cranberry	1 (2.7 oz)	90	2	0	176
Health Valley					
Apple Kiwi	1	180	0	0	190
Cinnamon Raisin	1	180	0	0	190

FOOD	PORTION	CALS	FAT	CHOL	SOD
Health Valley (cont.)					
Cranberry Orange	1	180	0	0	190
Mountain Blueberry	1	180	0	0	190
Pineapple Banana	1	180	0	0	190
take-out					
orange poppy	1 (3 oz)	260	6	30	400
raisin	1 (3 oz)	270	6	25	400
SEA BASS					
(*see* BASS)					
SEA TROUT					
(*see* TROUT)					
SEAWEED					
agar dried	1 oz	87	tr	0	29
agar fresh	1 oz	tr	tr	0	3
irishmoss fresh	1 oz	14	tr	0	19
kelp fresh	1 oz	12	tr	0	66
kombu fresh	1 oz	12	tr	0	66
laver fresh	1 oz	10	tr	0	14
nori fresh	1 oz	10	tr	0	14
spirulina dried	1 oz	83	2	0	309
spirulina fresh	1 oz	7	tr	0	28
tangle fresh	1 oz	12	tr	0	66
wakame fresh	1 oz	13	tr	0	249
SEITAN					
(*see* WHEAT)					
SEMOLINA					
dry	1 cup (5.9 oz)	601	2	0	2
SESAME					
seeds	1 tbsp	52	5	0	1
sesame butter	1 tbsp	95	8	0	2
tahini	1 tbsp	89	8	0	17
SESBANIA					
flowers	1 cup	5	tr	0	3
SHALLOTS					
dried	1 tbsp	3	0	0	1
raw chopped	1 tbsp	7	tr	0	1
SHARK					
batter-dipped & fried	3 oz	194	12	50	103
raw	3 oz	111	4	43	67
SHELLFISH					
(*see individual names,* SHELLFISH SUBSTITUTES)					
SHELLFISH SUBSTITUTES					
crab imitation	3 oz	87	1	17	715
scallop imitation	3 oz	84	tr	18	676
shrimp imitation	3 oz	86	1	31	599
Louis Kemp					
Crab Delights	1/2 cup (3 oz)	90	0	10	410

FOOD	PORTION	CALS	FAT	CHOL	SOD
Lobster Delights	1/2 cup (3 oz)	80	0	10	420
Scallop Delights	13 pieces (3 oz)	80	0	10	550
SHELLIE BEANS					
canned	1/2 cup	37	tr	0	408
SHERBET					
(*see also* ICES AND ICE POPS)					
Breyers					
Fat Free Orange	1/2 cup (3 oz)	110	0	0	25
Fat Free Rainbow	1/2 cup (3 oz)	110	0	0	25
Fat Free Raspberry	1/2 cup (3 oz)	120	0	0	20
Fat Free Tropical	1/2 cup (3 oz)	110	0	0	25
Orange	1/2 cup (3 oz)	120	1	5	25
Rainbow	1/2 cup (3 oz)	120	2	5	15
Raspberry	1/2 cup (3 oz)	120	2	5	15
Tropical	1/2 cup (3 oz)	120	1	5	15
SHRIMP					
canned					
canned	1 cup	154	3	222	216
fresh					
cooked	4 large	22	tr	43	49
frozen					
Gorton's					
Popcorn Garlic & Herb	22 pieces (3.6 oz)	270	14	90	600
Popcorn Original	20 pieces (3.2 oz)	240	13	65	780
take-out					
breaded & fried	6 to 8 (6 oz)	454	25	201	1447
jambalaya	3/4 cup	188	5	50	83
SMELT					
rainbow cooked	3 oz	106	3	76	65
SNACKS					
(*see also* CHIPS, FRUIT SNACKS, NUTS MIXED, POPCORN, POPCORN CAKES, PRETZELS, RICE CAKES)					
Baken-ets					
BBQ	9 (0.5 oz)	70	5	10	400
Hot N'Spicy	7 (0.5 oz)	70	5	20	440
Hot N'Spicy Cracklins	8 (0.5 oz)	80	5	20	320
Regular	9 (0.5 oz)	80	5	20	330
Regular Cracklins	8 (0.5 oz)	40	6	15	550
Barbara's					
Cheese Puffs Bakes	1 1/2 cups (1 oz)	160	11	0	190
Cheese Puffs Jalapeno	3/4 cup (1 oz)	150	9	0	250
Cheese Puffs Original	3/4 cup (1 oz)	150	10	0	130
Barbara's Bakery					
Cheese Puffs Bakes	1 1/2 cups (1 oz)	160	11	0	190
Cheese Puffs Jalapeno	3/4 cup (1 oz)	150	10	0	130
Cheese Puffs Original	3/4 cup (1 oz)	150	10	0	130

FOOD	PORTION	CALS	FAT	CHOL	SOD
Big Dipper					
Bagel Chips Lowfat Barbeque	12 (1 oz)	110	2	0	190
Bagel Chips Lowfat Garlic	12 (1 oz)	120	2	0	295
Bagel Chips Lowfat Original	12 (1 oz)	110	2	0	150
Bugles					
Baked Cheddar Cheese	1 1/2 cups (1 oz)	130	4	0	430
Baked Original	1 pkg (1.4 oz)	170	5	0	460
Nacho	1 1/3 cups (1 oz)	160	9	0	320
Nacho	1 pkg (0.9 oz)	130	7	0	280
Original	1 pkg (1.5 oz)	230	13	0	440
Original	1 1/3 cups (1 oz)	160	9	0	310
Ranch	1 1/3 cups (1 oz)	160	9	0	310
Smokin BBQ	1 1/3 cups (1 oz)	150	8	0	330
Sour Cream & Onion	1 1/3 cups (1 oz)	160	9	0	290
Cheetos					
Crunchy	21 pieces (1 oz)	160	10	0	290
Curls	15 pieces (1 oz)	150	10	0	290
Flamin' Hot	21 pieces (1 oz)	160	10	0	280
Nacho Cheese	23 pieces (1 oz)	160	10	0	260
Puffed Balls	38 pieces (1 oz)	150	10	0	300
Puffs	29 pieces (1 oz)	160	10	0	370
Zig Zags	17 pieces (1 oz)	170	11	<5	370
Chex Mix					
Bold'n Zesty	1 pkg (1.7 oz)	230	9	0	610
Cheddar Cheese	1 pkg (1.7 oz)	220	9	0	550
Hot'n Spicy	2/3 cup (1 oz)	130	5	0	410
Hot'n Spicy	1 pkg (1.7 oz)	210	7	0	90
Traditional	1 pkg (1.7 oz)	210	7	0	680
Dakota Gourmet					
Amazing Corn Classic	1 pkg (1 oz)	360	7	0	813
Amazing Corn Cool Ranch	1 pkg (1 oz)	367	9	2	1073
Amazing Corn Mesquite BBQ	1 pkg (1 oz)	369	8	0	725
Heart Smart Toasted Corn	1/3 cup (1 oz)	110	2	0	280
Toasted Corn Heart Smart	1 pkg (1.75 oz)	177	3	0	470
Trail Mix Heart Smart	1 pkg (1.75 oz)	172	0	0	156
Frito Lay					
Funyuns	13 (1 oz)	140	7	0	270
Munchos	16 (1 oz)	160	10	0	230
Munchos BBQ	14 (1 oz)	160	10	0	250
Health Valley					
Cheddar Lites Green Onion	1 3/4 cups	120	3	5	170
Cheddar Lites Original	1 3/4 cups	120	3	5	170
Corn Puffs Caramel	2 cups	120	2	0	80
Low Fat Potato Puffs Cheddar Cheese	1 1/2 cups	110	3	5	260
Low Fat Potato Puffs Garlic w/ Cheese	1 1/2 cups	260	3	0	260

FOOD	PORTION	CALS	FAT	CHOL	SOD
Low Fat Potato Puffs Zesty Ranch	1 1/2 cups	110	3	0	260
Innovative Foods					
Roasted Sweet Corn	1 pkg (0.8 oz)	76	0	0	5
Lance					
Cheese Balls	1 pkg (1 oz)	150	8	0	300
Crunchy Cheese Twists	1 pkg (1.25 oz)	190	4	0	280
Gold-N-Chees	1 pkg (1 oz)	130	5	0	290
Onion Rings	1 pkg (0.9 oz)	100	8	0	170
Pork Skins	1 pkg (0.4 oz)	65	4	10	230
Pork Skins BBQ	1 pkg (0.4 oz)	60	4	10	330
Old Dutch Foods					
Baked Cheese Curls	2 cups (1.1 oz)	180	12	0	340
Cheese Puffcorn Curls	2 cups (1.1 oz)	170	12	0	310
Pita Puffs					
Barbeque	35 (1 oz)	120	3	0	150
Lowfat Garlic	35 (1 oz)	110	1	0	125
Lowfat Original	35 (1 oz)	110	1	0	170
Lowfat Salsa	35 (1 oz)	110	1	0	290
Pizza	35 (1 oz)	120	2	0	230
Ranch	35 (1 oz)	120	2	0	195
Planters					
Cheez Mania Original	42 pieces (1 oz)	150	10	<5	300
Robert's American Gourmet					
Pirate's Booty Puffed Rice & Corn w/ Cheddar	1 oz	120	3	0	137
Snyder's Of Hanover					
Cheese Twists	1 oz	230	14	0	280
Fried Pork Skins	1 oz	80	4	30	115
Fried Pork Skins Barbecue	1 oz	80	4	20	106
Kruncheez	1.25 oz	200	10	0	210
Onion Toasters	1 oz	188	10	0	350
Utz					
Caramel Corn Clusters	1 1/8 cups (1 oz)	120	2	0	140
Cheese Balls	50 (1 oz)	150	9	0	260
Cheese Curls	18 (1 oz)	150	9	0	260
Cheese Curls Crunchy	30 (1 oz)	160	10	0	200
Cheese Curls Reduced Fat	32 (1 oz)	140	6	<5	300
Onion Rings	41 (1 oz)	140	7	0	340
Party Mix	3/4 cup (1 oz)	140	6	0	250
Pork Cracklins	0.5 oz	90	7	15	300
Pork Cracklins Hot & Spicy	0.5 oz	80	5	15	340
Pork Rinds	0.5 oz	80	5	15	230
Pork Rinds BBQ	0.5 oz	80	5	15	280
Weight Watchers					
Cheese Curls	1 pkg (0.5 oz)	70	3	0	85

FOOD	PORTION	CALS	FAT	CHOL	SOD
SNAIL					
cooked	3 oz	233	1	110	350
SNAPPER					
cooked	3 oz	109	1	40	48
SODA					
(see also DRINK MIXERS, ENERGY DRINKS, WATER)					
club	12 oz	0	0	0	75
cola	12 oz	151	tr	0	14
cream	12 oz	191	0	0	43
diet cola	12 oz	2	0	0	21
ginger ale	12 oz	124	0	0	25
grape	12 oz	161	0	0	57
lemon lime	12 oz	149	0	0	41
orange	12 oz	177	0	0	49
quinine	12 oz	125	0	0	15
root beer	12 oz	152	0	0	49
tonic water	12 oz	125	0	0	15
7 Up					
Original	1 can	140	0	0	75
A & W					
Root Beer	1 can	180	0	0	45
Barritts					
Ginger Beer	1 bottle (12 oz)	200	0	0	40
Best Health					
Root Beer	1 bottle (12 oz)	165	0	0	35
Vanilla Cream	1 bottle (12 oz)	170	0	0	30
Canada Dry					
Ginger Ale	1 can	120	0	0	40
Tonic Water	8 oz	90	0	0	15
Dr Pepper					
Original	1 can	150	0	0	55
Health Valley					
Ginger Ale	1 bottle	160	0	0	0
Rootbeer Old Fashioned	1 bottle	160	0	0	0
Sarsaparilla Rootbeer	1 bottle	160	0	0	0
IBC					
Root Beer	1 can	160	0	0	55
Saranac					
Diet Root Beer	1 bottle (12 oz)	35	0	0	55
Ginger Beer	1 bottle (12 oz)	160	0	0	55
Root Beer	1 bottle (12 oz)	180	0	0	55
Shasta					
Black Cherry	1 can (12 oz)	170	0	0	54
Caffeine Free Cola	1 can (12 oz)	160	0	0	45
Cherry Cola	1 can (12 oz)	160	0	0	45
Club Soda	1 can (12 oz)	0	0	0	90
Cola	1 can (12 oz)	170	0	0	45

FOOD	PORTION	CALS	FAT	CHOL	SOD
Creme	1 can (12 oz)	190	0	0	45
Diet Black Cherry	1 can (12 oz)	0	0	0	55
Diet Caffeine Free Cola	1 can (12 oz)	0	0	0	55
Diet Cherry Cola	1 can (12 oz)	0	0	0	55
Diet Cola	1 can (12 oz)	0	0	0	45
Diet Creme	1 can (12 oz)	0	0	0	55
Diet Doc Shasta	1 can (12 oz)	0	0	0	45
Diet Ginger Ale	1 can (12 oz)	0	0	0	55
Diet Grape	1 can (12 oz)	0	0	0	55
Diet Grapefruit	1 can (12 oz)	0	0	0	55
Diet Kiwi-Strawberry	1 can (12 oz)	0	0	0	45
Diet Lemon-Lime Twist	1 can (12 oz)	0	0	0	55
Diet Orange	1 can (12 oz)	0	0	0	55
Diet Pineapple-Orange	1 can (12 oz)	0	0	0	55
Diet Raspberry Creme	1 can (12 oz)	0	0	0	45
Diet Red Pop	1 can (12 oz)	0	0	0	55
Diet Root Beer	1 can (12 oz)	0	0	0	55
Diet Strawberry	1 can (12 oz)	0	0	0	55
Diet Strawberry-Peach	1 can (12 oz)	0	0	0	55
Doc Shasta	1 can (12 oz)	160	0	0	45
Fruit Punch	1 can (12 oz)	200	0	0	45
Ginger Ale	1 can (12 oz)	130	0	0	45
Grape	1 can (12 oz)	190	0	0	45
Kiwi-Strawberry	1 can (12 oz)	170	0	0	45
Lemon-Lime Twist	1 can (12 oz)	150	0	0	45
Moon Mist	1 can (12 oz)	180	0	0	45
Orange	1 can (12 oz)	200	0	0	45
Peach	1 can (12 oz)	170	0	0	45
Pineapple	1 can (12 oz)	200	0	0	45
Pineapple-Orange	1 can (12 oz)	180	0	0	45
Quinine/Tonic	1 can (12 oz)	130	0	0	45
Raspberry Creme	1 can (12 oz)	170	0	0	45
Red Pop	1 can (12 oz)	170	0	0	45
Root Beer	1 can (12 oz)	170	0	0	45
Strawberry	1 can (12 oz)	190	0	0	45
Strawberry-Peach	1 can (12 oz)	170	0	0	45
Sunkist					
Orange	1 can	190	0	0	45
SOLE					
fresh					
cooked	3 oz	99	1	58	89
take-out					
battered & fried	3.2 oz	211	11	31	484
SORBET					
(*see* ICES AND ICE POPS)					
SORGHUM					
sorghum	1 cup (6.7 oz)	651	6	0	12

FOOD	PORTION	CALS	FAT	CHOL	SOD
SOUFFLE					
lemon chilled	1 cup	176	tr	2	108
raspberry chilled	1 cup	173	tr	3	108
spinach	1 cup	218	18	184	763
SOUP					
canned					
black bean turtle soup	1 cup	218	1	0	922
cheese not prep	1 can (11 oz)	377	25	72	2331
vichyssoise	1 cup	148	6	22	1060
Butterball					
Chicken Broth Reduced Sodium 99% Fat Free	1 cup	10	0	0	620
Campbell					
98% Fat Free Cream Of Chicken as prep	1 cup	80	3	10	830
Bean With Bacon as prep	1 cup	168	4	3	891
Beef Barley as prep	1 cup	81	2	10	915
Beef Noodle as prep	1 cup	73	2	12	908
Cheddar Cheese	1 cup	130	8	15	950
Cheddar Cheese as prep	1 cup	134	8	19	1083
Chicken Vegetable as prep	1 cup	74	3	9	985
Chicken & Pasta With Garden Vegetables	1 cup (8.4 oz)	90	1	5	850
Chicken Gumbo as prep	1 cup	55	1	5	985
Clam Chowder New England as prep	1 cup	89	3	3	979
Classic Chicken Noodle	1 cup	70	2	15	890
Classic Chicken Rice	1 cup	80	2	5	850
Consomme as prep	1 cup	24	tr	tr	817
Cream Of Asparagus as prep	1 cup	72	4	2	749
Cream Of Mushroom as prep	1 cup	108	7	2	872
Cream Of Celery as prep	1 cup	107	7	2	903
Cream Of Chicken as prep	1 cup	102	6	9	935
Cream Of Potato as prep	1 cup	102	4	7	951
Fiesta Tomato as prep	1 cup	72	tr	1	856
Garden Vegetable as prep	1 cup	69	2	3	857
Green Pea as prep	1 cup	173	3	1	888
Healthy Request Chicken Noodle as prep	1 cup	60	2	10	450
Healthy Request Chicken Noodle as prep	1 cup	60	2	10	474
Healthy Request Cream Of Mushroom as prep	1 cup	66	2	4	475
Healthy Request Cream Of Chicken & Broccoli as prep	1 cup	78	3	6	460
Healthy Request Cream Of Chicken as prep	1 cup	72	2	7	441

FOOD	PORTION	CALS	FAT	CHOL	SOD
Healthy Request Hearty Pasta w/ Vegetables	1 cup	87	1	1	474
Healthy Request Tomato as prep	1 cup	91	2	1	456
Healthy Request Vegetable as prep	1 cup	84	1	1	473
Home Cookin' Chicken Vegetable	1 cup (8.4 oz)	130	4	10	820
Home Cookin' Chicken Rice	1 cup	110	1	10	920
Home Cookin' Chicken With Egg Noodles	1 cup (8.4 oz)	90	2	15	940
Home Cookin' Oriental Noodles w/ Vegetables	1 cup (8.4 oz)	100	1	10	890
Italian Tomato as prep	1 cup	105	tr	1	820
Low Sodium Chicken Broth	1 can (10.75 oz)	27	1	2	75
Low Sodium Chicken w/ Noodles	1 can (10.75 oz)	162	5	40	85
Low Sodium Chunky Vegetable Beef	1 can (10.75 oz)	159	4	39	64
Low Sodium Cream Of Mushroom	1 can (10.75 oz)	200	13	12	48
Low Sodium Green Pea	1 can (10.75 oz)	235	4	4	27
Low Sodium Tomato w/ Pieces	1 can (10.75 oz)	170	5	6	36
Minestrone as prep	1 cup	81	2	1	971
Plus! Hearty Minestrone	2 cup (8.4 oz)	130	1	0	670
Plus! Roasted Vegetable w/ Barley & Wild Rice	1 cup (8.4 oz)	130	1	<5	680
Ready To Serve Bean w/ Bacon 'N Ham	1 can (10.5 oz)	274	7	13	1299
Ready To Serve Chicken Noodle	1 can (10.5 oz)	134	4	23	1323
Ready To Serve Chicken w/ Rice	1 can (10.5 oz)	122	2	11	1132
Ready To Serve Vegetable Beef	1 can (10.5 oz)	143	1	10	1243
Savory Tomato & Dill as prep	1 cup	99	2	tr	811
Select Chicken & Pasta With Roasted Garlic	1 cup (8.4 oz)	110	2	10	800
Select Fiesta Vegetable	1 cup (8.4 oz)	120	1	0	810
Select Mushroom w/ White & Wild Rice	1 cup	90	1	0	820
Select Split Pea w/ Ham	1 cup (8.4 oz)	170	2	10	860
Select Tuscany-Style Minestrone	1 cup (8.4 oz)	190	9	5	870
Simply Home Chicken Noodle	1 cup (8.4 oz)	80	1	10	810
Simply Home Chicken With Rice	1 cup (8.4 oz)	100	1	5	810
Tomato as prep	1 cup	80	0	0	730

FOOD	PORTION	CALS	FAT	CHOL	SOD
Campbell (cont.)					
Vegetable Beef as prep	1 cup	68	2	8	897
Vegetarian Vegetable as prep	1 cup	79	2	0	844
Gold's					
Russian Borscht	8 oz	70	0	0	750
Health Valley					
5 Bean Vegetable	1 cup	250	0	0	250
Beef Broth Fat Free	1 cup	20	0	0	160
Beef Broth Fat Free No Salt	1 cup	20	0	0	160
Black Bean & Vegetable	1 cup	110	0	0	280
Chicken Broth	1 cup	45	2	25	250
Chicken Broth Fat Free	1 cup	30	0	0	170
Chicken Broth No Salt	1 cup	45	2	25	25
Country Corn & Vegetable	1 cup	70	0	0	135
Garden Vegetable	1 cup	80	0	0	250
Italian Plus Carotene	1 cup	80	0	0	240
Lentil & Carrot	1 cup	100	0	0	220
Organic Black Bean	1 cup	110	0	0	45
Organic Lentil No Salt	1 cup	90	0	0	40
Organic Minestrone	1 cup	100	0	0	190
Organic Mushroom Barley No Salt	1 cup	60	0	0	95
Organic Potato Leek	1 cup	70	0	0	230
Organic Potato Leek No Salt	1 cup	70	0	0	35
Organic Split Pea	1 cup	110	0	0	160
Organic Split Pea No Salt	1 cup	110	0	0	115
Organic Tomato	1 cup	90	0	0	250
Organic Vegetable No Salt	1 cup	80	0	0	80
Pasta Bolognese	1 cup	100	0	0	290
Pasta Cacciatore	1 cup	100	0	0	290
Pasta Romano	1 cup	100	0	0	290
Real Italian Minestrone	1 cup	90	0	0	210
Rotini & Vegetable	1 cup	100	0	0	290
Split Pea & Carrots	1 cup	110	0	0	230
Super Broccoli Carotene	1 cup	70	0	0	240
Tomato Vegetable	1 cup	80	0	0	240
Vegetable Barley	1 cup	90	0	0	210
Vegetable Power Carotene	1 cup	70	0	0	240
Healthy Choice					
Bean & Ham	1 cup (8.7 oz)	166	1	4	570
Beef & Potato	1 cup (8.5 oz)	116	1	5	452
Broccoli Cheddar	1 cup (8.4 oz)	116	2	4	304
Chicken Corn Chowder	1 cup (8.8 oz)	176	3	8	466
Chicken Pasta	1 cup (8.6 oz)	119	3	6	493
Chicken Rice	1 cup (8.4 oz)	119	2	6	324
Chili Beef	1 cup (9.1 oz)	189	2	12	441
Clam Chowder	1 cup (8.8 oz)	123	1	12	481
Classic Italian Bean and Pasta	1 cup (8 oz)	100	2	0	480

FOOD	PORTION	CALS	FAT	CHOL	SOD
Country Vegetable	1 cup (8.6 oz)	112	1	0	453
Cream Of Mushroom	1 cup (8.8 oz)	77	1	tr	450
Cream Of Celery as prep	1 cup	73	2	3	366
Cream Of Chicken Vegetable	1 cup (8.9 oz)	127	2	10	384
Cream Of Roasted Chicken as prep	1 cup	80	3	4	349
Cream Of Roasted Garlic as prep	1 cup	57	1	2	489
Garden Tomato Herbs as prep	1 cup	80	1	0	298
Garden Vegetable	1 cup (8.6 oz)	108	1	tr	454
Hearty Chicken	1 cup (8.7 oz)	136	3	21	482
Lentil	1 cup (8.7 oz)	135	1	tr	472
Minestrone	1 cup (8.6 oz)	107	1	1	370
Old Fashion Chicken Noodle	1 cup (8.8 oz)	137	3	9	402
Split Pea & Ham	1 cup (8.8 oz)	164	2	7	468
Tomato Garden	1 cup (8.6 oz)	101	1	1	468
Turkey Wild Rice	1 cup (8.4 oz)	72	1	3	407
Vegetable Beef	1 cup (8.8 oz)	96	1	2	433
Herb-Ox					
Beef Liquid	2 tsp (0.4 oz)	20	0	0	570
Chicken Liquid	2 tsp (0.4 oz)	15	0	0	620
Imagine					
Creamy Broccoli	1 serv (8 oz)	70	2	0	370
Creamy Butternut Squash	1 serv (8 oz)	120	2	0	370
Creamy Mushroom	1 serv (8 oz)	80	3	0	310
Creamy Potato Leek	1 serv (8 oz)	90	3	0	380
Creamy Sweet Corn	1 serv (8 oz)	100	3	0	540
Creamy Tomato	1 serv (8 oz)	90	2	0	520
Vegetable Broth	1 serv (8 oz)	45	1	0	500
Zesty Gazpacho	1 serv (8 oz)	80	0	0	720
Natural Choice					
Orangic Vegan Classic Tomato	1 cup	100	1	0	317
Organic Vegan Classic Mushroom	1 cup	50	2	0	435
Organic Vegan Country Corn	1 cup	100	1	0	377
Organic Vegan Kabocha Squash	1 cup	60	1	0	370
Organic Vegan Southern Greens	1 cup	80	3	0	399
Organic Vegan Split Pea	1 cup	120	1	0	420
Organic Vegan Vegetable Curry	1 cup	110	4	0	392
Progresso					
99% Fat Free Beef Barley	1 cup (8.5 oz)	140	2	20	470
99% Fat Free Beef Vegetable	1 cup (8.5 oz)	160	2	10	870
99% Fat Free Chicken Noodle	1 cup (8.3 oz)	90	2	20	950
99% Fat Free Chicken Rice w/ Vegetables	1 cup (8.4 oz)	110	2	10	780

FOOD	PORTION	CALS	FAT	CHOL	SOD
Progresso (cont.)					
99% Fat Free Creamy Mushroom Chicken	1 cup (8.3 oz)	90	2	10	840
99% Fat Free Lentil	1 cup (8.5 oz)	130	2	0	440
99% Fat Free Minestrone	1 cup (8.5 oz)	130	2	0	710
99% Fat Free Roasted Chicken w/ Italian Style Vegetable	1 cup (8 oz)	90	2	10	660
99% Fat Free Split Pea	1 cup (8.9 oz)	170	2	0	620
99% Fat Free Tomato Garden Vegetable	1 cup (8.6 oz)	100	2	0	660
99% Fat Free Vegetable	1 cup (8.4 oz)	70	1	0	870
99% Fat Free White Cheddar Potato	1 cup (8.6 oz)	140	3	5	930
Bean & Ham	1 cup (8.4 oz)	160	2	10	870
Beef Barley	1 cup (8.5 oz)	130	4	25	780
Beef Minestrone	1 cup (8.5 oz)	140	3	10	970
Beef Noodle	1 cup (8.5 oz)	140	4	30	950
Beef Vegetable & Rotini	1 cup (8.4 oz)	130	3	25	780
Cheese & Herb Tortellini Tomato	1 cup (8.6 oz)	140	3	<5	700
Chickarina	1 cup (8.3 oz)	130	5	20	1010
Chicken Minestrone	1 cup (8.4 oz)	110	2	15	890
Chicken Vegetable	1 cup (8.4 oz)	90	2	15	820
Chicken & Wild Rice	1 cup (8.4 oz)	100	2	15	850
Chicken Barley	1 cup (8.5 oz)	110	2	15	850
Chicken Broth	1 cup (8.2 oz)	20	2	0	920
Chicken Noodle	1 cup (8.4 oz)	90	2	25	950
Chicken Rice w/ Vegetable	1 cup (8.4 oz)	90	2	10	890
Clam & Rotini Chowder	1 cup (8.8 oz)	190	9	10	800
Escarole In Chicken Broth	1 cup (8.1 oz)	25	1	<5	930
Green Split Pea	1 cup (8.6 oz)	170	3	5	870
Hearty Black Bean	1 cup (8.5 oz)	170	2	<5	730
Hearty Penne In Chicken Broth	1 cup (8.4 oz)	80	1	0	1020
Hearty Tomato	1 cup (8.7 oz)	100	2	0	800
Herb Rotini Vegetable	1 cup (9.1 oz)	120	2	0	990
Homestyle Chicken w/ Vegetable	1 cup (8.4 oz)	90	2	15	900
Italian Herb Shells Minestrone	1 cup (9.1 oz)	120	2	0	1050
Lentil	1 cup (8.5 oz)	140	2	0	750
Macaroni & Bean	1 cup (8.6 oz)	160	4	<5	800
Manhattan Clam Chowder	1 cup (8.4 oz)	110	2	10	710
Meatballs & Pasta Pearls	1 cup (8.3 oz)	140	7	15	700
Minestrone	1 cup (8.4 oz)	120	2	0	960
Minestrone Parmesan	1 cup (8.3 oz)	100	3	0	700

FOOD	PORTION	CALS	FAT	CHOL	SOD
New England Clam Chowder	1 cup (8.4 oz)	190	10	15	920
Oregano Penne Italian Style Vegetable	1 cup (8.7 oz)	90	2	0	960
Peppercorn Penne Vegetable	1 cup (9.1 oz)	100	1	0	920
Potato Broccoli & Cheese	1 cup (8.8 oz)	160	6	<5	960
Potato Ham & Cheese	1 cup (8.6 oz)	170	7	10	860
Roasted Garlic Pasta Lentil	1 cup (9.3 oz)	120	2	0	960
Rotisserie Seasoned Chicken	1 cup (8.5 oz)	100	2	15	920
Spicy Chicken & Penne	1 cup (8.5 oz)	110	2	15	950
Split Pea w/ Ham	1 cup (8.4 oz)	150	4	15	830
Tomato	1 cup (8.5 oz)	100	2	0	790
Tomato Basil	1 cup (8.8 oz)	100	2	0	790
Tomato Vegetable	1 cup (8.5 oz)	90	2	0	990
Tortellini In Chicken Broth	1 cup (8.3 oz)	70	2	10	970
Turkey Noodle	1 cup (8.4 oz)	90	2	20	1080
Turkey Rice w/ Vegetables	1 cup (8.5 oz)	110	1	15	1040
Vegetable	1 cup (8.4 oz)	90	2	<5	810
White Meat Roasted Chicken Rotini	1 cup (8.1 oz)	80	2	15	970
Swanson					
Beef Broth	1 cup	19	1	tr	813
Beef Broth Onion Seasoned	1 cup (8.4 oz)	20	0	0	890
Chicken Broth	1 cup	19	1	1	985
Chicken Broth Seasoned w/ Italian Herbs	1 cup (8.4 oz)	20	1	<5	950
Vegetable Broth	1 cup	19	1	1	996
Ultra Slim-Fast					
Chicken Alfredo Pasta	1 cup (8.3 oz)	132	2	10	333
Weight Watchers					
Chicken & Rice	1 can (10.5 oz)	110	2	10	720
Chicken Noodle	1 can (10.5 oz)	150	2	30	740
Minestrone	1 can (10.5 oz)	130	2	5	760
Vegetable	1 can (10.5 oz)	130	1	0	680
mix					
Armour					
Bouillon Cubes Beef	1 (4 g)	5	0	0	920
Bouillon Cubes Chicken	1 (4 g)	5	0	0	910
Bean Cuisine					
Island Black Bean	1 cup (8.7 oz)	210	4	0	504
Cup-a-Soup					
Broccoli & Cheese as prep	1 serv (6 oz)	70	3	5	550
Chicken Vegetable as prep	1 serv (6 oz)	50	1	10	520
Chicken Broth as prep	1 serv (6 oz)	20	0	0	440
Chicken Broth w/ Pasta Fat Free as prep	1 serv (6 oz)	45	0	0	450
Chicken Noodle as prep	1 serv (6 oz)	50	1	10	540
Cream Of Chicken as prep	1 serv (6 oz)	70	2	0	640

FOOD	PORTION	CALS	FAT	CHOL	SOD
Cup-a-Soup (cont.)					
Creamy Chicken Vegetable as prep	1 serv (6 oz)	80	5	0	590
Creamy Mushroom as prep	1 serv (6 oz)	60	2	0	610
Green Pea as prep	1 serv (6 oz)	80	1	0	520
Hearty Chicken Noodle as prep	1 serv (6 oz)	60	1	15	590
Ring Noodle as prep	1 serv (6 oz)	50	1	10	560
Spring Vegetable as prep	1 serv (6 oz)	45	1	10	500
Tomato as prep	1 serv (6 oz)	100	1	5	510
Health Valley					
Chicken Noodles w/ Vegetables	1 serv	110	0	0	190
Corn Chowder w/ Tomatoes	1 serv	100	0	0	190
Creamy Potato w/ Broccoli	1 serv	70	0	0	190
Garden Split Pea w/ Carrots	1 serv	130	0	0	190
Lentil w/ Couscous	1 serv	130	0	0	190
Pasta Italiano	1 serv	140	0	0	190
Pasta Marinara	1 serv	100	0	0	190
Pasta Parmesan	1 serv	100	0	0	190
Spicy Black Bean w/ Couscous	1 serv	130	0	0	190
Zesty Black Bean w/ Rice	1 serv	100	0	0	190
Herb-Ox					
Beef Bouillon	1 cube (3.5 g)	5	0	0	900
Beef Instant Bouillon Powder	1 tsp (4 g)	5	0	0	1020
Beef Instant Broth & Seasoning Pack	1 pkg (4.5 g)	5	0	0	1020
Beef Instant Broth & Seasoning Pack Low Sodium	1 pkg (4 g)	10	0	0	5
Chicken Bouillon	1 cube (4 g)	5	0	0	1100
Chicken Instant Bouillon Powder	1 tsp (4 g)	5	0	0	1100
Chicken Instant Broth & Seasoning Pack	1 pkg (4 g)	5	0	0	1100
Chicken Instant Broth & Seasoning Pack Low Sodium	1 pkg (4 g)	10	0	0	5
Vegetable Bouillon	1 cube (4 g)	5	0	0	980
Hurst					
15 Bean Soup Beef	1 serv (6 oz)	120	1	0	310
15 Bean Soup Cajun	1 serv	120	1	0	100
15 Bean Soup Chicken	1 serv (6 oz)	120	1	0	250
15 Bean Soup Chili	1 serv (6 oz)	120	1	0	170
15 Bean Soup Ham	1 serv	120	1	0	70
HamBeens Great Northern Bean	1 serv	120	1	0	470
HamBeens Navy Bean	1 serv	120	1	0	470
Pasta Fagioli	1 serv	120	1	0	540

FOOD	PORTION	CALS	FAT	CHOL	SOD
Spanish American Pinto Bean	1 serv	120	1	0	350
Spanish-American Black Bean	1 serv	120	1	0	280
Lipton					
Chicken Noodle w/ White Chicken Meat as prep	1 cup	80	2	15	690
Extra Noodle w/ Chicken Broth as prep	1 cup	90	2	25	680
Giggle Noodle w/ Chicken Broth as prep	1 cup	70	2	20	750
Recipe Secrets Beefy Mushroom	1 1/2 tbsp (0.4 oz)	35	0	0	640
Recipe Secrets Beefy Onion	1 tbsp (0.3 oz)	25	1	0	610
Recipe Secrets Fiesta Herb w/ Red Pepper as prep	1 cup	30	0	0	560
Recipe Secrets Golden Herb w/ Lemon as prep	1 cup	35	1	0	510
Recipe Secrets Golden Onion	1 2/3 tbsp (0.5 oz)	50	1	0	700
Recipe Secrets Italian Herb w/ Tomato as prep	1 cup	40	1	0	510
Recipe Secrets Onion as prep	1 cup	20	0	0	610
Recipe Secrets Onion Mushroom as prep	1 cup	30	1	0	640
Recipe Secrets Savory Herb With Garlic as prep	1 cup	30	0	0	480
Recipe Secrets Vegetable as prep	1 cup	30	0	0	600
Ring-O-Noodle w/ Chicken Broth as prep	1 cup	70	2	15	720
Soup Secrets Chicken 'N Onion as prep	1 cup	120	2	5	740
Soup Secrets Chicken w/ Pasta & Beans as prep	1 cup	110	2	5	700
Soup Secrets Country Chicken w/ Pasta & Herbs as prep	1 cup	100	2	5	740
Soup Secrets Homestyle Lentil w/ Bow Tie Pasta as prep	1 cup	130	1	0	750
Soup Secrets Minestrone as prep	1 cup	110	1	0	750
Spiral Pasta w/ Chicken Broth as prep	1 cup	60	1	0	660
Morga					
Vegetable Bouillon No Salt Added	1/2 cube (5 g)	25	2	0	115
Vegetable Broth Fat Free	1 tsp (4 g)	10	0	0	710
Weight Watchers					
Instant Beef Broth	1 pkg (0.16 oz)	10	0	0	800
Instant Chicken Broth	1 pkg (0.16 oz)	10	0	0	830

FOOD	PORTION	CALS	FAT	CHOL	SOD
shelf-stable					
Hormel					
Micro Cup Bean & Ham	1 cup (7.5 oz)	190	4	15	680
Micro Cup Beef Vegetable	1 cup (7.5 oz)	90	1	10	790
Micro Cup Broccoli Cheese w/ Ham	1 cup (7.5 oz)	170	13	40	710
Micro Cup Chicken & Rice	1 cup (7.5 oz)	110	3	15	950
Micro Cup Chicken Noodle	1 cup (7.5 oz)	110	3	35	790
Micro Cup New England Clam Chowder	1 cup (7.5 oz)	130	5	25	820
Micro Cup Potato Cheese w/ Ham	1 cup (7.5 oz)	190	13	50	750
Lunch Bucket					
Chicken Noodle	1 pkg (7.25 oz)	80	2	10	830
Country Vegetable	1 pkg (7.25 oz)	60	1	0	750
take-out					
beef stew soup	1 cup (8.8 oz)	221	5	60	461
black bean turtle soup	1 cup	241	1	0	6
brunswick stew soup	1 cup (8.5 oz)	232	6	71	438
corn & cheese chowder	3/4 cup	215	12	66	386
gazpacho	1 cup	46	tr	0	63
greek	3/4 cup	63	2	83	386
hot & sour	1 serv (14 oz)	173	8	87	475
onion soup gratinee	1 serv	492	27	77	1325
pasta e fagioli	1 cup (8.8 oz)	194	5	3	790
ratatouille	1 cup (7.5 oz)	266	25	0	329
vietnamese pho beef noodle	1 serv (7.8 oz)	480	12	46	43
SOUR CREAM					
(*see also* SOUR CREAM SUBSTITUTES)					
sour cream	1 cup (8 oz)	493	48	102	123
sour cream	1 tbsp (0.4 oz)	26	3	5	6
Breakstone's					
Free	2 tbsp (1.1 oz)	35	0	<5	25
Reduced Fat	2 tbsp (1.1 oz)	45	4	15	20
Sour Cream	2 tbsp (1 oz)	60	5	20	15
Knudsen					
Free	2 tbsp (1.1 oz)	35	0	<5	25
Hampshire	2 tbsp (1 oz)	60	6	25	15
Light	2 tbsp (1.1 oz)	50	3	10	10
Land O'Lakes					
Fat Free	2 tbsp (1.1 oz)	25	0	<5	40
Light	2 tbsp (1 oz)	40	3	10	35
Sour Cream	2 tbsp (1 oz)	60	6	15	30
SOUR CREAM SUBSTITUTES					
nondairy	1 cup	479	45	0	235
SOURSOP					
fresh	1	416	2	0	87

FOOD	PORTION	CALS	FAT	CHOL	SOD
SOY					
(*see also* CHEESE SUBSTITUTES, ICE CREAM AND FROZEN DESSERTS, MILK SUBSTITUTES, MISO, SOY SAUCE, SOYBEANS, TEMPEH, TOFU, YOGURT FROZEN)					
Loma Linda					
Soyagen All Purpose	1/4 cup (1 oz)	130	6	0	150
Soyagen Carob	1/4 cup (1 oz)	130	6	0	170
Soyagen No Sucrose	1/4 cup (1 oz)	130	6	0	160
Natural Touch					
Roasted Soy Butter	2 tbsp (1.1 oz)	170	11	0	170
Tree Of Life					
Soy Wonder Spread	2 tbsp (1.1 oz)	170	11	0	170
SOY SAUCE					
shoyu	1 tbsp	9	tr	0	1029
soy sauce	1 tbsp	7	tr	0	1024
tamari	1 tbsp	11	tr	0	1005
Chun King					
Lite	1 tbsp (0.5 oz)	15	tr	0	542
Soy Sauce	1 tbsp (0.6 oz)	11	tr	0	1227
House Of Tsang					
Ginger Flavored	1 tbsp (0.6 oz)	20	0	0	730
Light	1 tbsp (0.6 oz)	5	0	0	900
Low Sodium	1 tbsp (0.6 oz)	5	0	0	280
Low Sodium Ginger	1 tbsp (0.6 oz)	10	0	0	280
Low Sodium Mushroom	1 tbsp (0.6 oz)	10	0	0	280
Just Rite					
Soy Sauce	1 tbsp (0.5 oz)	11	tr	0	1227
Kikkoman					
Soy Sauce	1 tbsp (0.5 oz)	10	0	0	920
La Choy					
Lite	1 tbsp (0.5 oz)	15	tr	0	542
Soy Sauce	1 tbsp (0.6 oz)	11	tr	0	1227
SOYBEANS					
(*see also* MILK SUBSTITUTES, MISO, SOY, SOY SAUCE, TEMPEH, TOFU)					
dried cooked	1 cup	298	15	0	1
green cooked	1/2 cup	127	6	0	13
honey toasted	1/4 cup (1 oz)	130	4	0	45
roasted	1/2 cup	405	22	0	140
sprouts steamed	1/2 cup	38	2	0	5
sprouts stir fried	1 cup	125	7	0	14
Dakota Gourmet					
Soy Nuts	1 oz	129	7	0	217
Seapoint Farms					
Edamame Organic	1/2 cup (2.6 oz)	100	3	0	30
Edamame In Pods frozen	1/2 cup (2.6 oz)	100	3	0	30
Edamame Rice Bowl Kung Pao Vegetable	1 pkg (12 oz)	420	6	0	960
Edamame Rice Bowl Szechwan Vegetables	1 pkg (12 oz)	420	4	0	510

FOOD	PORTION	CALS	FAT	CHOL	SOD
Seapoint Farms (cont.)					
Edamame Rice Bowl Teriyaki Vegetable	1 pkg (12 oz)	430	5	0	1130
Edamame Rice Bowl Vegetable Fried Rice	1 pkg (11 oz)	220	6	40	950
Seapoint Frams					
Edamane Shelled	1/2 cup (2.6 oz)	100	3	0	30
SPAGHETTI					
(*see* PASTA, PASTA DINNERS, PASTA SALAD, SPAGHETTI SAUCE)					
SPAGHETTI SAUCE					
(*see also* PIZZA SAUCE, TOMATO)					
jarred					
Colavita					
Garden Style	1/2 cup (4.4 oz)	60	3	0	290
Healthy Choice					
Chunky Italian Vegetable	1/2 cup (4.4 oz)	40	tr	0	299
Chunky Mushroom	1/2 cup (4.4 oz)	42	tr	0	297
Garlic & Herbs	1/2 cup (4.4 oz)	49	tr	0	337
Garlic Lovers Garlic & Mushroom	1/2 cup (4.4 oz)	44	tr	0	362
Garlic Lovers Roasted Garlic	1/2 cup (4.4 oz)	52	tr	0	293
Garlic Lovers Roasted Garlic & Sun Dried Tomato	1/2 cup (4.4 oz)	52	tr	0	357
Super Chunky Mushroom & Sweet Peppers	1/2 cup (4.4 oz)	43	tr	0	308
Super Chunky Tomato Mushroom & Garlic	1/2 cup (4.4 oz)	45	tr	0	372
Super Chunky Vegetable Primavera	1/2 cup (4.4 oz)	43	tr	0	327
Traditional	1/2 cup (4.4 oz)	48	tr	0	378
With Mushrooms	1/2 cup (4.4 oz)	48	tr	0	378
Hunt's					
Angela Mia Marinara	1/4 cup (2.2 oz)	24	1	0	252
Chunky	1/2 cup (4.4 oz)	38	1	0	467
Chunky Italian Sausage	1/2 cup (4.5 oz)	72	3	2	542
Chunky Italian Style Vegetable	1/2 cup (4.4 oz)	63	1	0	528
Chunky Marinara	1/2 cup (4.4 oz)	61	1	0	526
Chunky Tomato Garlic & Onion	1/2 cup (4.4 oz)	63	1	0	528
Classic Four Cheese	1/2 cup (4.4 oz)	50	1	0	600
Classic Garlic & Herb	1/2 cup (4.4 oz)	53	2	0	600
Classic Parmesan	1/2 cup (4.4 oz)	49	2	1	600
Classic Tomato & Basil	1/2 cup (4.4 oz)	48	1	0	563
Homestyle Meat Flavored	1/2 cup (4.4 oz)	51	2	0	600
Homestyle Mushrooms	1/2 cup (4.4 oz)	48	1	0	530
Homestyle Traditional	1/2 cup (4.4 oz)	49	1	0	598
Light Meat Flavored	1/2 cup (4.4 oz)	45	1	2	437
Light w/ Garlic & Herb	1/2 cup (4.5 oz)	40	1	0	380

FOOD	PORTION	CALS	FAT	CHOL	SOD
Original Meat Flavored	1/2 cup (4.4 oz)	68	2	1	600
Original Traditional	1/2 cup (4.4 oz)	67	2	0	477
Original w/ Mushrooms	1/2 cup (4.4 oz)	62	2	0	605
Original w/ Italian Cheese & Garlic	1/2 cup (4.5 oz)	64	2	1	622
Tomato Bits	1/2 cup (4.5 oz)	49	tr	0	607
Traditional Light	1/2 cup (4.4 oz)	40	tr	0	400
Newman's Own					
Marinara Ventian	1/2 cup (4.4 oz)	60	2	0	590
Marinara Ventian w/ Mushrooms	1/2 cup (4.4 oz)	60	2	0	590
Pasta Sauce Bambolina	1/2 cup (4.5 oz)	100	5	0	590
Pasta Sauce Roasted Garlic & Red & Green Peppers	1/2 cup (4.7 oz)	70	3	0	460
Pasta Sauce Say Cheese	1/2 cup (4.4 oz)	90	3	<5	510
Sockarooni	1/2 cup (4.4 oz)	60	2	0	590
Prego					
Pasta Bake Sauce Tomato Garlic & Basil	1 serv (3.4 oz)	80	4	0	530
Traditional	1/2 cup (4.2 oz)	140	5	0	610
Progresso					
Marinara	1/2 cup (4.3 oz)	80	5	<5	480
Meat Flavored	1/2 cup (4.4 oz)	100	5	5	610
Sauce	1/2 cup (4.4 oz)	100	5	<5	620
Ragu					
Chunky Garden Style Tomato Garlic & Onion	1/2 cup (4.5 oz)	110	3	0	520
mix					
Durkee					
Spaghetti Sauce as prep	1/2 cup	15	0	0	390
With Mushrooms as prep	1/2 cup	15	0	0	520
French's					
Italian as prep	1/2 cup	16	0	0	390
Mushroom as prep	1/2 cup	20	1	2	760
Thick as prep	1/2 cup	10	0	0	630
McCormick					
Alfredo Pasta Blend as prep	1/2 cup	60	2	10	680
Pasta Rosa Blend	1 tbsp (10 g)	40	2	<5	540
refrigerated					
Di Giorno					
Alfredo	1/4 cup (2.2 oz)	180	18	25	600
Basil Pesto	1/4 cup (2.2 oz)	320	31	15	530
Four Cheese	1/4 cup (2.2 oz)	160	15	30	410
Garlic Pesto	1/4 cup (2.1 oz)	340	33	15	540
Light Alfredo Sauce	1/4 cup (2.4 oz)	140	9	30	600
Marinara	1/2 cup (4.5 oz)	70	0	0	220
Plum Tomato Cream Sauce	1/2 cup (4.4 oz)	160	13	40	370
Plum Tomato & Mushroom	1/2 cup (4.4 oz)	60	0	0	260

FOOD	PORTION	CALS	FAT	CHOL	SOD
Di Giorno (cont.)					
Roasted Red Bell Pepper Cream Sauce	1/4 cup (2.3 oz)	140	10	35	510
SPANISH FOOD					
(*see also* BEANS, CHIPS, CHILI, DINNER, PEPPERS, SALSA, SAUCE, SNACKS, TORTILLA)					
canned					
Chi-Chi's					
Pico De Gallo	2 tbsp (1.2 oz)	10	0	0	170
Derby					
Tamales	3 (6.5 oz)	253	17	23	1034
Gebhardt					
Enchiladas	2 (5.7 oz)	258	19	25	687
Tamales	2 (5.7 oz)	268	21	28	770
Tamales Jumbo	2 (6.9 oz)	332	25	34	930
Hormel					
Tamales Beef	3 (7.5 oz)	280	21	35	1010
Tamales Chicken	3 (7.5 oz)	210	11	50	1020
Tamales Hot Spicy Beef	3 (7.5 oz)	280	21	35	1010
Tamales Jumbo Beef	2 (6.9 oz)	270	20	35	940
Rosarita					
Enchilada Sauce Mild	1/4 cup (2.1 oz)	23	1	0	409
Van Camp					
Tamales	2 (5 oz)	210	13	20	610
frozen					
Amy's Organic					
Black Bean Vegetable Enchilada	1 (4.75 oz)	130	4	0	390
Burritos Bean & Cheese	1 (6 oz)	280	8	10	460
Burritos Bean & Rice Non-Dairy	1 (6 oz)	250	5	0	450
Burritos Black Bean Vegetable	1 (6 oz)	320	8	0	480
Burritos Breakfast	1 (6 oz)	230	5	0	480
Cheese Enchilada	1 (4.7 oz)	210	9	20	390
Mexican Tamale Pie	1 (8 oz)	220	3	0	480
Pocket Sandwich Tamale	1 (4.5 oz)	250	7	10	580
Whole Meals Cheese Enchilada	1 pkg (9 oz)	330	14	30	680
Whole Meals Enchilada	1 pkg (10 oz)	250	8	0	680
Chi-Chi's					
Burro Beef	1 pkg (15.9 oz)	590	19	55	2060
Burro Chicken	1 pkg (15.9 oz)	540	14	55	2110
Chimichanga Beef	1 pkg (15.9 oz)	630	24	55	2050
Chimichanga Chicken	1 pkg (15.9 oz)	580	19	50	2100
Enchilada Chicken Suprema	1 pkg (15.9 oz)	600	20	70	2310
Enchilida Baja	1 pkg (15.9 oz)	590	20	50	1920
Health Is Wealth					
Burrito Munchees	10 (5 oz)	310	7	5	610
Mexican Munchees	2 (1 oz)	49	1	0	110

FOOD	PORTION	CALS	FAT	CHOL	SOD
Lean Cuisine					
Everyday Favorites Chicken Enchilada Suiza	1 pkg (9 oz)	280	5	25	520
Stouffer's					
Chicken Enchilada	1 serv (4.8 oz)	230	11	30	530
Tyson					
Beef Fajita	3 1/2 pieces (12.5 oz)	550	16	20	1130
Chicken Fajita	3 1/2 pieces (13.1 oz)	460	11	45	1220
Weight Watchers					
Smart Ones Chicken Enchiladas Suiza	1 pkg (9 oz)	270	9	50	660
Smart Ones Santa Fe Style Rice & Beans	1 pkg (10 oz)	290	8	20	590
mix					
Gebhardt					
Menudo Mix	1/4 tsp (0.4 g)	1	tr	0	52
Taco Bell					
Home Originals Chicken Fajita Dinner as prep	2 (6.9 oz)	340	9	40	1120
Home Originals Chicken Fajita Seasoning Mix	1 tbsp (8 g)	25	0	0	540
Home Originals Soft Taco Dinner as prep	2 (6.3 oz)	410	18	60	1090
Home Originals Taco Dinner as prep	2 (4.4 oz)	280	15	50	580
Home Originals Taco Seasoning Mix	2 tsp (6 g)	20	0	0	450
Home Originals Ultimate Bean Burrito Dinner as prep	1 (4.4 oz)	200	5	0	710
Home Originals Ultimate Nachos as prep	12 pieces (4.6 oz)	240	11	0	680
ready-to-eat					
Chi-Chi's					
Taco Shells White Corn	2 (1.2 oz)	170	8	0	0
Taco Shells Yellow Corn	2 shells (1.2 oz)	170	8	0	0
Gebhardt					
Taco Shells	3 (1.1 oz)	155	8	0	1
La Mexicana					
Flour Burritos	1 (1.6 oz)	160	5	0	580
Rosarita					
Taco Shells	3 (1.1 oz)	155	8	0	1
Tostada Shells	2 (1 oz)	125	5	37	20
Taco Bell					
Home Originals Taco Shells	3 (1.1 oz)	150	6	0	5

FOOD	PORTION	CALS	FAT	CHOL	SOD
SPARE RIBS					
(*see* PORK)					
SPICES					
(*see individual names,* HERBS/SPICES)					
SPINACH					
fresh					
cooked	1/2 cup	21	tr	0	63
malabar cooked	1 cup (1.5 oz)	10	tr	0	24
new zealand chopped cooked	1/2 cup	11	tr	0	97
new zealand raw	1/2 cup	4	tr	0	36
raw chopped	1/2 cup	6	tr	0	22
raw chopped	1 pkg (10 oz)	46	1	0	160
Dole					
Baby Spinach	3 1/2 cups (3 oz)	35	0	0	135
frozen					
cooked	1/2 cup	27	tr	0	82
Amy's Organic					
Pocket Sandwich Spinach Feta	1 (4.5 oz)	200	7	15	420
Birds Eye					
Creamed	1/2 cup (4.3 oz)	100	7	35	630
Whole Leaf	1 cup (2.8 oz)	20	0	0	110
Green Giant					
Butter Sauce	1/2 cup (3.4 oz)	40	2	<5	280
Creamed	1/2 cup (3.8 oz)	80	3	0	520
Cut Leaf	3/4 cup (2.6 oz)	25	0	0	65
Harvest Fresh	1/2 cup (3.5 oz)	25	0	0	240
Health Is Wealth					
Spinach Munchees	2 (1 oz)	60	3	0	105
Spinach Feta Munchees	2 (1 oz)	70	3	5	115
Stouffer's					
Creamed	1 serv (4.5 oz)	160	12	15	380
Souffle	1 serv (4 oz)	150	10	120	480
take-out					
indian saag	1 serv	28	2	0	44
spanakopita spinach pie	1 cup (6 oz)	196	3	30	590
SPINACH JUICE					
juice	3 1/2 oz	7	0	0	73
SPORTS DRINKS					
(*see also* ENERGY DRINKS)					
Gatorade					
Orange	1 cup (8 oz)	50	0	0	110
Powerade					
Lemon-Lime	8 oz	70	0	0	55
Ultra Fuel					
Lemon Lime	16 oz	400	0	0	55

FOOD	PORTION	CALS	FAT	CHOL	SOD
SPROUTS					
(see also ALFALFA)					
lentil sprouts	1/2 cup	40	tr	0	4
mung bean	1/2 cup	16	tr	0	3
pea	1/2 cup	77	tr	0	12
radish	1/2 cup	8	tr	0	1
Chun King					
Bean Sprouts	1 cup (3 oz)	11	tr	0	17
Fresh Alternatives					
BroccoSprouts	1/2 cup (1 oz)	10	0	0	0
Deli Blend	1/2 cup (1 oz)	10	0	0	0
Salad Blend	1/2 cup (1 oz)	10	0	0	0
Sandwich Blend	1/2 cup (1 oz)	5	0	0	0
La Choy					
Bean Sprouts	1 cup (2.9 oz)	11	tr	0	17
SQUAB					
boneless baked	3.5 oz	175	3	75	100
SQUASH					
(see also ZUCCHINI)					
fresh					
acorn cooked mashed	1/2 cup	41	tr	0	3
acorn cubed baked	1/2 cup	57	tr	0	4
butternut baked	1/2 cup	41	tr	0	4
crookneck sliced cooked	1/2 cup	18	tr	0	1
hubbard baked	1/2 cup	51	tr	0	8
hubbard cooked mashed	1/2 cup	35	tr	0	6
scallop sliced cooked	1/2 cup	14	tr	0	1
spaghetti cooked	1/2 cup	23	tr	0	14
seeds					
dried	1 oz	154	13	0	5
roasted	1 oz	148	12	0	5
salted & roasted	1 oz	148	12	0	5
SQUID					
fried	3 oz	149	6	221	260
SQUIRREL					
roasted	3 oz	147	4	103	102
STAR FRUIT					
fresh	1	42	tr	0	2
STRAWBERRIES					
canned					
in heavy syrup	1/2 cup	117	tr	0	5
fresh					
strawberries	1 pint	97	1	0	4
frozen					
sweetened sliced	1 cup	245	tr	0	8
unsweetened	1 cup	52	tr	0	3
Birds Eye					
Halves	1/2 cup (4.7 oz)	120	0	0	0

FOOD	PORTION	CALS	FAT	CHOL	SOD
Birds Eye (cont.)					
Halves In Lite Syrup	1/2 cup (4.6 oz)	70	0	0	0
Whole	1/2 cup (4.5 oz)	100	0	0	0
STRAWBERRY JUICE					
Capri Sun					
Strawberry Cooler Drink	1 pkg (7 oz)	90	0	0	20
Kool-Aid					
Drink as prep w/ sugar	1 serv (8 oz)	100	0	0	30
Drink Mix as prep	1 serv (8 oz)	60	0	0	0
Veryfine					
Juice-Ups	8 oz	140	0	0	15
STUFFING/DRESSING					
Kellogg's					
Croutettes Mix	1 cup (1.2 oz)	120	0	0	460
Pepperidge Farm					
Corn Bread	3/4 cup (1.5 oz)	170	2	0	480
Herb Seasoned	3/4 cup (1.5 oz)	170	2	0	600
Herb Seasoned Cubed	3/4 cup (1.3 oz)	140	2	0	530
One Step Chicken	1/2 cup (1.2 oz)	140	4	<5	440
One Step Southwestern Corn Bread	1/2 cup (1.2 oz)	150	5	0	440
One Step Turkey	1/2 cup (1.2 oz)	150	5	<5	500
Stove Top					
Chicken as prep w/ margarine	1/2 cup (3.6 oz)	170	9	0	510
Cornbread as prep w/ margarine	1/2 cup (3.6 oz)	170	8	0	580
Flexible Serve Chicken as prep w/ margarine	1/2 cup (3.3 oz)	170	8	0	520
Flexible Serve Cornbread as prep w/ margarine	1/2 cup (3.3 oz)	160	8	0	560
Flexible Serve Homestyle Herb as prep w/ margarine	1/2 cup (3.3 oz)	170	8	0	500
For Beef as prep w/ margarine	1/2 cup (3.7 oz)	180	9	0	540
For Pork as prep w/ margarine	1/2 cup (3.6 oz)	170	9	0	530
For Turkey as prep w/ margarine	1/2 cup (3.6 oz)	170	9	0	530
Long Grain & Wild Rice as prep w/ margarine	1/2 cup (3.7 oz)	180	9	0	500
Lower Sodium Chicken as prep w/ margarine	1/2 cup (3.6 oz)	180	9	0	340
Microwave Chicken as prep w/ margarine	1/2 cup (3.5 oz)	160	7	0	480
Microwave Homestyle Cornbread as prep w/ margarine	1/2 cup (3 oz)	160	7	0	480
Mushroom & Onion as prep w/ margarine	1/2 cup (3.6 oz)	180	9	0	480

FOOD	PORTION	CALS	FAT	CHOL	SOD
San Francisco Style as prep w/ margarine	1/2 cup (3.6 oz)	170	9	0	530
Savory Herb as prep w/ margarine	1/2 cup (3.6 oz)	170	9	0	530
Traditional Sage as prep w/ margarine	1/2 cup (3.6 oz)	180	9	0	530
take-out					
bread	1/2 cup (3 1/2 oz)	195	8	0	534
sausage	1/2 cup	292	11	12	258
SUCKER					
white baked	3 oz	101	3	45	44
SUGAR					
(see also FRUCTOSE, SUGAR SUBSTITUTES, SYRUP)					
brown packed	1 cup (7.7 oz)	828	0	0	86
maple	1 piece (1 oz)	100	tr	0	3
powdered	1 tbsp (0.3 oz)	31	0	0	0
white	1 cup (7 oz)	773	0	0	3
white	1 packet (6 g)	25	0	0	tr
white	1 tsp (4 g)	15	0	0	0
Maui Brand					
Raw Sugar	1 tsp	15	0	0	0
SUGAR SUBSTITUTES					
(see also FRUCTOSE)					
Mrs. Bateman's					
Sugarlike	1 tsp (4 g)	4	0	0	0
Weight Watchers					
Sweetener	1 serv (1 g)	5	0	0	30
SUGAR-APPLE					
fresh	1	146	tr	0	15
SUNDAE TOPPINGS					
(see ICE CREAM TOPPINGS)					
SUNFISH					
pumpkinseed baked	3 oz	97	1	73	87
SUNFLOWER					
seeds dried	1 oz	162	14	0	1
seeds toasted salted	1 oz	176	16	0	204
sunflower butter	1 tbsp	93	8	0	82
Dakota Gourmet					
Honey Roasted Kernels	1 pkg (1 oz)	158	12	0	56
Lightly Salted Kernels	1 pkg (1 oz)	168	14	0	85
Frito Lay					
Seeds	1 oz	180	15	0	25
Lance					
Seeds In Shell	2/3 cup (1.8 oz)	160	13	0	30
Seeds Roasted & Shelled	1 pkg (1 1/8 oz)	190	16	0	100

FOOD	PORTION	CALS	FAT	CHOL	SOD
SUSHI					
take-out					
california roll	1 piece (0.8 oz)	28	1	1	37
kim chi	1/3 cup (5.8 oz)	18	tr	0	2143
sashimi	1 serv (6 oz)	198	7	63	718
tuna roll	1 piece (0.7 oz)	23	tr	3	33
vegetable roll	1 piece (1.2 oz)	27	1	0	47
vinegared ginger	1/3 cup (1.6 oz)	48	tr	0	6
wasabi	2 tsp (0.3 oz)	5	tr	0	124
yellowtail roll	1 piece (0.6 oz)	25	1	0	32
SWAMP CABBAGE					
chopped cooked	1/2 cup	10	tr	0	60
SWEET POTATO					
(see also YAM)					
canned					
in syrup	1/2 cup	106	tr	0	38
pieces	1 cup	183	tr	0	107
fresh					
baked w/ skin	1 (3 1/2 oz)	118	tr	0	12
leaves cooked	1/2 cup	11	tr	0	4
mashed	1/2 cup	172	tr	0	21
frozen					
cooked	1/2 cup	88	tr	0	7
take-out					
candied	3 1/2 oz	144	3	0	73
SWEETBREADS					
lamb braised	3 oz	199	13	340	44
SWISS CHARD					
cooked	1/2 cup	18	tr	0	158
raw chopped	1/2 cup	3	tr	0	38
SWORDFISH					
cooked	3 oz	132	4	43	98
SYRUP					
(see also ICE CREAM TOPPINGS, PANCAKE/WAFFLE SYRUP)					
corn	2 tbsp	122	0	0	19
malt	1 tbsp (0.8 oz)	76	0	0	8
maple	1 tbsp (0.8 oz)	52	0	0	2
sorghum	1 tbsp (0.7 oz)	61	0	0	2
Estee					
Blueberry	1/4 cup	80	0	0	70
Hershey					
Strawberry	2 tbsp (1.4 oz)	100	0	0	10
Quik					
Strawberry	2 tbsp (1.5 oz)	110	0	0	0
TACO					
(see SPANISH FOOD)					

FOOD	PORTION	CALS	FAT	CHOL	SOD
TAHINI					
(*see* SESAME)					
TAMARIND					
fresh	1	5	tr	0	1
TANGERINE					
canned					
in light syrup	1/2 cup	76	tr	0	8
juice pack	1/2 cup	46	tr	0	7
fresh					
sections	1 cup	86	tr	0	3
tangerine	1	37	tr	0	1
TANGERINE JUICE					
canned sweetened	1 cup	125	1	0	2
fresh	1 cup	106	tr	0	2
frozen sweetened as prep	1 cup	110	tr	0	2
Fresh Samantha					
Fresh Juice	1 cup (8 oz)	110	0	0	0
TAPIOCA					
pearl dry	1/2 cup (2.7 oz)	272	tr	0	1
Minute					
Minute Tapioca	1 1/2 tsp (6 g)	20	0	0	0
TARO					
chips	10 (0.8 oz)	115	6	0	79
leaves cooked	1/2 cup	18	tr	0	2
sliced cooked	1/2 cup (2.3 oz)	94	tr	0	10
tahitian sliced cooked	1/2 cup	30	tr	0	37
TARRAGON					
ground	1 tsp	5	tr	0	1
TEA/HERBAL TEA					
(*see also* ICED TEA)					
herbal					
Celestial Seasonings					
Mandarin Orange Spice	1 tea bag	0	0	0	0
Lipton					
Bedtime Story	1 tea bag	0	0	0	0
Cinnamon Apple	1 tea bag	0	0	0	0
Gentle Orange	1 tea bag	0	0	0	0
Lemon Soother	1 tea bag	0	0	0	0
Peppermint	1 tea bag	0	0	0	0
Quietly Chamomile	1 tea bag	0	0	0	0
regular					
brewed tea	6 oz	2	0	0	5
instant unsweetened as prep w/ water	8 oz	2	0	0	8
General Foods					
International Instant Tea Decaffeinated English Breakfast Creme	1 serv (8 oz)	70	2	0	105

FOOD	PORTION	CALS	FAT	CHOL	SOD
General Foods (cont.)					
International Instant Tea Decaffeinated Viennese Cinnamon Creme	1 serv (8 oz)	70	2	0	105
International Instant Tea English Breakfast Creme as prep	1 serv (8 oz)	70	2	0	65
International Instant Tea English Raspberry Creme as prep	1 serv (8 oz)	70	2	0	65
International Instant Tea Island Orange Creme as prep	1 serv (8 oz)	70	2	0	65
International Instant Tea Viennese Cinnamon Creme as prep	1 serv (8 oz)	70	2	0	65
Lipton					
Brisk Tea as prep	1 serv	0	0	0	0
Decaffeinated Brisk Tea as prep	1 serv	0	0	0	0
English Blend as prep	1 cup	0	0	0	0
Flavored Decaffeinated Orange & Spice	1 tea bag	0	0	0	0
Green Tea	1 tea bag	0	0	0	0
Loose Tea	1 tsp (2 g)	0	0	0	0
Paradise					
Tropical Tea	8 oz	1	0	0	7
Tropical Tea Decafe	8 oz	1	0	0	7
Tropical Tea Passion Fruit	8 oz	1	0	0	7
Salada					
Green Tea	1 cup	0	0	0	0
Tetley					
Tea Bag as prep	1	0	0	0	0
TEMPEH					
tempeh	1/2 cup	165	6	0	5
Lightlife					
Garden Vege	4 oz	200	8	0	399
Quinoa Sesame	4 oz	220	8	0	0
Smokey Strips	3 slices (2 oz)	80	3	0	230
Soy	4 oz	210	8	0	0
Three Grain	4 oz	200	7	0	0
Wild Rice	4 oz	190	7	0	0
Turtle Island					
Five Grain	3 oz	190	6	0	10
Low Fat Millet	3 oz	130	2	0	10
Soy	3 oz	160	4	0	15
Wild Rice Rhapsody	3 oz	160	4	0	15

FOOD	PORTION	CALS	FAT	CHOL	SOD
THYME					
ground	1 tsp	4	tr	0	1
TOFU					
fresh fried	1 piece (0.5 oz)	35	3	0	2
fuyu salted & fermented	1 block (1/3 oz)	13	1	0	316
koyadofu dried frozen	1 piece (1/2 oz)	82	5	0	1
okara	1/2 cup	47	1	0	6
Galaxy					
Slices Hickory Smoked	1 slice (1 oz)	50	2	0	340
Slices Italian Garlic Herb	1 slice (1 oz)	50	2	0	390
Slices Original	1 slice (1 oz)	50	2	0	340
Slices Savory	1 slice (1 oz)	50	2	0	390
Hinoichi					
Firm	1 inch slice (3 oz)	60	3	0	10
Long Life					
Tofu	3 oz	60	3	0	10
Nasoya					
Chinise 5 Spice	1/4 block (3 oz)	68	4	0	121
Extra Firm	1/5 block (3.2 oz)	92	5	0	9
Firm	1/5 block (3.2 oz)	76	4	0	8
French Country	1/5 block (3 oz)	68	4	tr	130
Silken	1/5 block (3.2 oz)	48	2	0	12
Soft	1/5 block (3.2 oz)	63	3	0	6
Tree Of Life					
30% Reduced Fat Firm	1/5 block (3.2 oz)	90	4	0	5
Easymeal Pasta Primavera as prep	1 serv	460	16	10	790
Easymeal Southwest Medley as prep	1 serv	380	14	0	790
Easymeal Teriyaki Stir Fry as prep	1 serv	270	14	0	560
Easymeal Thai Stir Fry	1 serv	270	14	0	230
Organic Firm	1/5 block (3.2 oz)	100	5	0	5
Raw Firm	1/5 block (3.2 oz)	100	5	0	5
TOMATILLO					
fresh	1 (1.2 oz)	11	tr	0	0
fresh chopped	1/2 cup	21	1	0	1
TOMATO					
(*see also* PIZZA SAUCE, SPAGHETTI SAUCE)					
canned					
Amore					
Sun-Dried Tomato Paste	1 tsp (6 g)	15	1	0	115
Big R					
Cajun Stewed	1/2 cup (4.2 oz)	25	0	0	150
Diced w/ Chilies	1/2 cup (4.2 oz)	25	0	0	340
Mexican Stewed	1/2 cups (4.2 oz)	25	0	0	190
Stewed	1/2 cup (4.2 oz)	25	0	0	190
Whole	1/2 cup (4.2 oz)	25	0	0	190

FOOD	PORTION	CALS	FAT	CHOL	SOD
Contadina					
Recipe Ready Diced Roasted Garlic	1/2 cup (4.3 oz)	45	0	0	560
Del Monte					
Zesty Diced w/ Mild Green Chilies	1/2 cup (4.4 oz)	30	0	0	550
Hunt's					
Angela Mia Puree	1/4 cup (2.2 oz)	16	tr	0	21
Choice Cut	1/2 cup (4.2 oz)	23	tr	0	325
Choice Cut Diced Tomatoes & Italian Herb	1/2 cup (4.2 oz)	24	0	0	600
Choice Cut Diced Tomatoes & Roasted Garlic	1/2 cup (4.2 oz)	24	0	0	505
Choice Cut Diced Tomatoes w/ Red Pepper & Basil	1/4 cup (4.2 oz)	27	tr	0	396
Crushed Pear Tomatoes	1/2 cup (4.2 oz)	29	tr	0	286
Diced In Juice	1/2 cup (4.2 oz)	20	tr	0	477
Diced In Puree	1/2 cup (4.3 oz)	23	tr	0	304
Diced w/ Green Chilies	2 tbsp (0.4 oz)	1	tr	0	24
Paste	2 tbsp (1.2 oz)	30	tr	0	88
Paste Italian	2 tbsp (1.2 oz)	27	tr	0	264
Paste No Salt Added	2 tbsp (1.2 oz)	30	tr	0	7
Paste With Garlic	2 tbsp (1.2 oz)	28	tr	0	281
Puree	1/4 cup (2.2 oz)	24	tr	0	98
Ready Sauce Chunky Chili	1/4 cup (2.2 oz)	22	tr	0	320
Ready Sauce Chunky Italian	1/4 cup (2.2 oz)	30	1	0	179
Ready Sauce Chunky Mexican	1/4 cup (2.2 oz)	21	tr	0	390
Ready Sauce Chunky Salsa	1/4 cup (2.2 oz)	18	tr	0	357
Ready Sauce Chunky Tomato	1/4 cup (2.2 oz)	15	tr	0	403
Ready Sauce Garlic & Herb	1/4 cup (2.2 oz)	26	tr	0	202
Sauce	1/4 cup (2.2 oz)	16	tr	0	366
Sauce Herb	1/4 cup (2.2 oz)	32	1	0	271
Sauce Italian	1/4 cup (2.2 oz)	32	1	0	210
Sauce Meatloaf Fixins	1/4 cup (2.2 oz)	23	tr	0	600
Sauce No Salt Added	1/4 cup (2.2 oz)	16	tr	0	12
Sauce Special	1/4 cup (2.2 oz)	21	1	0	144
Stewed	1/2 cup (4.2 oz)	33	tr	0	357
Stewed No Salt Added	1/2 cup (4.2 oz)	33	tr	0	31
Whole Peeled	2 (5.2 oz)	24	tr	0	433
Whole Peeled No Salt Added	2 (4.8 oz)	21	tr	0	9
Progresso					
Crushed	1/4 cup (2.1 oz)	20	0	0	95
Italian Style Peeled	1/2 cup (4.2 oz)	20	0	0	220
Paste	2 tbsp (1.2 oz)	30	0	0	20
Puree	1/4 cup (2.2 oz)	25	0	0	15
Puree Thick Style	1/4 cup (2.2 oz)	20	0	0	15

FOOD	PORTION	CALS	FAT	CHOL	SOD
Sauce	1/4 cup (2.1 oz)	20	0	0	260
Whole Peeled	1/2 cup (4.2 oz)	25	0	0	220
Ro-Tel					
Diced Tomatoes & Green Chilies	1/2 cup (4.4 oz)	20	0	0	370
dried					
sun dried	1 cup	140	2	0	1131
sun dried	1 piece	5	tr	0	42
sun dried in oil	1 cup (4 oz)	235	15	0	293
sun dried in oil	1 piece (3 g)	6	tr	0	8
fresh					
cooked	1/2 cup	32	1	0	13
green	1	30	tr	0	16
red	1 (4.5 oz)	26	tr	0	11
red chopped	1 cup	35	tr	0	16
Eurofresh					
Tomatoes On The Vine	1 med (5.2 oz)	35	1	0	5
take-out					
stewed	1 cup	80	3	0	460
TOMATO JUICE					
Dole					
Juice	1 bottle (12 oz)	85	0	0	1000
Hunt's					
Juice	1 can (6 oz)	22	tr	0	452
No Salt Added	8 oz	34	tr	0	12
Mott's					
Tomato Juice	8 oz	40	0	0	850
TONGUE					
beef simmered	3 oz	241	18	91	51
lamb braised	3 oz	234	17	161	57
pork braised	3 oz	230	16	124	93
TOPPINGS					
(*see* ICE CREAM TOPPINGS)					
TORTILLA					
(*see also* CHIPS, SPANISH FOOD)					
La Mexicana					
Corn	1 (0.8 oz)	50	1	0	0
Flour	1 (0.8 oz)	80	3	0	260
Tortillas de Trigo	1 (1 oz)	140	7	0	75
Old El Paso					
Flour	1 (1.4 oz)	130	4	0	290
Tyson					
Flour	1 (1.7 oz)	150	4	0	310
Flour Heat Pressed	2 (2 oz)	170	4	0	410
White Corn	2 (1.8 oz)	100	1	0	70
Whole Wheat Heat Pressed	1 (1.4 oz)	120	3	0	240
Yellow Corn	3 (1.9 oz)	140	2	0	20

FOOD	PORTION	CALS	FAT	CHOL	SOD
TORTILLA CHIPS					
(see CHIPS)					
TREE FERN					
chopped cooked	1/2 cup	28	tr	0	3
TRITICALE					
dry	1 cup (6.7 oz)	645	4	0	10
TROUT					
rainbow cooked	3 oz	129	4	62	29
seatrout baked	3 oz	113	4	90	63
TRUFFLES					
fresh	3 1/2 oz	25	1	0	77
TUMERIC					
ground	1 tsp	8	tr	0	1
TUNA					
(see also TUNA DISHES)					
canned					
Bumble Bee					
Chunk Light In Water Pouch	2 oz	60	1	30	250
Solid White In Water	2 oz	70	1	25	250
Progresso					
In Olive Oil drained	1/4 cup (2 oz)	160	12	30	250
StarKist					
Chunk Light No Drain Package	1/4 cup (2 oz)	60	1	30	250
Solid White Albacore In Spring Water	1/4 cup (2 oz)	70	1	25	250
Tuna Fillet In Spring Water	1/4 cup (2 oz)	60	1	30	250
fresh					
bluefin cooked	3 oz	157	5	42	43
bluefin raw	3 oz	122	4	32	33
skipjack baked	3 oz	112	1	51	40
yellowfin baked	3 oz	118	1	49	40
TUNA DISHES					
mix					
Tuna Helper					
AuGratin 50% Less Fat Recipe as prep	1 cup	240	6	15	840
AuGratin as prep	1 cup	300	11	20	890
Cheesy Broccoli 50% Less Fat Recipe as prep	1 cup	240	5	15	820
Cheesy Broccoli as prep	1 cup	290	9	20	860
Cheesy Pasta 50% Less Fat Recipe as prep	1 cup	230	5	15	850
Cheesy Pasta as prep	1 cup	280	11	20	890
Creamy Broccoli 50% Less Fat Recipe as prep	1 cup	240	5	15	820
Creamy Broccoli as prep	1 cup	310	12	20	880

FOOD	PORTION	CALS	FAT	CHOL	SOD
Creamy Pasta 50% Less Fat Recipe as prep	1 cup	230	6	15	840
Creamy Pasta as prep	1 cup	300	13	20	910
Fettuccine Alfredo 50% Less Fat Recipe as prep	1 cup	240	6	15	870
Fettuccine Alfredo as prep	1 cup	310	14	15	950
Garden Cheddar 50% Less Fat Recipe as prep	1 cup	240	5	15	980
Garden Cheddar as prep	1 cup	290	11	20	1030
Pasta Salad Low Fat Recipe as prep	2/3 cup	230	2	10	790
Pasta Salad as prep	2/3 cup	380	27	10	730
Tetrazzini 50% Less Fat Recipe as prep	1 cup	230	5	20	980
Tetrazzini as prep	1 cup	300	12	20	1040
Tuna Melt Reduced Fat Recipe as prep	1 cup	240	6	15	850
Tuna Melt as prep	1 cup	300	12	20	900
Tuna Pot Pie as prep	1 cup	440	24	110	1080
Tuna Romanoff 50% Less Fat Recipe as prep	1 cup	240	3	20	740
Tuna Romanoff as prep	1 cup	280	8	20	800
ready-to-eat					
Wampler					
Salad	1/3 cup	180	12	20	450
Salad Chunky	1/3 cup	180	13	20	380
take-out					
tuna salad	1 cup	383	19	27	824
tuna salad	3 oz	159	8	11	342
TURKEY					
(*see also* DINNER, HOT DOG, TURKEY DISHES, TURKEY SUBSTITUTES)					
fresh					
breast w/ skin roasted	4 oz	212	8	83	70
dark meat w/ skin roasted	3.6 oz	230	12	93	79
dark meat w/o skin roasted	3 oz	170	7	78	72
ground cooked	3 oz	188	11	57	68
leg w/ skin roasted	1 (1.2 lbs)	1133	54	466	420
light meat w/ skin roasted	4.7 oz	268	11	103	85
light meat w/o skin roasted	4 oz	183	4	81	75
neck simmered	1 (5.3 oz)	274	11	186	84
skin roasted	from 1/2 turkey (9 oz)	1096	98	281	132
w/o skin roasted	1 cup (5 oz)	238	7	107	99
wing w/ skin roasted	1 (6.5 oz)	426	23	150	114
Louis Rich					
Ground	4 oz	190	12	90	140
Patties White	1 (4 oz)	170	10	65	440

FOOD	PORTION	CALS	FAT	CHOL	SOD
Shady Brook					
Cutlets	4 oz	130	1	70	55
Drumstick	4 oz	170	9	70	80
Ground Breast	4 oz	120	1	70	55
Ground Lean	4 oz	170	9	90	105
Ground Turkey 85%	4 oz	220	15	75	75
Mesquite Seasoned Tenderloin	4 oz	110	1	50	360
OnlyOne Boneless Breast Roast	4 oz	130	1	70	55
Split Breast	4 oz	190	9	70	60
Tenderloin	4 oz	130	1	70	55
Teriyaki Seasoned Tenderloin	4 oz	120	1	50	460
Thigh	4 oz	220	15	75	75
Turkey Burgers	4 oz	170	9	90	105
Turkey Meatloaf Lean	4 oz	150	7	95	400
Whole Breast	4 oz	190	9	70	60
Whole Turkey	4 oz	180	9	75	75
Wing	4 oz	220	14	80	60
Zesty Lemon Seasoned Tenderlion	4 oz	120	1	50	200
The Turkey Store					
Breakfast Sausage Patties Mild	2 patties (2.3 oz)	160	13	50	420
Seasoned Cuts Turkey Breast Roast	4 oz	110	1	45	530
Wampler					
Boneless Breast Roast	4 oz	160	6	35	25
Breast Half	4 oz	160	6	35	25
Breast Steaks	4 oz	120	1	70	55
Drumsticks	4 oz	180	10	75	45
Ground	4 oz	210	15	100	70
Ground Breast	4 oz	130	1	70	55
Ground Lean	4 oz	160	8	90	70
Thighs	4 oz	170	10	80	40
Wings	4 oz	220	14	80	60
Woodfire Grill Burger	1 (3 oz)	180	9	65	360
frozen					
roast boneless seasoned light & dark meat roasted	1 pkg (1.7 lbs)	1213	45	413	5320
Wampler					
Burger BBQ	1 (4 oz)	240	17	140	240
Seasoned Burgers Cracker Peppercorn & Garlic	1 (3 oz)	170	9	65	380
ready-to-eat					
bologna	1 oz	57	4	28	249
poultry salad sandwich spread	1 tbsp	109	2	4	49

FOOD	PORTION	CALS	FAT	CHOL	SOD
Alpine Lace					
Breast Fat Free	2 oz	45	0	25	350
Boar's Head					
Breast Cracked Pepper Smoked	2 oz	60	1	30	460
Breast Golden Skin On	2 oz	60	2	25	340
Breast Golden Skinless	2 oz	60	1	25	350
Breast Hickory Smoked	2 oz	70	2	25	340
Breast Low Sodium Skinless	2 oz	60	1	25	340
Breast Lower Sodium Skin On	2 oz	60	2	25	310
Breast Maple Glazed Honey Coat	2 oz	70	1	30	440
Breast Ovengold Skin On	2 oz	60	2	35	360
Breast Ovengold Skinless	2 oz	60	1	20	350
Breast Roasted Mesquite Smoked Skinless	2 oz	60	1	25	440
Breast Roasted Salsalito	2 oz	60	1	25	460
Pastrami Seasoned	2 oz	60	1	25	440
Carl Buddig					
Honey Roasted Turkey Breast	1 pkg (2.5 oz)	120	7	40	780
Lean Slices Honey Roasted Breast	1 pkg (2.5 oz)	70	1	30	980
Lean Slices Oven Roasted Breast	1 pkg (2.5 oz)	70	1	30	980
Lean Slices Smoked Breast	1 pkg (2.5 oz)	70	1	30	880
Oven Roasted Breast	1 pkg (2.5 oz)	110	7	40	780
Smoked Breast	1 pkg (2.5 oz)	110	7	40	780
Turkey Ham	1 pkg (2.5 oz)	100	5	40	1020
Hormel					
Light & Lean 97 Breast Sliced	1 slice (1 oz)	30	1	15	380
Light & Lean 97 Mesquite Smoked Breast	1 slice (1 oz)	30	1	15	370
turkey pepperoni	17 slices (1 oz)	80	4	40	550
Jordan's					
Healthy Trim Fat Free Oven Roasted Breast	1 slice (1 oz)	20	0	15	180
Healthy Trim Fat Free Oven Roasted Smoked Breast	1 slice (1 oz)	20	0	15	180
Louis Rich					
Bologna	1 slice (28 g)	50	4	20	270
Breaded Nuggets	4 (3.2 oz)	260	16	35	640
Breaded Patties	1 (3 oz)	220	13	35	530
Breaded Sticks	3 (3 oz)	230	15	35	580
Breast Skinless Hickory Smoked	2 oz	50	0	25	720
Breast Skinless Honey Roasted	2 oz	60	0	20	660
Breast Skinless Oven Roasted	2 oz	50	0	20	660

FOOD	PORTION	CALS	FAT	CHOL	SOD
Louis Rich (cont.)					
Breast Skinless Rotisserie	2 oz	50	0	20	670
Breast Slices Hickory Smoked	1 slice (2 oz)	50	0	25	720
Breast Slices Honey Roasted	1 slice (2 oz)	60	0	20	660
Breast Slices Oven Roasted	1 slice (2 oz)	50	0	20	660
Breast Slices Rotisserie	1 slice (2 oz)	50	0	20	670
Carving Board Hickory Smoked	2 slices (1.6 oz)	40	1	20	540
Carving Board Oven Roasted Thin	6 slices (2.1 oz)	60	1	25	710
Carving Board Oven Roasted Traditional	2 slices (1.6 oz)	40	1	20	540
Carving Board Rotisserie	2 slices (1.6 oz)	40	1	20	460
Cotto Salami	1 slice (28 g)	40	3	25	280
Deli-Thin Oven Roasted	4 slices (1.8 oz)	50	1	20	580
Deli-Thin Smoked	4 slices (1.8 oz)	50	2	20	480
Fat Free Hickory Smoked Breast	1 slice (1 oz)	25	0	10	300
Fat Free Oven Roasted Breast	1 slice (1 oz)	25	0	10	330
Fat Free Oven Roasted Deli-Thin Breast	4 slices (1.8 oz)	45	0	15	620
Fat Free Turkey Ham Honey	2 slices (1.7 oz)	35	0	15	600
Fat Free Turkey Ham Smoked	2 slices (1.7 oz)	35	0	15	580
Hickory Smoked	1 slice (1 oz)	30	1	10	260
Oven Roasted	1 slice (1 oz)	30	1	10	310
Pastrami	1 slice (1 oz)	30	1	20	380
Smoked	1 slice (1 oz)	30	1	15	280
Turkey Ham	1 slice (1 oz)	30	1	20	380
Turkey Ham Chopped	1 slice (1 oz)	45	3	20	350
Turkey Ham Honey Cured	1 slice (1 oz)	30	1	20	350
Oscar Mayer					
Free Oven Roasted Breast	4 slices (1.8 oz)	40	0	15	670
Free Smoked Breast	4 slices (1.8 oz)	40	0	15	570
Oven Roasted White	1 slice (1 oz)	30	1	10	300
Smoked White	1 slice (1 oz)	30	1	10	310
Shady Brook					
Black Forest Turkey Ham	2 oz	70	3	30	470
Browned Homestyle Oven Roasted Breast	2 oz	60	1	20	400
Browned Slow Roasted Breast	2 oz	60	0	20	400
Carved Breast Italian Seasoned	2 oz	60	0	20	490
Carved Breast Natural Roast	2 oz	60	0	20	470
Carved Breast Peppered	2 oz	60	0	20	450
Hickory Smoked Breast	2 oz	50	0	25	470
Honey Roasted Breast	2 oz	60	1	30	400
Honey Roasted Breast Covered w/ Cracked Pepper	2 oz	60	0	25	470

FOOD	PORTION	CALS	FAT	CHOL	SOD
Meatballs Italian Style	3 (3 oz)	130	7	45	350
Smoked Drumstick	3 oz	180	8	70	620
Smoked Neck	3 oz	150	6	65	700
Smoked Whole Turkey	3 oz	150	4	60	660
Smoked Wing	3 oz	200	10	65	680
Wampler					
Bologna	2 oz	130	11	50	550
Dark Cured	2 oz	80	5	30	600
Deli Roast Breast	2 oz	50	1	25	250
Deli Roast Classic Spiced Breast	2 oz	70	1	25	380
Deli Roast Pan Roasted Breast	2 oz	70	2	20	400
Deli Roast Pan Roasted Skinless Breast	2 oz	50	0	20	400
Deli Roast Peppered Breast	2 oz	40	0	20	520
Deli Roast Rotisserie Breast	2 oz	50	2	20	500
Pastrami	2 oz	90	5	40	220
Salami	2 oz	90	6	55	560
Turkey Ham	2 oz	60	3	40	590

TURKEY DISHES

(*see also* DINNER, TURKEY SUBSTITUTES)

canned

Dinty Moore

FOOD	PORTION	CALS	FAT	CHOL	SOD
Stew	1 cup (8.5 oz)	140	3	20	910

ready-to-eat

Shady Brook

FOOD	PORTION	CALS	FAT	CHOL	SOD
Meatloaf	1 serv (16 oz)	470	17	175	900

Wampler

FOOD	PORTION	CALS	FAT	CHOL	SOD
Turkey Ham Salad	1/3 cup	150	10	30	500

shelf-stable

Dinty Moore

FOOD	PORTION	CALS	FAT	CHOL	SOD
Microwave Cup Stew	1 pkg (7.5 oz)	130	3	10	760

TURKEY SUBSTITUTES

Lightlife

FOOD	PORTION	CALS	FAT	CHOL	SOD
Smart Deli Turkey	3 slices (1.5 oz)	40	0	0	290
Soy Is Us					
Turkey Not!	1/2 cup (1.75 oz)	140	2	0	5
Tofurkey					
Deli Slices Hickory	1.5 oz	120	2	0	286
Deli Slices Original	1.5 oz	120	2	0	286
Deli Slices Peppered	1.5 oz	120	2	0	286
Drummettes	1 (3 oz)	105	2	0	380
Giblet Gravy	1 serv (3.5 oz)	42	2	0	340
Stuffed Tofu Roast	1 serv (4 oz)	193	5	0	310
Worthington					
Smoked Turkey Meatless	3 slices (2 oz)	140	10	0	620
Turkee Slices	3 slices (3.3 oz)	130	14	0	580

FOOD	PORTION	CALS	FAT	CHOL	SOD
Yves					
Veggie Turkey Deli Slices	1 serv (2.2 oz)	85	0	0	480
TURNIPS					
canned					
greens	1/2 cup	17	tr	0	325
fresh					
cooked mashed	1/2 cup (4.2 oz)	47	tr	0	25
cubed cooked	1/2 cup (3 oz)	33	tr	0	17
greens chopped cooked	1/2 cup	15	tr	0	21
frozen					
Birds Eye					
Chopped Greens	1 cup (3.1 oz)	30	0	0	20
Greens w/ Diced Root	1 cup (3 oz)	25	0	0	20
VEAL					
(*see also* DINNER, VEAL DISHES)					
cutlet lean only braised	3 oz	172	4	115	57
cutlet lean only fried	3 oz	156	4	91	65
ground broiled	3 oz	146	6	87	70
loin chop w/ bone lean & fat braised	1 chop (2.8 oz)	227	14	94	64
shoulder w/ bone lean only braised	3 oz	169	5	110	83
sirloin w/ bone lean & fat roasted	3 oz	171	9	87	71
VEAL DISHES					
take-out					
parmigiana	4.2 oz	279	18	136	545
VEGETABLE JUICE					
Dole					
Vegetable Blend	1 bottle (12 oz)	90	0	0	820
Hunt's					
Cocktail	1 can (6 oz)	20	0	0	630
V8					
Splash Tropical Blend	8 oz	120	0	0	20
VEGETABLES MIXED					
(*see also* VEGETABLE JUICE)					
canned					
Chi-Chi's					
Diced Tomatoes & Green Chilies	1/4 cup (2.5 oz)	20	0	0	340
Chun King					
Chow Mein Vegetables	2/3 cup (3 oz)	14	tr	0	323
Green Giant					
Garden Medley	1/2 cup (4.2 oz)	40	0	0	360
Mixed	1/2 cup (4.3 oz)	60	0	0	460
Sweet Peas & Carrots	1/2 cup (4.3 oz)	50	0	0	410
Sweet Peas & Tiny Pearl Onion	1/2 cup (4.4 oz)	60	0	0	520

FOOD	PORTION	CALS	FAT	CHOL	SOD
House Of Tsang					
Vegetables & Sauce Cantonese Classic	1/2 cup (4.2 oz)	70	1	0	960
Vegetables & Sauce Hong Kong Sweet & Sour	1/2 cup (4.5 oz)	160	0	0	580
Vegetables & Sauce Szechuan Hot & Spicy	1/2 cup (4.2 oz)	70	1	0	1130
Vegetables & Sauce Tokyo Teriyaki	1/2 cup (4.4 oz)	100	0	0	1240
La Choy					
Chop Suey Vegetables	1/2 cup (2.2 oz)	10	tr	0	241
LeSueur					
Early Peas w/ Mushrooms & Pearl Onions	1/2 cup (4.3 oz)	60	0	0	380
frozen					
Amy's Organic					
Pocket Sandwich Mediterranean Vegetables	1 (4.5 oz)	220	7	15	540
Pocket Sandwich Roasted Vegetables	1 (4.5 oz)	220	8	0	480
Pocket Sandwich Vegetable Pie	1 (5 oz)	230	6	0	420
Birds Eye					
Baby Bean & Carrot Blend	1 cup (2.9 oz)	30	0	0	25
Broccoli Cauliflower Carrots w/ Cheese	1/2 cup (3.9 oz)	70	4	5	460
Brussels Sprouts Cauliflower Carrots	1/2 cup (3.1 oz)	30	0	0	20
Chicken Voila Pesto	2 1/4 cups (6.6 oz)	250	9	25	720
Chicken Voila Three Cheese	1 3/4 cups (6.2 oz)	240	9	25	630
Farm Fresh Broccoli Carrots Water Chestnuts	1/2 cup (3.3 oz)	30	0	0	30
Farm Fresh Broccoli Cauliflower	1/2 cup (3.2 oz)	20	0	0	20
Farm Fresh Broccoli Cauliflower Carrots	1/2 cup (3.2 oz)	25	0	0	30
Farm Fresh Broccoli Cauliflower Red Peppers	1/2 cup (3.3 oz)	20	0	0	20
Farm Fresh Broccoli Corn Red Peppers	1/2 cup (3.6 oz)	50	0	0	15
Farm Fresh Broccoli Red Peppers Onions Mushrooms	1/2 cup (3.5 oz)	25	0	0	20
Farm Fresh Brussels Sprouts Cauliflower Carrots	1/2 cup (3.1 oz)	30	0	0	20
Farm Fresh Cauliflower Carrots Snow Pea Pods	1/2 cup (3.2 oz)	30	0	0	25

FOOD	PORTION	CALS	FAT	CHOL	SOD
Birds Eye (cont.)					
For Soup	2/3 cup (3 oz)	45	0	0	45
For Stew	3/4 cup (2.9 oz)	40	0	0	40
Gumbo Blend	3/4 cup (3 oz)	40	0	0	30
Internationals Bavarian Style	1 cup (5.5 oz)	150	8	30	460
Internationals California Style	1/2 cup (3 oz)	100	5	10	240
Internationals French Country Style	2/3 cup (4.4 oz)	110	6	10	290
Internationals Italian Style	1 cup (5.8 oz)	150	10	15	380
Internationals New England Style	1 pkg (9 oz)	260	14	15	480
Internationals Oriental Style	1/2 cup (3 oz)	60	4	10	260
Internationals Stir Fry Style	1/2 cup (3.6 oz)	60	4	10	270
Peas & Carrots	2/3 cup (3 oz)	50	0	0	65
Peas & Pearl Onions	2/3 cup (4.2 oz)	90	1	0	520
Peas & Potatoes In Cream Sauce	1/2 cup (4.4 oz)	90	3	10	350
Seasoning Blend	3/4 cup (2.9 oz)	20	0	0	25
Stir Fry Asparagus	2 cups (5.8 oz)	90	1	0	35
Stir Fry Broccoli	1 cup (3.3 oz)	30	0	0	30
Stir Fry Pepper	1 cup (2.9 oz)	25	0	0	15
Stir Fry Sugar Snap	3/4 cup (2.6 oz)	35	0	0	20
Stir Fry Whole Green Bean	1 3/4 cup (5.3 oz)	100	1	0	30
Green Giant					
American Mixtures Broccoli Carrots Cauliflower	3/4 cup (2.6 oz)	25	0	0	30
American Mixtures Broccoli Carrots Water Chestnuts	3/4 cup (3 oz)	30	0	0	30
American Mixtures Carrots Green Bean Cauliflower	3/4 cup (2.7 oz)	25	0	0	20
American Mixtures Cauliflower Broccoli Sugar Snap & Sweet Pea	3/4 cup (2.8 oz)	35	0	0	45
American Mixtures Corn Broccoli Red Pepper	3/4 cup (3.1 oz)	60	0	0	10
American Mixtures Green Beans Potatoes Onions Red Peppers	3/4 cup (2.8 oz)	45	1	0	15
American Mixtures Sweet Peas Potatoes Carrots	2/3 cup (3 oz)	70	2	0	70
Butter Sauce Broccoli Cauliflower Carrots Corn Sweet Peas	3/4 cup (3.6 oz)	60	2	<5	300
Butter Sauce Broccoli Pasta Sweet Peas Corn Red Peppers	3/4 cup (3.5 oz)	70	2	<5	280
Butter Sauce Mixed	3/4 cup (3.6 oz)	70	2	<5	240

FOOD	PORTION	CALS	FAT	CHOL	SOD
Cheese Sauce Broccoli Cauliflower Carrots	2/3 cup (4.3 oz)	80	3	<5	560
Harvest Fresh Broccoli Cauliflower Carrots	1 cup (3.4 oz)	30	0	0	125
Harvest Fresh Mixed Vegetables	2/3 cup (3.1 oz)	50	0	0	125
Harvest Fresh Sweet Peas & Pearl Onions	1/2 cup (2.7 oz)	55	0	0	170
Mixed	3/4 cup (2.9 oz)	50	0	0	35
Select Sweet Peas & Pearl Onions	2/3 cup (3.1 oz)	60	0	0	125
Health Is Wealth					
Veggie Munchees	2 (1 oz)	50	1	0	170
La Choy					
Fancy Chinese Mixed Vegetables	1/2 cup (2.9 oz)	9	tr	0	31
take-out					
buddha's delight	1 serv (16 oz)	174	5	35	1368
gyoza potstickers vegetable	8 (4.9 oz)	210	4	0	500
ratatouille	1 serv (3.5 oz)	96	7	0	812
succotash	1/2 cup	111	1	0	16
VENISON					
roasted	3 oz	134	3	95	46
VINEGAR					
Progresso					
Balsamic	2 tbsp (0.5 oz)	10	0	0	0
Victoria					
Balsamic	1 tbsp (0.5 oz)	5	0	0	0
White House					
Apple Cider	1 tbsp (0.5 oz)	0	0	0	0
White	1 tbsp (0.5 oz)	0	0	0	0
WAFFLES					
frozen					
Eggo					
Apple Cinnamon	2 (2.7 oz)	220	8	20	450
Banana Bread	2 (2.7 oz)	200	7	0	280
Blueberry	2 (2.7 oz)	220	9	20	460
Buttermilk	2 (2.7 oz)	220	8	25	460
Golden Oat	2 (2.7 oz)	150	3	0	340
Homestyle	2 (2.7 oz)	220	8	25	480
Minis Cinnamon Toast	12 (3.2 oz)	290	10	25	470
Minis Homestyle	12 (3.3 oz)	260	9	25	600
Nut & Honey	2 (2.7 oz)	240	10	25	450
Nutri-Grain	2 (2.7 oz)	190	6	0	450
Nutri-Grain Multi-Bran	2 (2.7 oz)	180	6	0	410
Nutri-Grain Raisin & Bran	2 (2.9 oz)	210	6	0	430
Special K	2 (2 oz)	120	0	0	280
Strawberry	2 (2.7 oz)	220	8	20	460

FOOD	PORTION	CALS	FAT	CHOL	SOD
Kellogg's					
Homestyle Low Fat	2 (2.7 oz)	180	3	20	340
Nutri-Grain Low Fat	2 (2.7 oz)	160	3	0	480
Nutri-Grain Low Fat Blueberry	2 (2.7 oz)	160	2	0	460
Van's					
7 Grain Belgian	2	152	4	0	160
Belgian Original	2	145	4	0	108
Belgian Original Toaster	2	145	4	0	92
Blueberry Toaster	2	157	4	0	92
Blueberry Wheat Free Toaster	2	225	5	0	390
Fat Free	2	155	2	0	230
Mini	4	107	4	0	275
Multigrain Toaster	2	160	4	0	135
Organic Whole Wheat	2	190	5	0	230
Organic Whole Wheat Blueberry	2	190	5	0	230
Wheat Free Cinnamon Apple Toaster	2	220	5	0	390
Wheat Free Toaster	2	220	5	0	390
mix					
plain as prep	1 7 in diam (2.6 oz)	218	10	39	458
ready-to-eat					
Thomas'					
Buttermilk	1 (1.6 oz)	130	5	0	490
WALNUTS					
black dried chopped	1 cup	759	71	0	2
english dried chopped	1 cup	770	74	0	12
halves	14 (1 oz)	190	19	0	tr
WASABI					
root raw	1 (5.9 oz)	184	1	0	29
WATER					
Absopure					
Natural Spring	8 oz	0	0	0	0
Aquess					
Purified Water w/ Soluble Fiber	1 bottle (18 oz)	30	0	0	0
Crystal Geyser					
Spring Water	8 oz	0	0	0	0
Dasani					
Purfied Water	8 oz	0	0	0	0
Gerolsteiner					
Sparling Mineral	8 oz	0	0	0	30
Glaceau					
Vitamin Water Tropical Citrus	1 cup (8 oz)	40	0	0	0
Glacier Springs					
Drinking Water	8 oz	0	0	0	0
LaCroix					
Spring	1 bottle (12 oz)	0	0	0	<8

FOOD	PORTION	CALS	FAT	CHOL	SOD
Meridian					
Clear All Flavors	8 oz	100	0	0	0
Mt Shasta					
Natural Spring	1 bottle (20 oz)	0	0	0	<13
San Pellegrino					
Acqua Panna	8 oz	0	0	0	0
Saratoga					
Spring	8 oz	0	0	0	0
Snapple					
Natural Spring	8 oz	0	0	0	0
Veryfine					
Fruit 2 0 Lemon	8 oz	0	0	0	5
Water Joe					
Caffeine Enhanced	8 oz	0	0	0	0
WATER CHESTNUTS					
Chun King					
Sliced	2 tbsp (0.8 oz)	11	tr	0	3
Whole	2 (0.7 oz)	10	tr	0	2
La Choy					
Chopped	2 tbsp (0.6 oz)	9	tr	0	2
Sliced	2 tbsp (0.8 oz)	11	tr	0	3
Whole	2 (0.7 oz)	10	tr	0	2
WATERCRESS					
(*see also* CRESS)					
raw chopped	1/2 cup	2	tr	0	7
WATERMELON					
cut up	1 cup	50	1	0	3
seeds dried	1 oz	158	13	0	28
wedge	1/16	152	2	0	10
WATERMELON JUICE					
Kool-Aid					
Splash Drink	1 serv (8 oz)	110	0	0	35
WHEAT					
(*see also* BULGUR, BRAN, CEREAL, COUSCOUS, FLOUR, WHEAT GERM)					
sprouted	1 cup (3.8 oz)	214	1	0	17
Lightlife					
Savory Seitan Barbecue	4 oz	160	2	0	360
Savory Seitan Teriyaki	4 oz	160	2	0	320
WHEAT GERM					
plain toasted	1/4 cup (1 oz)	108	3	0	1
Kretschmer					
Original Toasted	2 tbsp (0.5 oz)	50	1	0	0
WHIPPED TOPPINGS					
(*see also* CREAM)					
cream pressurized	1 cup (2.1 oz)	154	13	46	78
cream pressurized	1 tbsp (3 g)	8	tr	2	4
Cool Whip					
Extra Creamy	2 tbsp (0.3 oz)	25	2	0	5

FOOD	PORTION	CALS	FAT	CHOL	SOD
Cool Whip (cont.)					
Free	2 tbsp (0.3 oz)	15	0	0	5
Lite	2 tbsp (0.3 oz)	20	1	0	0
Original	2 tbsp (0.3 oz)	25	2	0	0
Dream Whip					
Mix as prep	2 tbsp (0.3 oz)	20	1	0	5
Estee					
Whipped Topping	1 serv	10	1	0	5
Kraft					
Dairy Whip Light Cream	2 tbsp (0.2 oz)	10	1	<5	0
Fat Free	1 tbsp (0.3 oz)	15	0	0	5
WHITE BEANS					
canned					
Progresso					
Cannellini	1/2 cup (4.6 oz)	100	1	0	270
dried					
regular cooked	1 cup	249	1	0	11
WHITEFISH					
baked	3 oz	146	6	65	56
smoked	3 oz	92	1	28	866
WHITING					
cooked	3 oz	98	1	71	113
WILD RICE					
cooked	1 cup (5.7 oz)	166	1	0	5
WINE					
red	3 1/2 oz	74	0	0	6
rosé	3 1/2 oz	73	0	0	5
sweet dessert	2 oz	90	0	0	5
white	3 1/2 oz	70	0	0	5
WINGED BEANS					
dried cooked	1 cup	252	10	0	22
WOLFFISH					
atlantic baked	3 oz	105	3	50	93
WRAPS					
(*see* BREAD)					
YAM					
(*see also* SWEET POTATO)					
fresh					
mountain yam hawaii cooked	1/2 cup	59	tr	0	9
yam cubed cooked	1/2 cup	79	tr	0	6
YAMBEAN					
cooked	3/4 cup	38	tr	0	4
YARDLONG BEANS					
dried cooked	1 cup	202	1	0	9
YAUTIA (TANNIER)					
raw sliced	1 cup (4.7 oz)	132	1	0	28
root raw	1 (10.7 oz)	299	1	0	64

FOOD	PORTION	CALS	FAT	CHOL	SOD
YEAST					
baker's compressed	1 cake (0.6 oz)	18	tr	0	5
brewer's dry	1 tbsp	25	tr	0	10
YELLOW BEANS					
canned	1/2 cup	13	tr	0	170
canned low sodium	1/2 cup	13	tr	0	1
dried cooked	1 cup	254	2	0	8
fresh cooked	1/2 cup	22	tr	0	2
YOGURT					
(see also YOGURT FROZEN)					
Breyers					
Blended Blueberry	4.4 oz	130	1	10	60
Blended Peach	4.4 oz	130	1	10	65
Blended Strawberry	4.4 oz	130	1	10	60
Light Nonfat Apple Pie A La Mode	8 oz	120	0	10	105
Light Nonfat Berry Banana Split	8 oz	120	0	10	105
Light Nonfat Black Cherry Jubilee	8 oz	120	0	10	100
Light Nonfat Blueberries 'N Cream	8 oz	120	0	10	100
Light Nonfat Cherry Bon-Bon	8 oz	120	0	10	105
Light Nonfat Cherry Vanilla Cream	8 oz	120	0	10	105
Light Nonfat Classic Strawberry	8 oz	120	0	10	100
Light Nonfat Key Lime Pie	8 oz	120	0	10	100
Light Nonfat Lemon Chiffon	8 oz	120	0	10	100
Light Nonfat Peaches 'N Cream	8 oz	120	0	10	115
Light Nonfat Raspberries 'N Cream	8 oz	120	0	10	105
Light Nonfat Strawberry Cheesecake	8 oz	120	0	10	100
Lowfat Black Cherry	8 oz	240	3	15	125
Lowfat Blueberry	8 oz	230	3	15	125
Lowfat Mixed Berry	8 oz	320	3	15	125
Lowfat Peach	8 oz	240	3	15	125
Lowfat Pineapple	8 oz	240	3	15	125
Lowfat Red Raspberry	8 oz	230	3	15	125
Lowfat Strawberry	8 oz	230	3	15	125
Lowfat Strawberry Banana	8 oz	240	3	15	125
Lowfat Vanilla	8 oz	220	3	20	135
Smooth & Creamy Apple Cobbler	8 oz	230	2	20	140
Smooth & Creamy Black Cherry Parfait	4.4 oz	130	1	10	70

FOOD	PORTION	CALS	FAT	CHOL	SOD
Breyers (cont.)					
Smooth & Creamy Black Cherry Parfait	8 oz	240	2	20	130
Smooth & Creamy Blueberries 'N Cream	8 oz	240	2	20	125
Smooth & Creamy Blueberries 'N Cream	4.4 oz	130	1	10	70
Smooth & Creamy Classic Strawberry	4.4 oz	130	1	10	70
Smooth & Creamy Classic Strawberry	8 oz	230	2	20	125
Smooth & Creamy Orange Vanilla Cream	8 oz	230	2	20	125
Smooth & Creamy Peaches 'N Cream	8 oz	230	2	20	125
Smooth & Creamy Peaches 'N Cream	4.4 oz	130	1	10	70
Smooth & Creamy Raspberries 'N Cream	8 oz	230	2	20	135
Smooth & Creamy Strawberry Banana Split	8 oz	240	2	10	125
Smooth & Creamy Strawberry Cheesecake	8 oz	240	2	20	125
Dannon					
Chunky Fruit Nonfat Apple Cinnamon	6 oz	160	0	5	100
Chunky Fruit Nonfat Blueberry	6 oz	160	0	5	110
Chunky Fruit Nonfat Cherry Vanilla	6 oz	160	0	5	100
Chunky Fruit Nonfat Peach	6 oz	160	0	5	100
Chunky Fruit Nonfat Strawberry	6 oz	160	0	5	105
Chunky Fruit Nonfat Strawberry Banana	6 oz	160	0	5	105
Danimals Lowfat Blueberry	4.4 oz	130	1	5	100
Danimals Lowfat Grape Lemonade	4.4 oz	120	1	5	90
Danimals Lowfat Lemon Ice	4.4 oz	120	1	5	100
Danimals Lowfat Orange Banana	4.4 oz	130	1	5	90
Danimals Lowfat Strawberry	4.4 oz	130	1	5	90
Danimals Lowfat Tropical Punch	4.4 oz	130	1	5	95
Danimals Lowfat Vanilla	4.4 oz	120	1	5	90
Danimals Lowfat Wild Raspberry	4.4 oz	120	1	5	90
Double Delights Banana Creme Strawberry	6 oz	160	1	10	100

FOOD	PORTION	CALS	FAT	CHOL	SOD
Double Delights Bavarian Creme Raspberry	6 oz	170	1	10	125
Double Delights Cheesecake Cherry	6 oz	170	1	10	100
Double Delights Cheesecake Strawberry	6 oz	170	1	10	100
Double Delights Chocolate Cheesecake	6 oz	220	1	10	150
Double Delights Chocolate Dipped Strawberry	6 oz	210	1	10	150
Double Delights Chocolate Eclair	6 oz	220	1	10	150
Double Delights Vanilla Strawberry	6 oz	170	1	10	100
Double Delights Vanilla Peach & Apricot	6 oz	170	1	10	100
Fruit On The Bottom Lowfat Apple Cinnamon	8 oz	240	3	15	140
Fruit On The Bottom Lowfat Blueberry	8 oz	240	3	15	140
Fruit On The Bottom Lowfat Boysenberry	8 oz	240	3	15	150
Fruit On The Bottom Lowfat Cherry	8 oz	240	3	15	135
Fruit On The Bottom Lowfat Minipack Mixed Berry	4.4 oz	130	2	10	80
Fruit On The Bottom Lowfat Minipack Strawberry	4.4 oz	130	2	10	75
Fruit On The Bottom Lowfat Mixed Berries	8 oz	240	3	15	150
Fruit On The Bottom Lowfat Orange	8 oz	240	3	15	135
Fruit On The Bottom Lowfat Peach	8 oz	240	3	15	140
Fruit On The Bottom Lowfat Raspberry	8 oz	240	3	15	150
Fruit On The Bottom Lowfat Strawberry	8 oz	240	3	15	135
Fruit On The Bottom Lowfat Strawberry Banana	8 oz	240	3	15	140
LaCreme Vanilla	1 pkg (4.4 oz)	140	5	20	75
Light 'N Crunchy Mint Chocolate Chip	8 oz	140	0	5	150
Light 'N Crunchy Nonfat Caramel Apple Crunch	8 oz	140	0	<5	340
Light 'N Crunchy Nonfat Lemon Blueberry Cobbler	8 oz	140	0	<5	135

FOOD	PORTION	CALS	FAT	CHOL	SOD
Dannon (cont.)					
Light 'N Crunchy Nonfat Mocha Cappuccino	8 oz	140	0	<5	150
Light 'N Crunchy Nonfat Raspberry w/ Granola	8 oz	140	0	<5	120
Light 'N Crunchy Nonfat Vanilla Chocolate Crunch	8 oz	130	0	<5	140
Light Duets Cherry Cheesecake	6 oz	90	0	0	70
Light Duets Peaches 'N Cream	6 oz	90	0	0	70
Light Duets Raspberry Royale	6 oz	90	0	0	75
Light Duets Strawberry Cheesecake	6 oz	90	0	0	70
Light Nonfat Banana Cream Pie	8 oz	100	0	<5	120
Light Nonfat Blueberry	8 oz	100	0	<5	115
Light Nonfat Cappuccino	8 oz	100	0	5	120
Light Nonfat Cherry Vanilla	8 oz	100	0	<5	120
Light Nonfat Coconut Cream Pie	8 oz	100	0	5	120
Light Nonfat Creme Caramel	8 oz	100	0	<5	120
Light Nonfat Lemon Chiffon	8 oz	100	0	5	120
Light Nonfat Mint Chocolate Cream Pie	8 oz	100	0	<5	120
Light Nonfat Peach	8 oz	100	0	<5	115
Light Nonfat Raspberry	8 oz	100	0	<5	120
Light Nonfat Strawberry	8 oz	100	0	<5	115
Light Nonfat Strawberry Banana	8 oz	100	0	<5	120
Light Nonfat Strawberry Kiwi	8 oz	100	0	5	120
Light Nonfat Tangerine Chiffon	8 oz	100	0	5	120
Light Nonfat Vanilla	8 oz	100	0	<5	120
Lowfat Coffee	8 oz	210	3	15	160
Lowfat Cranberry Raspberry	8 oz	210	3	15	160
Lowfat Lemon	8 oz	210	3	15	160
Lowfat Vanilla	8 oz	210	3	15	160
Minipack Blended Nonfat Blueberry	4.4 oz	120	0	5	80
Minipack Blended Nonfat Cherry	4.4 oz	110	0	5	80
Minipack Blended Nonfat Peach	4.4 oz	120	0	5	80
Minipack Blended Nonfat Raspberry	4.4 oz	120	0	5	80
Minipack Blended Nonfat Strawberry	4.4 oz	120	0	5	85
Minipack Blended Nonfat Strawberry Banana	4.4 oz	120	0	5	85

FOOD	PORTION	CALS	FAT	CHOL	SOD
Sprinkl'ins Cherry Vanilla	1 (4.1 oz)	130	2	5	85
Sprinkl'ins Strawberry	1 (4.1 oz)	130	2	5	85
Sprinkl'ins Strawberry Banana	1 (4.1 oz)	130	2	5	80
Sprinkl'ins Vanilla w/ Cherry Crystals	1 (4.1 oz)	110	1	5	85
Sprinkl'ins Vanilla w/ Orange Crystals	1 (4.1 oz)	110	1	5	85
Horizon Organic					
Fat Free Apricot Mango	3/4 cup (6 oz)	120	0	<5	100
Fat Free Honey	1 cup (8 oz)	160	0	<5	135
Jell-O					
Lowfat Cherry	4.4 oz	130	1	10	65
Lowfat Grape	4.4 oz	130	1	10	65
Lowfat Raspberry	4.4 oz	130	1	10	65
Lowfat Tropical Berry Twist	4.4 oz	130	1	10	65
Lowfat Tropical Punch	4.4 oz	130	1	10	65
Lowfat Watermelon	4.4 oz	130	1	10	65
Lowfat Wild Berry	4.4 oz	130	1	10	65
Lowfat Wild Strawberry	4.4 oz	130	1	10	65
Light N'Lively					
Free Blueberry	4.4 oz	70	0	5	55
Free Peach	4.4 oz	70	0	5	65
Free Strawberry	4.4 oz	70	0	5	55
Free Strawberry Banana Cream	4.4 oz	70	0	5	55
Free Strawberry Fruit Cup	4.4 oz	70	0	5	55
Lowfat Blueberry	4.4 oz	130	1	10	60
Lowfat Peach	4.4 oz	130	1	10	65
Lowfat Pineapple	4.4 oz	130	1	10	60
Lowfat Red Raspberry	4.4 oz	120	1	10	65
Lowfat Strawberry	4.4 oz	130	1	10	60
Lowfat Strawberry Banana Cream	4.4 oz	130	1	10	60
Lowfat Strawberry Fruit Cup	4.4 oz	130	1	10	60
Oberweis					
Peach	1 pkg (8 oz)	210	3	15	140
Pascual					
Nonfat Cherries & Berries	1 pkg (4.4 oz)	100	0	0	70
Nonfat Peach	1 pkg (4.4 oz)	100	0	0	70
Stonyfield Farm					
Creamy Maple	1 pkg	160	6	25	90
Mocho-Ccino	1 pkg	170	6	20	95
Nonfat Apricot Mango	1 pkg (8 oz)	160	0	0	125
Nonfat Black Cherry	1 pkg (8 oz)	160	0	0	130
Nonfat Cappuccino	1 pkg (8 oz)	160	0	0	135
Nonfat Cherry Vanilla	1 pkg (8 oz)	190	0	0	120
Nonfat Chocolate Underground	1 pkg (8 oz)	200	0	0	135

FOOD	PORTION	CALS	FAT	CHOL	SOD
Stonyfield Farm (cont.)					
Nonfat French Vanilla	1 pkg (8 oz)	180	0	0	135
Nonfat Lotsa Lemon	1 pkg (8 oz)	160	0	0	140
Nonfat Peach	1 pkg (8 oz)	150	0	0	130
Nonfat Plain	1 pkg (8 oz)	100	08	<5	150
Nonfat Raspberry	1 pkg (8 oz)	160	0	0	130
Nonfat Strawberry	1 pkg (8 oz)	180	0	0	130
Organic French Vanilla	1 pkg	170	6	20	85
Organic Wild Blueberry	1 pkg	160	6	20	85
Organic Lowfat Blueberry	1 pkg (6 oz)	130	2	5	90
Organic Lowfat Luscious Lemon	1 pkg (6 oz)	130	2	5	115
Organic Lowfat Maple Vanilla	1 pkg (6 oz)	120	2	6	90
Organic Lowfat Mocha Latte	1 pkg (6 oz)	120	2	5	85
Organic Lowfat Plain	1 cup (8 oz)	110	2	10	135
Organic Lowfat Raspberry	1 pkg (6 oz)	130	2	5	100
Organic Lowfat Strawberry	1 pkg (6 oz)	130	2	5	115
Organic Lowfat Vanilla	1 pkg (6 oz)	120	2	5	100
Strawberries & Cream	1 pkg	160	5	20	110
Vanilla Truffle	1 pkg	220	5	20	100
YoSelf Organic Chocolate	1 (4 oz)	110	1	0	65
YoSelf Organic Creme Carmel	1 (4 oz)	110	1	5	65
Yosqueeze Strawberry	1 tube (2 oz)	60	1	5	30
Yoplait					
99% Fat Free Blueberry	6 oz	180	2	10	80
99% Fat Free Boysenberry	6 oz	180	2	10	80
99% Fat Free Cherry	6 oz	180	2	10	80
99% Fat Free Harvest Peach	6 oz	120	1	5	55
99% Fat Free Key Lime Pie	6 oz	180	2	10	80
99% Fat Free Lemon	6 oz	180	2	10	80
99% Fat Free Mixed Berry	6 oz	180	2	10	80
99% Fat Free Mixed Berry	6 oz	120	1	5	55
99% Fat Free Orange	6 oz	180	2	10	80
99% Fat Free Pina Colada	6 oz	180	2	10	80
99% Fat Free Pineapple	6 oz	180	2	10	80
99% Fat Free Raspberry	6 oz	180	2	10	80
99% Fat Free Strawberry	6 oz	180	2	10	80
99% Fat Free Strawberry Banana	6 oz	180	2	10	80
99% Fat Free Strawberry Cheesecake	6 oz	180	2	10	80
Custard Style Banana	6 oz	190	4	15	100
Custard Style Blueberry	6 oz	190	4	15	100
Custard Style Cherry Vanilla	6 oz	190	4	15	100
Custard Style Key Lime Pie	6 oz	190	4	15	100
Custard Style Lemon	6 oz	190	4	15	100
Custard Style Peaches'n Cream	6 oz	190	4	15	100

FOOD	PORTION	CALS	FAT	CHOL	SOD
Custard Style Raspberry	6 oz	190	4	15	100
Custard Style Raspberry Cheesecake	6 oz	190	4	15	100
Custard Style Strawberry	6 oz	190	4	15	100
Custard Style Strawberry Banana	6 oz	190	4	15	100
Custard Style Strawberry Vanilla	4 oz	120	2	10	70
Custard Style Vanilla	6 oz	190	4	15	95
Go-Gurt Strawberry Banana Burst	1 pkg (2.25 oz)	80	2	5	40
Go-Gurt Watermelon Meltdown	1 pkg (2.25 oz)	80	2	5	40
Light Amaretto Cheesecake	6 oz	90	0	5	95
Light Apricot Mango	6 oz	90	0	5	75
Light Banana Cream	6 oz	90	0	5	95
Light Blueberry	6 oz	90	0	5	75
Light Boston Cream Pie	6 oz	90	0	5	95
Light Caramel Apple	6 oz	90	0	5	95
Light Cherry	6 oz	90	0	5	75
Light Key Lime Pie	6 oz	90	0	5	95
Light Lemon Cream Pie	6 oz	90	0	5	95
Light Peach	6 oz	90	0	5	75
Light Peach Melba	6 oz	90	0	5	75
Light Raspberry	6 oz	90	0	5	75
Light Strawberry	6 oz	90	0	5	75
Light Strawberry Banana	6 oz	90	0	5	75
Light White Chocolate Strawberry	6 oz	90	0	5	75
Original Cafe Au Lait	6 oz	170	2	10	80
Original Coconut Cream Pie	6 oz	200	4	10	80
Original French Vanilla	6 oz	180	2	10	90
Trix Rainbow Punch	6 oz	190	2	10	85
Trix Raspberry Rainbow	6 oz	190	2	10	85
Trix Strawberry Banana Bash	6 oz	190	2	10	85
Trix Strawberry Punch	4 oz	130	2	5	55
Trix Triple Cherry	6 oz	190	2	10	85
Trix Watermelon Burst	4 oz	130	2	5	55
Trix Wild Berry Blue	4 oz	130	2	5	55
YOGURT FROZEN					
Ben & Jerry's					
Cherry Garcia	1/2 cup	170	3	20	80
Chocolate Cherry Garcia	1/2 cup	190	4	15	65
Chocolate Chip Cookie Dough	1/2 cup	200	5	10	120
Chocolate Fudge Brownie	1/2 cup	190	3	5	105
Chocolate Heath Bar Crunch	1/2 cup	210	6	10	115
Chunky Monkey	1/2 cup	200	6	5	65
Pop Cherry Garcia	1	260	14	15	70

FOOD	PORTION	CALS	FAT	CHOL	SOD
Breyers					
Chocolate	1/2 cup (2.6 oz)	130	3	10	45
Fat Free Chocolate	1/2 cup (2.6 oz)	100	0	<5	40
Fat Free Cookies N Cream	1/2 cup (2.6 oz)	110	0	0	75
Fat Free Peach	1/2 cup (2.6 oz)	90	0	0	40
Fat Free Strawberry	1/2 cup (2.6 oz)	100	0	0	40
Fat Free Take Two Vanilla Chocolate	1/2 cup (2.6 oz)	100	0	0	45
Fat Free Vanilla	1/2 cup (2.6 oz)	100	0	0	50
Fat Free Vanilla Fudge Twirl	1/2 cup (2.6 oz)	110	0	0	45
Vanilla	1/2 cup (2.6 oz)	120	3	10	40
Vanilla Chocolate Strawberry	1/2 cup (2.6 oz)	120	3	10	40
Dannon					
Light Cappuccino	1/2 cup (2.8 oz)	80	0	0	60
Light Cherry Vanilla Swirl	1/2 cup (2.8 oz)	90	0	0	55
Light Chocolate	1/2 cup (2.7 oz)	80	0	0	55
Light Mint Chocolate Fudge	1/2 cup (2.8 oz)	90	0	0	60
Light Peach Raspberry Melba	1/2 cup (2.8 oz)	90	0	0	60
Light Strawberry Cheesecake	1/2 cup (2.8 oz)	90	0	0	70
Light Vanilla	1/2 cup (2.8 oz)	80	0	0	60
Light Duets Strawberry Sundae	6 oz	90	0	0	70
Light'N Crunchy Banana Cream Pie	1/2 cup (2.8 oz)	110	1	0	65
Light'N Crunchy Carmel Toffee Crunch	1/2 cup (2.8 oz)	110	1	0	75
Light'N Crunchy Mocha Chocolate Chunk	1/2 cup (2.8 oz)	110	1	0	60
Light'N Crunchy Peanut Chocolate Crunch	1/2 cup (2.8 oz)	110	1	0	65
Light'N Crunchy Rocky Road	1/2 cup (2.8 oz)	110	1	0	60
Light'N Crunchy Triple Chocolate	1/2 cup (2.8 oz)	110	1	0	60
Light'N Crunchy Vanilla Streusel	1/2 cup (2.8 oz)	110	1	0	80
ZUCCHINI					
canned					
Progresso					
Italian Style	1/2 cup (4.2 oz)	50	2	0	400
fresh					
baby raw	1 (0.5 oz)	3	tr	0	0
raw sliced	1/2 cup	9	tr	0	2
sliced cooked	1/2 cup	14	tr	0	2
take-out					
indian paalkora	1 serv	46	2	1	141

Part 2

Restaurant Chains

You Should Know

During 2001, Americans purchased an average of 137 restaurant meals per person.

FOOD	PORTION	CALS	FAT	CHOL	SOD
APPLEBEE'S					
desserts					
Apple Betty Cobbler Ala Mode	1 serv	598	22	31	197
Fudge Brownie Sundae	1 serv	739	40	66	332
Low Fat Bikini Banana Strawberry Shortcake	1 serv	248	2	8	223
Low Fat Brownie Sundae	1 serv	415	2	3	417
Low Fat Marble Cheesecake	1 serv	261	2	10	378
main menu selections					
Applebee's Burger w/ Fries	1 serv	1274	79	263	2713
Basic Hamburger w/ Fries	1 serv	980	58	118	1814
Beef Fajita Quesadilla	1 serv	1205	86	159	2969
Bourbon Street Steak w/ Fried New Potatoes	1 serv	1115	94	168	3542
Low Fat Asian Chicken Salad	1 med serv (2.5 oz)	370	6	40	1431
Low Fat Asian Chicken Salad	1 serv (5 oz)	623	9	76	2487
Low Fat Blackened Chicken Salad	1 serv (5 oz)	411	5	82	2188
Low Fat Blackened Chicken Salad	1 med serv (2.5 oz)	287	3	43	1763
Low Fat Garlic Chicken Pasta	1 serv	587	8	39	1551
Low Fat Lemon Chicken Pasta	1 serv	528	11	50	2438
Low Fat Quesadilla Chicken Fajita	1 serv	518	11	35	2244
Low Fat Quesadilla Veggie	1 serv	344	8	8	1138
Mozzarella Stix	8 pieces	963	57	64	1990
Quesadillas	1 serv	684	46	99	2175
Riblet Basket w/ Fries	1 serv	1317	92	219	2697
Salad Dinner w/o Dressing	1 serv	303	18	277	661
Salad Santa Fe Chicken	1 med	724	42	96	2409
Sandwich Bacon Cheese Chicken Grill w/o Fries	1	746	46	133	1722
Sandwich Gyro	1	880	69	15	2015
Stir Fry Chicken	1 serv	566	7	76	2470
ARBY'S					
breakfast selections					
Add Egg To Breakfast	1 serv (2 oz)	110	9	175	170
Add Swiss Cheese Slice	1 slice (0.5 oz)	45	3	10	220
Biscuit w/ Bacon	1 (3.4 oz)	360	24	10	220
Biscuit w/ Butter	1 (2.9 oz)	280	17	0	780
Biscuit w/ Ham	1 (4.3 oz)	330	20	30	830
Biscuit w/ Sausage	1 (4.2)	460	33	25	300
Croissant w/ Bacon	1 (2.7 oz)	340	23	30	520
Croissant w/ Ham	1 (3.7 oz)	310	19	11	1130
Croissant w/ Sausage	1 (3.6 oz)	440	32	45	600
Maple Syrup	1 serv (0.5 oz)	130	0	0	45
Sourdough w/ Bacon	1 (5.1 oz)	420	10	10	960
Sourdough w/ Ham	1 (6.1 oz)	390	6	30	1570

FOOD	PORTION	CALS	FAT	CHOL	SOD
Sourdough w/ Sausage	1 (5.9 oz)	520	19	25	1040
Toastix w/o Syrup	6 pieces (4.4 oz)	370	17	0	440
desserts					
Apple Turnover Iced	1 (4.5 oz)	420	16	0	230
Cherry Turnover Iced	1 (4.5 oz)	410	16	0	250
main menu selections					
Arby's Sauce	1 serv (0.5 oz)	15	0	0	180
Au Jus Sauce	1 serv (3 oz)	5	tr	0	386
BBQ Dipping Sauce	1 serv (1 oz)	40	0	0	350
Baked Potato Broccoli'N Cheddar	1 (14 oz)	540	24	50	680
Baked Potato Deluxe	1 (13 oz)	650	34	90	750
Baked Potato w/ Butter & Sour Cream	1 (11.2 oz)	500	24	55	170
Bronco Berry Sauce	1 serv (1.5 oz)	90	0	0	35
Caesar Salad w/o Dressing	1 serv (8 oz)	90	4	10	170
Cheddar Curly Fries	1 serv (6 oz)	460	24	5	1290
Chicken Finger 4-Pak	1 serv (6.77 oz)	640	38	70	1590
Chicken Finger Salad w/o Dressing	1 serv (13 oz)	570	34	65	1300
Chicken Finger Snack	1 serv (6.4 oz)	580	32	35	1450
Curly Fries	1 med (4.5 oz)	400	20	0	990
Curly Fries	1 lg (7 oz)	620	30	0	1540
Curly Fries	1 sm (3.8 oz)	310	15	0	770
German Mustard	1 pkg (0.25 oz)	5	0	0	60
Grilled Chicken Caesar Salad w/o Dressing	1 serv (12 oz)	230	8	80	920
Homestyle Fries	1 med (5 oz)	370	16	0	710
Homestyle Fries	1 sm (4 oz)	300	13	0	570
Homestyle Fries	1 lg (7.5 oz)	560	24	0	1070
Homestyle Fries Child-Size	1 serv (3 oz)	220	10	0	430
Honey Mustard	1 serv (1 oz)	130	12	10	160
Horsey Sauce	1 pkg (0.5 oz)	60	5	0	150
Jalapeno Bites	1 serv (4 oz)	330	21	40	670
Ketchup	1 pkg (0.3 oz)	10	0	0	100
Light Grilled Chicken Salad	1 (16.3 oz)	210	5	65	800
Marinara Sauce	1 serv (1.5 oz)	35	1	0	260
Mayonnaise	1 pkg (0.4 oz)	90	10	10	65
Mayonnaise Light Cholesterol Free	1 pkg (0.4 oz)	20	2	0	110
Mozzarella Sticks	1 serv (4.8 oz)	470	29	60	1330
Onion Petals	1 serv (4 oz)	410	24	0	300
Potato Cakes	2 (3.5 oz)	250	16	0	490
Roast Beef Sandwich Arby's Melt w/ Cheddar	1 (5.2 oz)	320	14	45	850
Roast Beef Sandwich Arby-Q	1 (6.4 oz)	360	14	70	1530

FOOD	PORTION	CALS	FAT	CHOL	SOD
Roast Beef Sandwich Beef'N Cheddar	1 (6.9 oz)	460	23	50	1170
Roast Beef Sandwich Big Montana	1 (11 oz)	560	27	50	1900
Roast Beef Sandwich Giant	1 (7.9 oz)	440	20	45	1330
Roast Beef Sandwich Junior	1 (4.4 oz)	290	12	40	700
Roast Beef Sandwich Regular	1 (5.4 oz)	330	14	45	890
Roast Beef Sandwich Super	1 (8.5 oz)	450	21	45	1060
Sandwich Chicken Bacon'N Swiss	1 (7.4 oz)	610	33	110	1550
Sandwich Chicken Breast Fillet	1 (7.2 oz)	550	30	90	1160
Sandwich Chicken Cordon Bleu	1 (8.4 oz)	630	35	120	1820
Sandwich Grilled Chicken Deluxe	1 (8.7 oz)	450	22	110	1050
Sandwich Hot Ham 'N Swiss	1 (5.9 oz)	340	13	90	1450
Sandwich Light Roast Chicken Deluxe	1 (7.2 oz)	260	5	40	1010
Sandwich Light Roast Turkey Deluxe	1 (7.2 oz)	260	5	40	1030
Sandwich Market Fresh Roast Beef & Swiss	1 (12.5 oz)	780	40	80	1690
Sandwich Market Fresh Roast Chicken Caesar	1 (12.7 oz)	820	38	140	2160
Sandwich Market Fresh Roast Ham & Swiss	1 (12.5 oz)	730	34	125	2180
Sandwich Market Fresh Roast Turkey & Swiss	1 (12.5 oz)	760	33	135	1920
Sandwich Roast Chicken Club	1 (8.4 oz)	520	28	115	1440
Sub Sandwich French Dip	1 (10 oz)	410	16	45	1200
Sub Sandwich Hot Ham'N Swiss	1 (9.7 oz)	530	27	110	1860
Sub Sandwich Italian	1 (11 oz)	780	53	120	2440
Sub Sandwich Philly Beef'N Swiss	1 (10.8 oz)	670	40	75	1850
Sub Sandwich Roast Beef	1 (11.6 oz)	730	46	76	2140
Sub Sandwich Turkey	1 (10.6 oz)	630	37	100	2170
Tangy Southwest Sauce	1 serv (1.5 oz)	250	26	30	290
salad dressings					
Bleu Cheese	1 serv (2 oz)	300	31	45	580
Buttermilk Ranch	1 serv (2 oz)	360	39	5	490
Buttermilk Ranch Reduced Calorie	1 serv (2 oz)	60	0	0	750
Caesar	1 serv (2 oz)	310	34	60	470
Honey French	1 serv (2 oz)	290	24	0	410

FOOD	PORTION	CALS	FAT	CHOL	SOD
Italian Reduced Calorie	1 serv (2 oz)	25	1	0	1030
Thousand Island	1 serv (2 oz)	290	28	35	480
salads and salad bars					
Croutons Seasoned	1 serv (0.25 oz)	30	1	0	70
Garden Salad	1 (12.3 oz)	70	1	0	45
Light Roast Chicken Salad	1 (14.8 oz)	160	3	40	700
Light Grilled Chicken Sandwich	1 (7.5 oz)	280	5	55	1170
Side Salad	1 (6.1 oz)	30	0	0	20
Turkey Club Salad w/o Dressing	1 serv (12 oz)	350	21	90	860
AU BON PAIN					
baked selections					
Apple Coffee Cake	1 piece (4.6 oz)	480	24	96	285
Bagel Chocolate Chip	1 (5 oz)	380	7	5	480
Bagel Dutch Apple w/ Walnut Streusel	1 (5 oz)	360	5	0	480
Baguette Loaf	1 slice (1.8 oz)	140	5	0	350
Biscotti	1 (1.5 oz)	200	10	35	45
Biscotti Chocolate	1 (1.7 oz)	240	13	35	50
Braided Roll	1 (1.8 oz)	170	5	0	320
Cinnamon Roll	1 (7 oz)	710	26	100	740
Cookie Chocolate Chip	1 (2.1 oz)	280	13	40	85
Cookie Oatmeal Raisin	1 (2.1 oz)	250	10	30	240
Cookie Shortbread	1 (2.4 oz)	390	25	65	190
Croissant Almond	1 (4.3 oz)	560	37	105	260
Croissant Apple	1 (3.4 oz)	280	10	25	180
Croissant Chocolate	1 (3.4 oz)	440	23	30	230
Croissant Cinnamon Raisin	1 (3.7 oz)	380	13	35	290
Croissant Plain	1 (2.1 oz)	270	15	40	240
Croissant Raspberry Cheese	1 (3.5 oz)	380	19	60	300
Croissant Sweet Cheese	1 (3.6 oz)	390	22	75	330
Danish Cheese Swirl	1 (3.8 oz)	450	28	95	410
Danish Lemon Swirl	1 (4 oz)	450	24	80	410
Four Grain Loaf	1 slice (1.8 oz)	130	1	0	280
French Sandwich Roll	1 (1.8 oz)	120	5	0	320
Hazelnut Fudge Brownie	1 (4 oz)	380	18	100	150
Holiday Cookie Cranberry Almond Macaroon	1 (1.5 oz)	160	8	0	115
Holiday Cookie Cranberry Almond Macaroon w/ Chocolate	1 (1.9 oz)	210	11	0	120
Holiday Cookie English Toffee	1 (1.8 oz)	220	12	45	110
Holiday Cookie Ginger Pecan	1 (2 oz)	260	15	40	115
Mochaccino Bar	1 (4 oz)	404	24	37	294
Muffin Blueberry	1 (4.5 oz)	410	15	85	380
Muffin Carrot	1 (5 oz)	480	23	55	650

FOOD	PORTION	CALS	FAT	CHOL	SOD
Muffin Chocolate Chip	1 (4.5 oz)	490	20	35	560
Muffin Corn	1 (4.6 oz)	470	18	65	570
Muffin Pumpkin w/ Streusel Topping	1 (5.5 oz)	470	18	60	550
Muffin Low Fat Chocolate Cake	1 (4 oz)	290	3	20	630
Muffin Low Fat Triple Berry	1 (4.2 oz)	270	3	25	560
Multigrain Loaf	1 slice (1.8 oz)	130	1	0	340
Parisienne Loaf	1 slice (1.8 oz)	120	5	0	300
Pear Ginger Tea Cake	1 piece (4 oz)	380	20	0	202
Pecan Roll	1 (6.8 oz)	900	48	50	480
Roll 3 Seed Pecan Raisin	1 (2.7 oz)	250	6	0	240
Roll Hearth Sandwich	1 (2.8 oz)	220	2	0	410
Rolls Petit Pan	1 (2.5 oz)	200	1	0	570
Rye Loaf	1 slice (1.8 oz)	110	2	0	310
Scone Cinnamon	1 (4.1 oz)	520	28	145	230
Scone Currant	1 (3.7 oz)	430	23	155	230
Scone Orange	1 (4.1 oz)	440	23	155	240
Sourdough Bagel Asiago Cheese	1 (4.2 oz)	380	6	15	690
Sourdough Bagel Cinnamon Raisin	1 (4.5 oz)	390	1	0	550
Sourdough Bagel Cranberry Walnut	1 (5 oz)	460	4	0	590
Sourdough Bagel Everything	1 (4.2 oz)	360	3	0	710
Sourdough Bagel Honey 8 Grain	1 (4.2 oz)	360	2	0	580
Sourdough Bagel Mocha Chip Swirl	1 (5 oz)	370	4	0	480
Sourdough Bagel Plain	1 (4 oz)	350	1	0	540
Sourdough Bagel Sesame	1 (4.2 oz)	380	4	0	540
Sourdough Bagel Wild Blueberry	1 (4.5 oz)	380	2	0	570
Valentine Cookie Chocolate Dipped Shortbread	1 (2.8 oz)	410	27	55	160
Valentine Cookie Red Sugar Shortbread Heart	1 (2.4 oz)	350	22	60	170
Valentine Cookie Shortbread	1 (2.4 oz)	340	22	60	170
salad dressings					
Bleu Cheese	1 serv (3 oz)	370	41	40	910
Buttermilk Ranch	1 serv (3 oz)	310	32	35	270
Caesar	1 serv (3 oz)	380	39	25	410
Fat Free Tomato Basil	1 serv (3 oz)	70	0	0	650
Greek	1 serv (3 oz)	440	50	0	820
Lemon Basil Vinaigrette	1 serv (3 oz)	330	32	0	460
Lite Honey Mustard	1 serv (3 oz)	280	17	40	560
Lite Italian	1 serv (3 oz)	230	20	0	570
Sesame French	1 serv (3 oz)	370	30	0	1010

FOOD	PORTION	CALS	FAT	CHOL	SOD
salads and salad bars					
Caesar	1 serv (8.9 oz)	270	10	20	800
Chicken Caesar	1 serv (11.4 oz)	360	11	65	910
Garden	1 lg (10.6 oz)	160	2	0	290
Garden	1 sm (7.5 oz)	100	1	0	150
Mozzarella & Roasted Pepper Salad	1 serv (13.7 oz)	340	18	60	135
Pesto Chicken Salad	1 serv (10.7 oz)	230	11	45	250
Tuna	1 serv (15 oz)	490	27	45	750
sandwiches and fillings					
Bagel Spreads Lite Strawberry	1 serv (2 oz)	150	11	35	210
Bagel Spreads Lite Vanilla Hazelnut	1 serv (2 oz)	150	11	35	210
Cheddar	1/2 serv (1.5 oz)	170	14	45	260
Chicken Tarragon	1 serv (4 oz)	240	17	65	170
Club Sandwich Hot Roasted Turkey	1 (14.9 oz)	950	50	135	2240
Country Ham	1 serv (3.7 oz)	150	7	55	1370
Cracked Pepper Chicken	1 serv (3.9 oz)	140	2	72	184
Cream Cheese Lite	1 serv (2 oz)	130	12	35	230
Cream Cheese Lite Honey Walnut	1 serv (2 oz)	260	12	20	260
Cream Cheese Lite Raspberry	1 serv (2 oz)	200	8	20	280
Cream Cheese Lite Sun-Dried Tomato	1 serv (2 oz)	130	11	35	230
Cream Cheese Plain	1 serv (2 oz)	190	18	55	210
Cream Cheese Veggie Lite	1 serv (2 oz)	100	10	20	300
Grilled Chicken	1 serv (3.9 oz)	140	2	72	184
Hot Croissant Ham & Cheese	1 (4.2 oz)	380	20	70	690
Hot Croissant Spinach & Cheese	1 (3.6 oz)	270	16	40	330
Provolone	1/2 serv (1.5 oz)	150	11	30	370
Roast Beef	1 serv (3.7 oz)	140	5	50	550
Sandwich Arizona Chicken	1 (12.7 oz)	720	33	125	1190
Sandwich Buffalo Chicken	1 (13.7 oz)	640	19	85	1650
Sandwich California Chicken	1 (13.2 oz)	820	44	135	1200
Sandwich Fresh Mozzarella Tomato & Pesto	1 (10.5 oz)	650	30	55	1090
Sandwich Honey Dijon Chicken	1 (15.3 oz)	730	18	135	1990
Sandwich Parmesan Chicken	1 (11.1 oz)	740	24	70	1620
Sandwich Steak & Cheese Melt	1 (11.7 oz)	750	32	90	1600
Sandwich Thai Chicken	1 (8.3 oz)	420	6	20	1320
Swiss	1/2 serv (1.5 oz)	160	12	40	110

FOOD	PORTION	CALS	FAT	CHOL	SOD
Tuna Salad	1 serv (4.5 oz)	360	29	50	520
Turkey Breast	1 serv (3.7 oz)	120	1	20	1110
Wraps Chicken Caesar	1 (9.9 oz)	630	31	80	1140
Wraps Southwestern Tuna	1 (14.4 oz)	950	64	110	1230
Wraps Summer Turkey	1 (11.7 oz)	340	9	35	1380
soups					
Beef Barley	1 serv (8 oz)	75	2	15	660
Beef Barley	1 serv (16 oz)	150	4	25	1310
Beef Barley	1 serv (12 oz)	112	3	18	980
Bohemian Cabbage	1 serv (8 oz)	70	3	0	650
Bohemian Cabbage	1 serv (16 oz)	140	6	0	1280
Bohemian Cabbage	1 serv (12 oz)	110	5	0	960
Bread Bowl	1 (9 oz)	640	4	0	1950
Caribbean Black Bean	1 serv (16 oz)	250	2	10	1540
Caribbean Black Bean	1 serv (12 oz)	180	2	10	1150
Caribbean Black Bean	1 serv (8 oz)	120	1	5	770
Chicken Chili	1 serv (8 oz)	240	12	45	1350
Chicken Chili	1 serv (12 oz)	350	18	65	2030
Chicken Chili	1 serv (16 oz)	470	24	90	2700
Chicken Noodle	1 serv (12 oz)	120	2	25	1000
Chicken Noodle	1 serv (16 oz)	170	3	35	1340
Chicken Noodle	1 serv (8 oz)	80	2	15	670
Clam Chowder	1 serv (12 oz)	400	29	95	1090
Clam Chowder	1 serv (16 oz)	540	39	125	1460
Clam Chowder	1 serv (8 oz)	270	19	65	730
Cream Of Broccoli	1 serv (16 oz)	440	37	80	1550
Cream Of Broccoli	1 serv (12 oz)	330	28	60	1160
French Onion	1 serv (16 oz)	170	7	0	2550
French Onion	1 serv (8 oz)	80	4	0	1280
French Onion	1 serv (12 oz)	120	5	0	1910
In A Bread Bowl Beef Barley	1 serv (21 oz)	760	7	20	2940
In A Bread Bowl Caribbean Black Bean	1 serv (21 oz)	830	5	10	3100
In A Bread Bowl Chicken Chili	1 serv (21 oz)	990	22	65	3970
In A Bread Bowl Chicken Noodle	1 serv (21 oz)	760	6	20	2950
In A Bread Bowl Clam Chowder	1 serv (21 oz)	1050	32	100	3040
In A Bread Bowl Cream of Broccoli	1 serv (21 oz)	970	31	60	3100
In A Bread Bowl French Onion	1 serv (21 oz)	760	8	0	3860
In A Bread Bowl New England Potato & Cheese w/ Ham	1 serv (21 oz)	860	15	40	3170
In A Bread Bowl Tomato Florentine	1 serv (21 oz)	760	5	10	3490
In A Bread Bowl Vegetarian Chili	1 serv (21 oz)	870	7	0	3550
Louisiana Beans & Rice	1 serv (16 oz)	360	9	20	1320

FOOD	PORTION	CALS	FAT	CHOL	SOD
Louisiana Beans & Rice	1 serv (12 oz)	280	7	15	960
Louisiana Beans & Rice	1 serv (8 oz)	180	5	10	660
New England Potato & Cheese w/ Ham	1 serv (8 oz)	150	8	25	820
New England Potato & Cheese w/ Ham	1 serv (12 oz)	220	12	40	1220
New England Potato & Cheese w/ Ham	1 serv (16 oz)	290	15	55	1630
Potato Leek	1 serv (12 oz)	320	20	70	1700
Potato Leek	1 serv (8 oz)	200	13	45	1060
Potato Leek	1 serv (16 oz)	400	25	85	2120
Sante Fe Chicken Tortilla	1 serv (8 oz)	150	7	15	950
Sante Fe Chicken Tortilla	1 serv (16 oz)	300	13	30	1900
Sante Fe Chicken Tortilla	1 serv (12 oz)	230	10	25	1430
Tomato Florentine	1 serv (8 oz)	61	1	5	1030
Tomato Florentine	1 serv (12 oz)	90	2	5	1550
Tomato Florentine	1 serv (16 oz)	122	2	5	2070
Vegetarian Chili	1 serv (16 oz)	278	5	0	2150
Vegetarian Chili	1 serv (8 oz)	139	3	0	1070
Vegetarian Chili	1 serv (12 oz)	210	4	0	1610
Vegetarian Corn & Green Chili Bisque	1 serv (12 oz)	300	16	45	1830
Vegetarian Corn & Green Chili Bisque	1 serv (8 oz)	190	10	30	1140
Vegetarian Corn & Green Chili Bisque	1 serv (16 oz)	380	20	60	2290
AUNTIE ANNE'S					
Caramel Dip	1 serv (1.5 oz)	135	3	5	110
Cheese Sauce	1 serv (1 oz)	70	5	15	400
Chocolate Dip	1 serv (1.25 oz)	130	4	2	65
Cream Cheese Light	1 serv (.75 oz)	45	4	15	105
Cream Cheese Pineapple	1 serv (.75 oz)	70	6	20	70
Cream Cheese Strawberry	1 serv (.75 oz)	70	6	20	70
Dutch Ice Kiwi Banana	1 (18 oz)	250	0	0	40
Dutch Ice Kiwi Banana	1 (12 oz)	160	0	0	25
Dutch Ice Lemonade	1 (12 oz)	270	0	0	0
Dutch Ice Lemonade	1 (18 oz)	405	0	0	0
Dutch Ice Mocha	1 (12 oz)	340	9	0	90
Dutch Ice Mocha	1 (18 oz)	500	14	0	135
Dutch Ice Orange Creme	1 (18 oz)	360	0	0	45
Dutch Ice Orange Creme	1 (12 oz)	240	0	0	30
Dutch Ice Raspberry	1 (18 oz)	220	0	0	40
Dutch Ice Raspberry	1 (12 oz)	150	0	0	25
Dutch Ice Strawberry	1 (12 oz)	190	0	0	35
Dutch Ice Strawberry	1 (18 oz)	280	0	0	50
Marinara Sauce	1 serv (1 oz)	10	0	0	130
Pretzel Almond w/ Butter	1	400	8	20	400
Pretzel Almond w/o Butter	1	350	2	0	390

FOOD	PORTION	CALS	FAT	CHOL	SOD
Pretzel Cinnamon Raisin w/o Butter	1	350	2	0	410
Pretzel Cinnamon Sugar w/ Butter	1	450	9	25	430
Pretzel Garlic w/ Butter	1	350	5	10	850
Pretzel Garlic w/o Butter	1	320	1	0	830
Pretzel Glazein' Raisin w/ Butter	1	510	4	10	480
Pretzel Glazin' Raisin w/o Butter	1	470	1	0	460
Pretzel Jalapeno w/ Butter	1	310	5	10	940
Pretzel Jalapeno w/o Butter	1	270	1	0	780
Pretzel Original w/ Butter	1	370	4	10	930
Pretzel Original w/o Butter	1	340	1	0	900
Pretzel Sesame w/ Butter	1	410	12	15	860
Pretzel Sesame w/o Butter	1	350	6	0	840
Pretzel Sour Cream & Onion w/Butter	1	340	5	10	930
Pretzel Sour Cream & Onion w/o Butter	1	310	1	0	920
Pretzel Whole Wheat w/ Butter	1	370	5	10	1120
Pretzel Whole Wheat w/o Butter	1	350	2	0	1100
Sweet Mustard	1 serv (1 oz)	60	2	40	120
BASKIN-ROBBINS					
frozen yogurt					
Maui Brownie Madness	1/2 cup	140	3	5	80
Perils Of Pauline	1/2 cup	140	3	5	105
ice cream					
Banana Strawberry	1/2 cup	130	7	25	40
Baseball Nut	1/2 cup	160	9	30	55
Black Walnut	1/2 cup	160	11	30	45
Cherries Jubilee	1/2 cup	140	7	30	40
Chocolate	1/2 cup	150	9	30	60
Chocolate Almond	1/2 cup	180	11	30	55
Chocolate Chip	1/2 cup	150	10	35	45
Chocolate Chip Cookie Dough	1/2 cup	170	9	35	70
Chocolate Fudge	1/2 cup	160	9	30	80
Chocolate Mousse Royale	1/2 cup	170	10	25	60
Chocolate Raspberry Truffle	1/2 cup	180	9	30	60
Chunky Heath Bar	1/2 cup	170	10	30	70
Cookies N Cream	1/2 cup	170	11	30	80
Dirt'N Worms	1/2 cup	160	8	25	80
Egg Nog	1/2 cup	150	8	40	45
Everybody's Favorite Candy Bar	1/2 cup	170	9	30	30
French Vanilla	1/2 cup	160	10	70	45

FOOD	PORTION	CALS	FAT	CHOL	SOD
Fudge Brownie	1/2 cup	170	11	25	75
German Chocolate Cake	1/2 cup	180	10	25	75
Gold Medal Ribbon	1/2 cup	150	8	30	95
Jamoca	1/2 cup	140	9	35	45
Jamoca Almond Fudge	1/2 cup	140	9	25	40
Lemon Custard	1/2 cup	150	8	45	55
Lowfat Carmel Apple AlaMode	1/2 cup	100	2	5	75
Lowfat Espresso'N Cream	1/2 cup	100	3	5	60
Mint Chocolate Chip	1/2 cup	150	10	35	35
No Sugar Added Call Me Nuts	1/2 cup	110	2	5	55
No Sugar Added Cherry Cordial	1/2 cup	100	2	5	55
No Sugar Added Mad About Chocolate	1/2 cup	100	2	5	40
No Sugar Added Pineapple Coconut	1/2 cup	90	2	5	60
No Sugar Added Thin Mint	1/2 cup	100	3	5	65
Nonfat Berry Innocent Cheese	1/2 cup	110	0	0	100
Nonfat Check-It-Out Cherry	1/2 cup	100	0	0	90
Nonfat Jamoca Swirl	1/2 cup	110	0	5	105
Ocean Commotion	1/2 cup	150	7	25	40
Old Fashion Butter Pecan	1/2 cup	160	11	35	35
Oregon Blueberry	1/2 cup	140	8	30	50
Peanut Butter N Chocolate	1/2 cup	180	12	30	95
Pink Bubblegum	1/2 cup	150	8	30	40
Pistachio Almond	1/2 cup	170	12	30	45
Pralines N Cream	1/2 cup	160	9	30	85
Pumpkin Pie	1/2 cup	130	7	30	50
Quarterback Crunch	1/2 cup	160	10	30	75
Reeses Peanut Butter	1/2 cup	180	11	30	70
Rocky Road	1/2 cup	170	10	30	60
Rum Raisin	1/2 cup	140	7	30	40
Strawberry Cheesecake	1/2 cup	150	9	35	65
Triple Chocolate Passion	1/2 cup	180	11	35	70
Vanilla	1/2 cup	140	8	40	40
Very Berry Strawberry	1/2 cup	130	7	25	40
Winter White Chocolate	1/2 cup	150	9	25	50
World Class Chocolate	1/2 cup	160	9	30	55
ices and ice pops					
Daiquiri Ice	1/2 cup	110	0	0	10
Sherbet Blue Raspberry	1/2 cup	120	2	5	30
Sherbet Orange	1/2 cup	120	2	5	25
Sherbet Rainbow	1/2 cup	120	2	5	25
Sorbet Pink Raspberry Lemon	1/2 cup	120	0	0	10
The Mask Ice	1/2 cup	120	0	0	10
Watermelon Ice	1/2 cup	110	0	0	10

FOOD	PORTION	CALS	FAT	CHOL	SOD
BEN & JERRY'S					
Sugar Cone	1	48	tr	0	42
frozen yogurt					
Cherry Garcia	1/2 cup (3.3 oz)	150	3	15	60
Chocolate Cherry Garcia	1/2 cup (3.3 oz)	170	4	5	55
Chocolate Fudge Brownie	1/2 cup (3.3 oz)	180	3	15	100
No Fat Black Raspberry	1/2 cup (3.4 oz)	140	0	5	60
No Fat Coffee Fudge	1/2 cup (3.4 oz)	140	0	0	65
No Fat Vanilla	1/2 cup (3.4 oz)	140	0	5	75
No Fat Vanilla Fudge Swirl	1/2 cup (3.4 oz)	130	0	0	70
ice cream					
Bovinity Divinity	1/2 cup (3.1 oz)	240	14	30	50
Butter Pecan	1/2 cup (3.1 oz)	270	21	60	105
Cherry Garcia	1/2 cup (3.1 oz)	210	12	55	45
Chocolate Chip Cookie Dough	1/2 cup (3.1 oz)	180	11	55	45
Chocolate Fudge Brownie	1/2 cup (3.1 oz)	230	11	35	80
Chubby Hubby	1/2 cup (3.1 oz)	280	17	50	135
Chunky Monkey	1/2 cup (3.1 oz)	220	13	50	45
Coconut Almond Fudge Chip	1/2 cup (3.1 oz)	250	18	30	60
Coffee Coffee Buzz Buzz	1/2 cup (3.1 oz)	240	16	55	60
Coffee Ole	1/2 cup (3.1 oz)	200	13	65	50
Coffee w/ Heath Bar Crunch	1/2 cup (3.1 oz)	250	16	30	105
Deep Dark Chocolate	1/2 cup (3.1 oz)	210	12	40	40
Dilbert's World Totally Nuts	1/2 cup (3.1 oz)	260	18	30	85
Low Fat Blackberry Cobbler	1/2 cup (3.2 oz)	160	2	10	60
Low Fat Chocolate Comfort	1/2 cup (3.2 oz)	150	2	10	80
Low Fat Coconut Creme Pie	1/2 cup (3.2 oz)	160	3	15	75
Low Fat Mocha Latte	1/2 cup (3.2 oz)	150	2	10	65
Low Fat Rockin Road	1/2 cup (3.2 oz)	180	3	5	65
Low Fat Smore's	1/2 cup (3.2 oz)	180	2	5	80
Low Fat Vanilla & Chocolate Mint Patty	1/2 cup (3.2 oz)	170	3	20	65
Maple Walnut	1/2 cup (3.1 oz)	240	13	55	40
Mint Chocolate Chunk	1/2 cup (3.1 oz)	240	16	60	55
Mint Chocolate Cookie	1/2 cup (3.1 oz)	230	14	60	110
New York Super Fudge Chunk	1/2 cup (3.1 oz)	250	16	35	45
Peanut Butter Cup	1/2 cup (3.1 oz)	270	18	55	95
Phish Food	1/2 cup (3.1 oz)	230	12	30	70
Pistachio Pistachio	1/2 cup (3.1 oz)	190	13	35	45
Praline Pecan	1/2 cup (3.1 oz)	230	14	30	105
Southern Pecan Pie	1/2 cup (3.1 oz)	240	16	35	80
Strawberry	1/2 cup (3.1 oz)	180	10	50	40
Sweet Cream Cookie	1/2 cup (3.1 oz)	230	14	60	110
Triple Caramel Chunk	1/2 cup (3.1 oz)	240	13	30	95
Vanilla Caramel Fudge	1/2 cup (3.1 oz)	230	13	60	85
Vanilla Chocolate Chunk	1/2 cup (3.1 oz)	240	16	60	55

FOOD	PORTION	CALS	FAT	CHOL	SOD
Vanilla World's Best	1/2 cup (3.1 oz)	200	13	65	50
Vanilla w/ Heath Toffee Crunch	1/2 cup (3.1 oz)	250	16	35	105
Wavy Gravy	1/2 cup (3.1 oz)	260	17	50	75
White Russian	1/2 cup (3.1 oz)	200	13	65	45
sorbets					
Doonesberry	1/2 cup (3.2 oz)	100	0	0	10
Lemon Swirl	1/2 cup (3.2 oz)	100	0	0	10
Purple Passion Fruit	1/2 cup (3.2 oz)	100	0	0	10
Strawberry Kiwi	1/2 cup (3.2 oz)	110	0	0	10
BIG BOY					
desserts					
Frozen Yogurt Fat Free	1 serv	118	0	0	60
Frozen Yogurt Shake	1	156	1	2	120
main menu selections					
Baked Cod w/ Salad Baked Potato Roll & Margarine	1 meal	744	21	76	655
Baked Potato	1	163	2	0	7
Breast of Chicken Pita w/ Mozzarella & Ranch Dressing	1	361	11	84	369
Breast of Chicken w/ Mozzarella Salad Baked Potato Roll & Margarine	1 meal	697	20	76	613
Cabbage Soup	1 bowl	40	5	0	347
Cabbage Soup	1 cup	34	4	0	295
Cajun Cod w/ Salad Baked Potato Roll & Margarine	1 meal	736	21	76	745
Chicken & Pasta Primavera w/ Salad Roll & Margarine	1 meal	676	14	65	875
Chicken 'n Vegetable Stir Fry w/ Salad Baked Potato Roll & Margarine	1 meal	795	18	65	845
Dinner Roll	1	210	5	0	340
Plain Egg Beaters Omelette w/ Whole Wheat Bread & Margarine	1 meal	305	10	0	603
Promise Margarine	1 pat	25	3	0	35
Rice Pilaf	1 serv	153	4	10	688
Scrambled Egg Beaters w/ Whole Wheat Bread & Margarine	1 meal	305	10	0	603
Southwest Chicken w/ Salad Baked Potato Roll & Margarine	1 meal	702	18	76	948
Spaghetti Marinara w/ Salad Roll & Margarine	1 meal	754	11	8	754

FOOD	PORTION	CALS	FAT	CHOL	SOD
Turkey Pita w/ Ranch Dressing	1	245	6	83	938
Vegetable Stir Fry w/ Salad Baked Potato Roll & Margarine	1 meal	616	14	0	774
Vegetarian Egg Beaters Omelette w/ Whole Wheat Bread & Margarine	1 meal	330	10	0	618
salad dressings					
Italian Fat Free	1 oz	11	0	0	191
Lo Cal Oriental	1 oz	20	2	0	189
Lo Cal Ranch	1 oz	41	3	8	151
salads and salad bars					
Chicken Breast Salad w/ Roll & Margarine	1 serv	523	16	73	654
Oriental Chicken Breast Salad w/ Dinner Roll & Margarine	1 serv	660	20	65	855
Tossed Salad	1	35	2	0	71
BLIMPIE					
6 inch sub					
5 Meatball	1 (7.8 oz)	500	22	25	970
Blimpie Best	1 (8.5 oz)	410	13	50	1480
Cheese Trio	1 (8.2 oz)	510	23	60	1060
Club	1 (9.8 oz)	450	13	40	1350
Grilled Chicken	1 (9.1 oz)	400	9	30	950
Ham & Swiss	1 (8.2 oz)	400	13	35	970
Ham Salami Provolone	1 (9.8 oz)	590	28	70	1880
Roast Beef	1 (8.5 oz)	340	5	20	870
Steak & Cheese	1 (7.1 oz)	550	26	70	1080
Tuna	1 (10.2 oz)	570	32	50	790
Turkey	1 (8.2 oz)	320	5	10	890
salads and salad bars					
Grilled Chicken Salad	1 serv (16.2 oz)	350	12	140	1190
BOJANGLES					
baked selections					
Biscuit	1	243	12	2	663
Multi-Grain Roll	1	150	3	0	210
Sweet Biscuit Apple Cinnamon	1	330	13	tr	540
Sweet Biscuit Bo*Berry	1	220	10	tr	410
Sweet Biscuit Cinnamon	1	320	18	tr	560
main menu selections					
Biscuit Sandwich Bacon	1	290	17	10	810
Biscuit Sandwich Bacon Egg & Cheese	1	550	42	160	1250
Biscuit Sandwich Cajun Filet	1	454	21	41	949
Biscuit Sandwich Country Ham	1	270	15	20	1010

FOOD	PORTION	CALS	FAT	CHOL	SOD
Biscuit Sandwich Egg	1	400	30	120	630
Biscuit Sandwich Sausage	1	350	23	20	810
Biscuit Sandwich Smoked Sausage	1	380	26	20	940
Biscuit Sandwich Steak	1	649	49	34	1126
Bo Rounds	1 serv	235	11	13	328
Buffalo Bites	1 serv	180	5	105	720
Cajun Pintos	1 serv	110	0	0	480
Cajun Roast Skinfree Breast	1 serv	143	5	84	562
Cajun Roast Skinfree Leg	1 serv	161	8	125	566
Cajun Roast Skinfree Thigh	1 serv	215	15	95	428
Cajun Roast Wing	1 serv	231	15	117	617
Cajun Spiced Breast	1 serv	278	17	75	565
Cajun Spiced Leg	1 serv	310	23	67	465
Cajun Spiced Thigh	1 serv	264	16	96	530
Cajun Spiced Wing	1 serv	355	25	94	630
Chicken Supremes	1 serv	337	16	58	629
Corn On The Cob	1 serv	140	2	0	20
Dirty Rice	1 serv	166	6	10	762
Green Beans	1 serv	25	0	0	710
Macaroni & Cheese	1 serv	198	14	26	418
Marinated Cole Slaw	1 serv	136	3	0	454
Potatoes w/o Gravy	1 serv	80	1	0	380
Sandwich Cajun Filet w/ Mayonnaise	1	437	22	55	506
Sandwich Cajun Filet w/o Mayonnaise	1	337	11	45	401
Sandwich Cajun Steak w/ Horseradish Sauce & Pickles	1	434	26	55	985
Sandwich Grilled Filet w/ Mayonnaise	1	335	16	61	645
Seasoned Fries	1 serv	344	19	13	480
Southern Style Breast	1 serv	261	16	76	702
Southern Style Leg	1 serv	254	15	94	446
Southern Style Thigh	1 serv	308	21	78	630
Southern Style Wing	1 serv	337	21	86	684
BOSTON MARKET					
baked selections					
Brownie	1 (3.3 oz)	450	27	80	190
Cinnamon Apple Pie	1/5 pie (4.8 oz)	390	23	0	250
Cookie Chocolate Chip	1 (2.8 oz)	340	17	25	240
main menu selections					
1/2 Chicken w/ Skin	1 serv (9.7 oz)	590	33	280	1010
1/4 Dark Meat Chicken No Skin	1 serv (3.3 oz)	190	10	115	440
1/4 Dark Meat Chicken w/ Skin	1 serv (4.4 oz)	320	21	155	500

FOOD	PORTION	CALS	FAT	CHOL	SOD
1/4 White Meat Chicken No Skin Or Wing	1 serv (4.9 oz)	170	4	85	480
1/4 White Meat Chicken w/ Skin And Wing	1 serv (5.3 oz)	280	12	135	510
BBQ Baked Beans	3/4 cup (7.1 oz)	270	5	0	540
BBQ Chicken Sandwich	1 (9.9 oz)	540	9	75	1690
Baked Sweet Potato Low Fat	1 (12.5 oz)	460	7	0	510
Black Beans And Rice	1 cup (8 oz)	300	10	0	1050
Boston Hearth Ham Lean	1 serv (5 oz)	210	9	75	1490
Broccoli Cauliflower Au Gratin	3/4 cup (6.1 oz)	200	11	20	600
Broccoli Rice Casserole	3/4 cup (6 oz)	240	12	40	800
Broccoli With Red Peppers	3/4 cup (3.4 oz)	60	4	0	130
Butternut Squash Low Fat	3/4 cup (6.8 oz)	160	6	15	580
Chicken Gravy	1 serv (1 oz)	15	1	0	170
Chicken Salad Sandwich	1 (11.5 oz)	680	30	120	1360
Chicken Sandwich w/ Cheese & Sauce	1 (12.4 oz)	750	33	135	1860
Chicken Sandwich w/o Cheese & Sauce Low Fat	1 (10 oz)	430	5	65	910
Chunky Chicken Salad	3/4 cup (5.5 oz)	370	27	120	800
Chunky Cinnamon Apple Sauce No Fat	3/4 cup (6.4 oz)	250	0	0	30
Cole Slaw	3/4 cup (6.5 oz)	300	19	20	540
Corn Bread	1 (2.4 oz)	200	6	25	390
Coyote Bean Salad	3/4 cup (5.3 oz)	190	9	0	210
Cranberry Relish Low Fat	3/4 cup (7.9 oz)	370	5	0	5
Creamed Spinach	3/4 cup (6.4 oz)	260	20	55	740
Fruit Salad Low Fat	3/4 cup (5.5 oz)	70	1	0	10
Green Bean Casserole	3/4 cup (6 oz)	130	9	20	440
Green Beans	3/4 cup (3 oz)	80	6	0	200
Ham Sandwich w/ Cheese & Sauce	1 (11.8 oz)	760	34	100	1730
Ham Sandwich w/o Cheese & Sauce	1 (9.3 oz)	440	8	45	1450
Homestyle Mashed Potatoes & Gravy	3/4 cup (6.6 oz)	210	10	25	740
Honey Glazed Carrots	3/4 cup (5.4 oz)	280	15	0	80
Hot Cinnamon Apples	3/4 cup (6.4 oz)	250	5	0	45
Macaroni & Cheese	3/4 cup (6.7 oz)	280	11	30	830
Mashed Potatoes	2/3 cup (5.6 oz)	190	9	25	570
Meat Loaf & Brown Gravy	1 serv (7 oz)	390	22	120	1040
Meat Loaf & Chunky Tomato Sauce	1 serv (8 oz)	370	18	120	1170
Meat Loaf Sandwich w/ Cheese	1 (13.8 oz)	860	33	165	2270
Meat Loaf Sandwich w/o Cheese	1 (12.3 oz)	690	21	120	1610

FOOD	PORTION	CALS	FAT	CHOL	SOD
New Potatoes Low Fat	3/4 cup (4.6 oz)	130	3	0	150
Old Fashioned Potato Salad	3/4 cup (6.2 oz)	340	24	30	870
Open Face Turkey Sandwich	1 (13.4 oz)	500	12	80	2170
Original Chicken Pot Pie	1 pie (14.9 oz)	780	46	135	1480
Oven Roasted Potato Planks Low Fat	5 pieces (5.8 oz)	180	5	0	370
Pastry Sandwich BBQ Chicken	1 (7.2 oz)	640	39	60	1260
Pastry Sandwich Broccoli Chicken Cheddar	1 (7.2 oz)	690	47	85	1050
Pastry Sandwich Ham & Cheddar	1 (6.6 oz)	640	41	60	1560
Pastry Sandwich Italian Chicken	1 (7.2 oz)	630	41	60	910
Red Beans And Rice Low Fat	1 cup (8 oz)	260	5	5	1050
Rice Pilaf	2/3 cup (5.1 oz)	180	5	0	600
Rotisserie Turkey Breast Skinless Low Fat	1 serv (5 oz)	170	1	100	850
Savory Stuffing	3/4 cup (6.1 oz)	310	12	0	1140
Southwest Savory Chicken	1 serv (9.6 oz)	400	15	100	1670
Squash Casserole	3/4 cup (6.6 oz)	330	24	70	1110
Steamed Vegetables Low Fat	2/3 cup (3.7 oz)	35	1	0	35
Sweet Potato Casserole	3/4 cup (6.4 oz)	280	18	10	190
Tabasco BBQ Drumstick	1 (2.4 oz)	130	6	50	190
Tabasco BBQ Wing	1 (1.8 oz)	110	7	30	170
Teriyaki Chicken 1/4 White w/ Skin	1 serv (6.8 oz)	340	12	135	890
Teriyaki Chicken 1/4 w/ Skin	1 serv (5.9 oz)	380	21	155	870
Tossed Salad w/ Caesar Dressing	1 serv (8 oz)	380	31	15	810
Triple Topped Chicken	1 serv (9.2 oz)	470	22	155	1350
Turkey Club Sandwich	1 (11.1 oz)	650	26	105	1590
Turkey Sandwich w/ Cheese & Sauce	1 (11.8 oz)	710	28	110	1390
Turkey Sandwich w/o Cheese & Sauce	1 (9.3 oz)	400	4	60	1070
Whole Kernel Corn	3/4 cup (5.8 oz)	180	4	0	170
Zucchini Marinara Low Fat	3/4 cup (6.6 oz)	60	3	0	330
salads and salad bars					
Caesar Salad Entree	1 serv (10 oz)	510	42	35	1130
Caesar Salad w/o Dressing	1 serv (8 oz)	230	12	20	500
Caesar Side Salad	1 (4 oz)	200	17	15	450
Chicken Caesar Salad	1 serv (13 oz)	650	45	105	1580
Tossed Salad w/ Fat Free Ranch	1 serv (8 oz)	160	3	0	940
Tossed Salad w/ Old Venice Dressing	1 serv (8 oz)	340	27	0	1110
soups					
Chicken Chili	1 cup (8.7 oz)	220	7	40	1000
Chicken Noodle	1 cup (8.4 oz)	130	5	40	1310

FOOD	PORTION	CALS	FAT	CHOL	SOD
Chicken Tortilla	1 cup (8.4 oz)	220	11	35	1410
Potato	1 cup (8 oz)	270	16	40	1020
Tomato Bisque	1 cup (8 oz)	280	23	50	1280
BROWN'S CHICKEN					
Breadsticks w/ Garlic Butter	1	199	4	tr	2213
Breast	3.5 oz	284	15	67	529
Coleslaw	3.5 oz	131	10	6	211
Corn Fritters	3.5 oz	415	25	4	552
Corn On Cob	1 ear (3 inch)	126	3	1	23
Fettucini Alfredo	1 serv (12 oz)	1507	64	51	3018
French Fries	3.5 oz	503	22	1	235
Gizzard	3.5 oz	387	20	88	795
Leg	3.5 oz	287	16	52	542
Liver	3.5 oz	341	19	147	704
Mostaccioli w/ Meat	1 serv (12 oz)	835	14	17	898
Mostaccioli w/o Meat	1 serv (12 oz)	792	10	0	842
Mushrooms	3.5 oz	289	16	1	671
Potato Salad	3.5 oz	94	4	11	639
Ravioli w/ Meat	1 serv (12 oz)	865	20	17	934
Ravioli w/o Meat	1 serv (12 oz)	822	16	0	878
Shrimp	3.5 oz	277	10	31	778
Thigh	3.5 oz	355	24	63	574
Wing	3.5 oz	385	25	81	654
BRUEGGER'S BAGELS					
Blueberry	1 (3.5 oz)	300	2	0	480
Cinnamon Raisin	1 (3.5 oz)	290	2	0	400
Egg	1 (3.5 oz)	280	1	25	510
Everything	1 (3.6 oz)	290	2	0	700
Garlic	1 (3.6 oz)	280	2	0	440
Honey Grain	1 (3.6 oz)	300	3	0	390
Onion	1 (3.6 oz)	280	2	0	430
Orange Cranberry	1 (3.5 oz)	290	1	0	470
Pesto	1 (3.5 oz)	280	2	0	480
Plain	1 (3.5 oz)	280	2	0	430
Poppy Seed	1 (3.6 oz)	280	2	0	440
Pumpernickel	1 (3.5 oz)	280	2	0	390
Salt	1 (3.6 oz)	270	2	0	1670
Sesame	1 (3.6 oz)	290	3	0	440
Spinach	1 (3.5 oz)	280	1	0	490
Sun Dried Tomato	1 (3.5 oz)	280	2	0	490
Wheat Bran	1 (3.5 oz)	280	2	0	410
BURGER KING					
breakfast selections					
AM Express Grape Jam	1 serv (0.4 oz)	30	0	0	0
AM Express Strawberry Jam	1 serv (0.4 oz)	30	0	0	0
AM Express Dip	1 serv (1 oz)	80	0	0	20
Bacon	3 strips (0.3 oz)	40	3	10	170
Biscuit	1 (3.3 oz)	300	15	0	830

FOOD	PORTION	CALS	FAT	CHOL	SOD
Biscuit w/ Bacon Egg & Cheese	1 (6.6 oz)	620	43	185	1650
Biscuit w/ Egg	1 (4.6 oz)	380	21	140	1010
Biscuit w/ Sausage	1 (4.6 oz)	490	33	35	1240
Cini-Minis w/o Icing	4 (3.8 oz)	440	23	25	710
Croissan'wich Sausage Egg & Cheese	1 (5.3 oz)	530	41	185	1120
Croissan'wich w/ Sausage & Cheese	1 (3.7 oz)	450	35	45	940
French Toast Sticks	5 sticks (4 oz)	440	23	2	490
Ham	1 serv (1.2 oz)	35	1	15	770
Hash Browns	1 sm (2.6 oz)	240	15	0	440
Land O'Lakes Whipped Classic Blend	1 serv (0.4 oz)	65	7	0	75
Vanilla Icing Cini-Minis	1 serv (1 oz)	110	3	0	40
main menu selections					
American Cheese	2 slices (0.9 oz)	90	8	25	420
BK Big Fish Sandwich	1 (8.8 oz)	720	43	80	1180
BK Broiler Chicken Breast Patty	1 (3.5 oz)	140	4	90	570
BK Broiler Chicken Sandwich	1 (8.7 oz)	530	16	105	1060
BK Broiler Chicken Sandwich w/o Mayo	1 (8.7 oz)	370	9	105	1060
Bacon Cheeseburger	1 (4.9 oz)	400	22	70	940
Bacon Double Cheeseburger	1 (7.2 oz)	630	38	125	1230
Big King Sandwich	1 (7.6 oz)	640	42	125	980
Bull's Eye Barbecue Sauce	1 serv (0.5 oz)	20	0	0	140
Cheeseburger	1 (4.7 oz)	360	19	60	760
Chick'N Crisp Sandwich	1 (4.9 oz)	460	27	35	890
Chick'N Crisp Sandwich w/o Mayo	1 (4.9 oz)	360	16	35	890
Chicken Sandwich	1 (8 oz)	710	43	60	1400
Chicken Sandwich w/o Mayo	1 (8 oz)	500	20	60	1400
Chicken Tenders	8 (4.3 oz)	350	22	65	940
Chicken Tenders	4 (2.2 oz)	180	11	30	470
Chicken Tenders	5 (2.7 oz)	230	14	40	590
Dipping Sauce Barbecue	1 serv (1 oz)	35	0	0	400
Dipping Sauce Honey	1 serv (1 oz)	90	0	0	10
Dipping Sauce Honey Mustard	1 serv (1 oz)	90	6	10	150
Dipping Sauce Ranch	1 serv (1 oz)	170	17	0	200
Dipping Sauce Sweet & Sour	1 serv (1 oz)	45	0	0	50
Double Cheeseburger	1 (6.9 oz)	580	36	120	1060
Double Whopper	1 (12.2 oz)	920	59	155	980
Double Whopper w/ Cheese	1 (13.1 oz)	1010	67	180	1460
Double Whopper w/o Mayo	1 (13.1 oz)	850	50	180	1460
Dutch Apple Pie	1 serv (4 oz)	300	15	0	230
French Fries No Salt	1 med (4.1 g)	400	21	0	760

FOOD	PORTION	CALS	FAT	CHOL	SOD
French Fries No Salt	1 sm (2.6 oz)	250	13	0	480
French Fries No Salt	1 king size (6 oz)	590	30	0	1110
French Fries Salted	1 med (4.1 oz)	400	21	0	820
French Fries Salted	1 sm (2.6 oz)	250	13	0	550
French Fries Salted	1 king size (6 oz)	590	30	0	1180
Hamburger	1 (4.2 oz)	320	15	50	520
Hamburger Bun	1 (4.6 oz)	130	2	0	250
Hamburger Patty	1 (1.9 oz)	170	13	50	55
Hash Browns	1 lg (4.5 oz)	410	26	0	750
Ketchup	1 serv (0.5 oz)	15	0	0	180
King Sauce	1 serv (0.5 oz)	70	7	4	70
Lettuce	1 leaf (0.7 oz)	0	0	0	0
Mustard	1 serv (3 g)	0	0	0	40
Onion	1 serv (0.5 oz)	5	0	0	0
Onion Rings	1 med serv (3.3 oz)	380	19	2	550
Onion Rings	1 king serv (5.3 oz)	600	30	4	880
Pickles	4 slices (0.5 oz)	0	0	0	140
Tartar Sauce	1 serv (1.5 oz)	260	29	20	330
Tomato	2 slices (1 oz)	5	0	0	0
Whopper	1 (9.5 oz)	660	40	85	900
Whopper Bun	1 (2.7 oz)	220	4	0	370
Whopper Jr.	1 (5.5 oz)	400	24	55	530
Whopper Jr. w/ Cheese	1 (6 oz)	450	28	65	770
Whopper Jr. w/ Cheese w/o Mayo	1 (6 oz)	370	19	65	770
Whopper Jr. w/o Mayo	1 (5.5 oz)	320	15	55	530
Whopper Patty	1 (2.8 oz)	250	19	70	85
Whopper w/ Cheese	1 (10.4 oz)	760	48	110	1380
Whopper w/ Cheese w/o Mayo	1 (10.4 oz)	600	31	110	1380
Whopper w/o Mayo	1 (9.5 oz)	510	23	85	900
CARVEL					
ice cream					
Brown Bonnet Cone	1 (4.7 oz)	380	21	40	150
Cake	1 pkg (7 oz)	450	23	45	230
Cake	1 pkg (4 oz)	270	14	30	160
Cake Cheesecake	1 serv (4 oz)	280	14	30	190
Cake Chocolate Vanilla Chocolate Crunchies	1/15 cake (3.4 oz)	230	12	35	95
Cake Cookies & Cream	1 serv (4 oz)	270	14	35	160
Cake Fudge Drizzle	1/8 cake (4 oz)	310	17	30	170
Cake Fudgie The Whale	1/14 cake (3.6 oz)	290	16	30	180
Cake Holiday	1/15 cake (3.4 oz)	240	12	30	100
Cake S'mores	1 serv (4 oz)	270	14	25	150
Cake Sinfully Chocolate	1 serv (4 oz)	280	14	25	150
Cake Strawberries & Cream	1/8 cake (3.8 oz)	240	12	35	100
Chocolate	4 oz	190	10	25	100
Chocolate No Fat	4 oz	120	0	0	40

FOOD	PORTION	CALS	FAT	CHOL	SOD
Flying Saucer Chocolate	1 (4 oz)	230	9	30	140
Flying Saucer Chocolate w/ Sprinkles	1 (4 oz)	330	14	30	150
Flying Saucer Low Fat Chocolate	1 (4 oz)	190	3	0	130
Flying Saucer Low Fat Vanilla	1 (4 oz)	180	3	0	140
Flying Saucer Vanilla	1 (4 oz)	240	10	40	150
Flying Saucer Vanilla w/ Sprinkles	1 (4 oz)	340	14	40	160
Lil'Love Cake All Vanilla	1 piece (4.4 oz)	330	16	35	200
Lil'Love Cake Chocolate & Vanilla	1 piece (4 oz)	260	13	30	140
Nature's Crunch	1 (4.2 g)	450	25	20	240
Olde Fashion Sundae Butterscotch	1 (8 oz)	500	17	60	340
Olde Fashion Sundae Chocolate	1 (8 oz)	470	19	55	280
Olde Fashion Sundae Strawberry	1 (8 oz)	420	15	55	230
Sheet Cake Chocolate Vanilla Chocolate Crunchies	1/26 cake (3.3 oz)	230	12	35	100
Sinful Love Bar	1 (4.2 oz)	460	29	20	240
Thick Shake Chocolate	1 (16 oz)	719	31	116	418
Thick Shake Low Fat Chocolate	1 (16 oz)	490	1	15	330
Thick Shake Low Fat Strawberry	1 (16 oz)	460	1	15	290
Thick Shake Low Fat Vanilla	1 (16 oz)	460	1	15	280
Thick Shake No Fat Chocolate	1 (16 oz)	524	8	36	346
Thick Shake No Fat Strawberry	1 (16 oz)	453	7	36	285
Thick Shake No Fat Vanilla	1 (16 oz)	462	7	36	278
Thick Shake Strawberry	1 (16 oz)	648	30	116	358
Thick Shake Vanilla	1 (16 oz)	657	30	116	350
Vanilla	4 oz	200	10	40	110
Vanilla No Fat	4 oz	120	0	0	55
sherbet					
Black Raspberry	1/2 cup (3.4 oz)	150	1	5	35
Blueberry	1/2 cup (3.4 oz)	150	1	5	30
Lemon	1/2 cup (3.5 oz)	150	1	5	30
Lime	1/2 cup (3.5 oz)	150	1	5	30
Mango	1/2 cup (3.5 oz)	140	1	5	25
Orange	1/2 cup (3.5 oz)	150	1	5	30
Peach	1/2 cup (3.4 oz)	150	1	5	35
Pineapple	1/2 cup (3.5 oz)	150	1	5	40
Strawberry	1/2 cup (3.5 oz)	150	1	5	35

FOOD	PORTION	CALS	FAT	CHOL	SOD
CHICK-FIL-A					
desserts					
Cheesecake + One Side	1 slice (3.1 oz)	300	21	115	200
Fudge Nut Brownie	1 (2.6 oz)	350	16	30	650
Icedream Cone	1 sm (4.5 oz)	140	4	40	240
Lemon Pie	1 slice (3.5 oz)	280	22	5	550
main menu selections					
Barbecue Sauce	1 serv (1 oz)	45	0	0	190
Carrot & Raisin Salad	1 sm (2.7 oz)	150	2	6	650
Chargrilled Chicken Club Sandwich	1 (8.2 oz)	390	12	70	980
Chargrilled Chicken Garden Salad	1 serv (9.8 oz)	190	5	83	800
Chargrilled Chicken Sandwich	1 (5.3 oz)	280	3	40	640
Chick-n-Strips	4 (4.2 oz)	230	8	20	380
Chick-n-Strips Salad	1 serv (11.7 oz)	370	17	113	725
Chicken Sandwich	1 (5.9 oz)	290	9	50	870
Chicken Caesar Salad	1 serv (8.1 oz)	230	10	85	940
Chicken Salad Sandwich	1 (5.9 oz)	320	5	10	810
Cole Slaw	1 sm (2.8 oz)	130	6	15	430
Dijon Honey Sauce	1 serv (0.4 oz)	60	1	5	70
Hearty Breast of Chicken Soup	1 cup (7.6 oz)	110	1	45	760
Honey Mustard Sauce	1 serv (1 oz)	45	0	0	150
Nuggets	8 (3.9 oz)	290	14	60	770
Polynesian Sauce	1 serv (1 oz)	110	6	0	210
Side Salad	1 serv (4.6 oz)	70	0	0	0
Waffle Potato Fries	1 sm (3 oz)	290	10	5	960
salad dressings					
Basil Vinaigrette	1 serv (1.5 oz)	250	26	0	190
Blue Cheese	1 serv (1.5 oz)	230	24	30	450
Buttermilk Ranch	1 serv (1.5 oz)	220	24	10	420
Fat Free Dijon Honey Mustard	1 serv (1.5 oz)	70	1	0	230
House	1 serv (1.6 oz)	190	17	5	380
Light Italian	1 serv (1.5 oz)	20	1	0	770
Spicy	1 serv (1.2 oz)	210	22	10	170
Thousand Island	1 serv (1.5 oz)	210	20	20	360
CHURCH'S CHICKEN					
Apple Pie	1 serv (3.1 oz)	280	12	<5	340
Biscuit	1 (2.1 oz)	250	16	<5	640
Breast	1 serv (2.8 oz)	200	12	65	510
Cajun Rice	1 serv (3.1 oz)	130	7	5	260
Cole Slaw	1 serv (3 oz)	92	6	0	230
Corn On The Cob	1 serv (5.7 oz)	139	3	0	15
French Fries	1 serv (2.7 oz)	210	11	0	60
Leg	1 serv (2 oz)	140	9	45	160
Okra	1 serv (2.8 oz)	210	16	0	520
Potatoes & Gravy	1 serv (3.7 oz)	90	3	0	520

FOOD	PORTION	CALS	FAT	CHOL	SOD
Tender Strip	1 (1.1 oz)	80	4	15	140
Thigh	1 serv (2.8 oz)	230	16	80	520
Wing	1 serv (3.1 oz)	250	16	60	540
DAIRY QUEEN					
food selections					
Chicken Breast Fillet Sandwich	1 (6.7 oz)	430	20	55	760
Chicken Strip Basket	1 serv (14.5 oz)	1000	50	55	2510
Chili 'n' Cheese Dog	1 (5 oz)	330	21	45	1090
DQ Homestyle Bacon Double Cheeseburger	1 (8.9 oz)	610	36	130	1380
DQ Homestyle Cheeseburger	1 (5.3 oz)	340	17	55	850
DQ Homestyle Double Cheeseburger	1 (7.7 oz)	540	31	115	1130
DQ Homestyle Hamburger	1 (4.8 oz)	290	12	45	630
DQ Ultimate Burger	1 (9.4 oz)	670	43	135	1210
French Fries	1 med (3.9 oz)	440	23	0	1110
French Fries	1 sm (4 oz)	350	18	0	880
Grilled Chicken Sandwich	1 (6.5 oz)	310	10	50	1040
Hot Dog	1 (3.5 oz)	240	14	25	730
Onion Rings	1 serv (4 oz)	320	16	0	180
The Great Steakmelt Basket	1 serv (13.2 oz)	770	38	75	2290
ice cream					
Banana Split	1 (12.9 oz)	510	12	30	180
Blizzard Chocolate Sandwich Cookie	1 sm (12 oz)	520	18	40	380
Blizzard Chocolate Sandwich Cookie	1 med (11.4 oz)	640	23	45	500
Blizzard Chocolate Chip Cookie Dough	1 med (15.4 oz)	950	36	75	660
Blizzard Chocolate Chip Cookie Dough	1 sm (12 oz)	660	24	55	440
Breeze Heath	1 sm (10.2 oz)	470	10	10	380
Breeze Heath	1 med (14.2 oz)	710	18	20	580
Breeze Strawberry	1 med (13.4 oz)	460	1	10	270
Breeze Strawberry	1 sm (12 oz)	320	1	5	190
Buster Bar	1 (5.2 oz)	450	28	15	280
Chocolate Malt	1 sm (14.7 oz)	650	16	55	370
Chocolate Malt	1 med (19.9 oz)	880	22	70	500
Cone Chocolate	1 sm (5 oz)	240	8	20	115
Cone Chocolate	1 med (6.9 oz)	340	11	30	160
Cone Vanilla	1 lg (8.9 oz)	410	12	40	200
Cone Vanilla	1 sm (5 oz)	230	7	20	115
Cone Vanilla	1 med (6.9 oz)	330	9	30	160
Cone Yogurt	1 med (6.9 oz)	260	1	5	160
Cone Dipped	1 med (7.7 oz)	490	24	30	190
Cone Dipped	1 sm (5.5 oz)	340	17	20	130
Cup Of Yogurt	1 med (6.7 oz)	230	1	5	150

FOOD	PORTION	CALS	FAT	CHOL	SOD
DQ 8 Inch Round Cake Undecorated	1/8 of cake (6.2 oz)	340	13	25	280
DQ Fudge Bar No Sugar Added	1 (2.3 oz)	50	0	0	70
DQ Lemon Freez'r	1/2 cup (3.2 oz)	80	0	0	10
DQ Nonfat Frozen Yogurt	1/2 cup (3 oz)	100	0		70
DQ Sandwich	1 (2.1 oz)	200	6	10	140
DQ Soft Serve Chocolate	1/2 cup (3.3 oz)	150	5	15	75
DQ Soft Serve Vanilla	1/2 cup (3.3 oz)	140	5	15	70
DQ Treatzza Pizza Heath	1/8 of pie (2.4 oz)	180	7	5	160
DQ Treatzza Pizza M&M	1/8 of pie (2.4 oz)	190	7	5	160
DQ Vanilla Orange Bar No Sugar Added	1 (2.3 oz)	60	0	0	40
Dilly Bar Chocolate	1 (3 oz)	210	13	10	75
Frozen Hot Chocolate	1 (20.9 oz)	860	35	50	350
Misty Slush	1 sm (15.9 oz)	220	0	0	20
Misty Slush	1 med (20.9 oz)	290	0	0	30
Peanut Buster Parfait	1 (10.7 oz)	730	31	35	400
Pecan Mudslide Treat	1 (4.6 oz)	650	30	35	420
S'more Galore Parfait	1 (10.7 oz)	730	30	30	340
Shake Chocolate	1 sm (13.9 oz)	560	15	50	310
Shake Chocolate	1 med (18.9 oz)	770	20	70	420
Starkiss	1 (3 oz)	80	0	0	10
Strawberry Shortcake	1 (8.5 oz)	430	14	60	360
Sundae Chocolate	1 med (8.2 oz)	400	10	30	210
Sundae Chocolate	1 sm (5.7 oz)	280	7	20	140
Yogurt Sundae Strawberry	1 med (8.2 oz)	280	1	5	160
D'ANGELO'S SANDWICH SHOP					
salads and salad bars					
Antipasto Salad w/o Dressing	1	420	14	40	1400
Caesar Salad w/ Dressing	1	740	45	70	2270
Caesar Salad w/o Dressing	1	490	20	15	1310
Chicken Caesar Salad w/ Dressing	1	860	48	130	2820
Chicken Caesar Salad w/o Dressing	1	600	23	70	1870
Chicken Salad D'Lite	1	325	4	49	980
Chicken Salad w/o Dressing	1	390	5	60	1200
Greek Salad w/ Dressing	1	940	71	50	1320
Greek Salad w/ Tuna & Dressing	1	1010	72	65	1510
Greek Salad w/ Tuna w/o Dressing	1	490	15	65	1510
Greek Salad w/o Dressing	1	420	15	50	1310
Roast Beef Salad D'Lite	1	350	5	63	890
Roast Beef Salad w/o Dressing	1	400	6	50	920
Tossed Garden Salad w/o Dressing	1	270	2	0	650
Tuna Salad D'Lite	1	305	2	32	805

FOOD	PORTION	CALS	FAT	CHOL	SOD
Tuna Salad w/o Dressing	1	330	3	15	840
Turkey Salad w/o Dressing	1	400	3	80	700
sandwiches					
BLT w/ Cheese	1	1170	62	165	3310
BLT w/ Cheese Medium Sub	1	870	47	125	2490
BLT w/ Cheese Pokket	1	570	31	90	1690
BLT w/ Cheese Small Sub	1	600	33	90	1730
Barbecue Curls	1	480	19	70	650
Buffalo Chicken Wrap w/ Blue Cheese Dressing	1	621	28	93	1831
Buffalo Chicken Wrap w/o Dressing	1	417	13	78	1551
Caesar Salad w/ Dressing Pokket	1	590	26	40	1690
Caesar Salad w/o Dressing Pokket	1	460	13	10	1210
Caesar Salad w/ Chicken w/ Dressing Pokket	1	570	16	70	1760
Caesar Wrap w/ Dressing	1	484	15	10	2135
Caesar Wrap w/ Fat Free Dressing	1	484	15	10	2135
Capicola Ham & Cheese Large Sub	1	740	23	85	2540
Capicola Ham & Cheese Medium Sub	1	550	17	65	1900
Capicola Ham & Cheese Pokket	1	350	11	45	1260
Capicola Ham & Cheese Small Sub	1	390	13	45	1310
Cheeseburger Large Sub	1	1060	49	165	2090
Cheeseburger Medium Sub	1	780	37	125	1560
Cheeseburger Pokket	1	490	23	80	1000
Cheeseburger Small Sub	1	530	25	80	1040
Chicken Salad Large Sub	1	1370	78	155	1570
Chicken Salad Medium Sub	1	970	55	110	1120
Chicken Salad Pokket	1	650	38	80	740
Chicken Salad Small Sub	1	690	39	80	790
Chicken Stir Fry D'Lite Pokket	1	360	5	70	1240
Chicken Stir Fry D'Lite Sub	1	280	6	70	1280
Chicken Stir Fry Large Sub	1	800	12	160	2730
Chicken Stir Fry Medium Sub	1	560	9	110	1890
Chicken Stir Fry Pokket	1	360	5	70	1240
Chicken Stir Fry Small Sub	1	380	6	70	1280
Classic Vegetable D'Lite Pokket	1	340	10	23	960
Classic Vegetable Large Sub	1	860	33	80	2450
Classic Vegetable Medium Sub	1	610	23	55	1700
Classic Vegetable Pokket	1	400	15	40	1180
Classic Vegetable Small Sub	1	430	15	40	1220

FOOD	PORTION	CALS	FAT	CHOL	SOD
Crunchy Vegetable D'Lite Pokket	1	350	10	23	1000
Crunchy Vegetable D'Lite Small Sub	1	385	11	23	1045
Crunchy Vegetable Large Sub	1	880	33	80	2520
Crunchy Vegetable Medium Sub	1	620	23	55	1750
Crunchy Vegetable Pokket	1	410	15	40	1220
Crunchy Vegetable Small Sub	1	440	16	40	1260
Ginger Chicken Stir Fry D'Lite Pokket	1	400	5	72	1240
Greek Pokket	1	910	71	50	1120
Grilled Spicy Steak D'Lite Pokket	1	425	11	41	735
Grilled Steak Cheese Large Sub	1	1160	54	195	1970
Grilled Steak Cheese Medium Sub	1	820	38	135	1460
Grilled Steak Cheese Pokket	1	550	26	100	1010
Grilled Steak Cheese Small Sub	1	580	28	100	1050
Grilled Steak Combo Large Sub	1	1170	54	195	2200
Grilled Steak Combo Medium Sub	1	830	38	135	1630
Grilled Steak Combo Pokket	1	550	26	100	1120
Grilled Steak Combo Small Sub	1	590	28	100	1170
Grilled Steak D'Lite Pokket	1	390	11	41	735
Grilled Steak Large Sub	1	990	40	155	1320
Grilled Steak Medium Sub	1	680	27	105	940
Grilled Steak Mushrooms Large Sub	1	1000	40	155	1570
Grilled Steak Mushrooms Medium Sub	1	690	27	105	1120
Grilled Steak Mushrooms Pokket	1	450	18	70	720
Grilled Steak Mushrooms Small Sub	1	480	19	70	770
Grilled Steak Onion Large Sub	1	1000	40	155	1330
Grilled Steak Onion Medium Sub	1	700	27	105	940
Grilled Steak Onion Pokket	1	450	17	70	600
Grilled Steak Onion Small Sub	1	480	19	70	650
Grilled Steak Peppers	1	690	27	105	940
Grilled Steak Peppers Large Sub	1	1000	40	155	1330
Grilled Steak Peppers Pokket	1	540	17	70	600
Grilled Steak Pokket	1	440	17	70	600
Grilled Steak Small Sub	1	470	19	70	650

FOOD	PORTION	CALS	FAT	CHOL	SOD
Ham & Cheese Large Sub	1	760	25	105	3030
Ham & Cheese Medium Sub	1	550	19	75	2170
Ham & Cheese Pokket	1	370	13	55	1550
Ham & Cheese Small Sub	1	400	14	55	1600
Ham Salami & Cheese Large Sub	1	870	36	110	3000
Ham Salami & Cheese Medium Sub	1	630	27	80	2190
Ham Salami & Cheese Pokket	1	420	18	60	1500
Ham Salami & Cheese Small Sub	1	450	20	60	1550
Hamburger Large Sub	1	920	38	130	1570
Hamburger Medium Sub	1	680	28	95	1150
Hamburger Pokket	1	430	18	65	740
Hamburger Small Sub	1	460	19	65	780
Italian Cold Cut Large Sub	1	1130	61	155	3580
Italian Cold Cut Medium Sub	1	820	44	110	2600
Italian Cold Cut Pokket	1	550	30	80	1790
Italian Cold Cut Small Sub	1	580	32	80	1830
Meatball Large Sub	1	1010	42	135	2600
Meatball Medium Sub	1	750	32	100	1980
Meatball Pokket	1	480	20	65	1360
Meatball Small Sub	1	520	21	65	1400
Meatball w/ Cheese Large Sub	1	1170	54	165	3000
Meatball w/ Cheese Medium Sub	1	880	41	125	2300
Meatball w/ Cheese Pokket	1	580	28	85	1600
Meatball w/ Cheese Small Sub	1	620	29	85	1650
Pastrami Large Sub	1	1250	69	175	2920
Pastrami Medium Sub	1	860	46	115	2010
Pastrami Pokket	1	550	30	75	1310
Pastrami Small Sub	1	580	31	75	1350
Pastrami w/ Cheese Large Sub	1	1640	102	270	4420
Pastrami w/ Cheese Medium Sub	1	1170	73	195	3210
Pastrami w/ Cheese Pokket	1	780	49	135	2210
Pastrami w/ Cheese Small Sub	1	820	51	135	2250
Roast Beef D'Lite Pokket	1	330	6	48	710
Roast Beef D'Lite Small Sub	1	365	7	48	755
Roast Beef Large Sub	1	710	14	95	1510
Roast Beef Medium Sub	1	520	10	70	1100
Seafood Salad Large Sub	1	1210	68	50	2890
Seafood Salad Medium Sub	1	860	48	35	2050
Seafood Salad Pokket	1	570	33	25	1400
Seafood Salad Small Sub	1	610	34	25	1440
Stuffed Turkey D'Lite Pokket	1	510	8	82	880
Stuffed Turkey D'Lite Small Sub	1	545	9	82	920
Stuffed Turkey Large Sub	1	1070	19	165	1850

FOOD	PORTION	CALS	FAT	CHOL	SOD
Stuffed Turkey Medium Sub	1	790	14	120	1360
Tuna Salad Large Sub	1	1510	102	120	2200
Tuna Salad Medium Sub	1	1070	72	85	1570
Tuna Salad Pokket	1	720	50	60	1060
Turkey D'Lite Pokket	1	330	2	79	490
Turkey D'Lite Small Sub	1	365	4	79	535
Turkey Large Sub	1	710	7	160	1070
Turkey Medium Sub	1	520	5	115	780
Turkey Club Large Sub	1	860	20	180	1470
Turkey Club Medium Sub	1	630	15	130	1080
Turkey Club Pokket	1	400	9	90	690
Turkey Club Small Sub	1	430	10	90	740

DELTACO

breakfast selections

Burrito Breakfast	1 (3.8 oz)	250	11	160	520
Burrito Egg & Cheese	1 (7.5 oz)	450	24	530	740
Burrito Macho Bacon & Egg	1 (15.9 oz)	1030	60	790	1760
Burrito Steak & Egg	1 (9 oz)	580	34	560	1270
Quesadilla Bacon & Egg	1 (6.1 oz)	450	23	260	920
Side of Bacon	2 strips (0.3 oz)	50	4	10	170

main menu selections

Beans 'n Cheese Cup	1 serv (7.7 oz)	260	3	5	1810
Burrito Combo	1 (8.2 oz)	490	21	55	1380
Burrito Del Beef	1 (8 oz)	550	30	90	1090
Burrito Del Classic Chicken	1 (8.5 oz)	580	38	70	1100
Burrito Deluxe Combo	1 (10.7 oz)	530	25	60	1390
Burrito Deluxe Del Beef	1 (10.5 oz)	590	33	95	1110
Burrito Green	1 (5 oz)	280	8	15	1030
Burrito Macho Beef	1 (18.9 oz)	1170	62	190	2190
Burrito Macho Combo	1 (19.4 oz)	1050	44	115	2760
Burrito Red	1 (5 oz)	270	8	15	1020
Burrito Red Regular	1 (7.5 oz)	390	12	20	1439
Burrito Regular Green	1 (7.5 oz)	400	12	10	1450
Burrito Spicy Chicken	1 (8.7 oz)	480	16	40	1620
Burrito The Works	1 (10.2 oz)	480	18	25	1500
Cheeseburger	1 (4.6 oz)	330	13	35	870
Del Cheeseburger	1 (5.6 oz)	430	25	45	710
Double Del Cheeseburger	1 (7.1 oz)	560	35	85	960
Fries	1 sm (3 oz)	210	14	0	160
Fries	1 reg (5 oz)	350	23	0	270
Fries Best Value	1 serv (7 oz)	490	32	0	380
Fries Chili Cheese	1 serv (10.5 oz)	670	46	45	880
Fries Deluxe Chili Cheese	1 serv (11.9 oz)	710	49	50	880
Get A Lot Meals #1 Combo Burrito Fries Drink	1 meal	980	44	55	1670
Get A Lot Meals #2 Del Classic Chicken Burrito Fries Drink	1 meal	1080	61	70	1390

FOOD	PORTION	CALS	FAT	CHOL	SOD
Get A Lot Meals #3 Regular Red Burrito Fries Drink	1 meal	890	35	20	1710
Get A Lot Meals #4 Two Chicken Soft Tacos Fries Drink	1 meal	910	46	60	1330
Get A Lot Meals #5 Taco Combo Burrito Drink	1 meal	790	31	75	1540
Get A Lot Meals #6 Two Tacos Quesadilla Drink	1 meal	960	47	115	1170
Get A Lot Meals #7 Macho Combo Burrito Drink	1 meal	1530	67	115	3050
Get A Lot Meals #8 Two Big Fat Tacos Fries Drink	1 meal	802	45	70	1640
Get A Lot Meals #9 Double Del Cheeseburger Fries Drink	1 meal	1050	58	85	1250
Nachos	1 serv (4 oz)	380	24	5	630
Nachos Macho	1 serv (17 oz)	1200	66	55	2720
Quesadilla Chicken	1 (6.8 oz)	580	31	104	1240
Quesadilla Regular	1 (5.3 oz)	500	27	75	860
Quesadilla Spicy Jack Chicken	1 (6.8 oz)	570	30	105	1300
Quesadilla Spicy Jack Regular	1 (5.3 oz)	490	26	75	920
Rice Cup	1 serv (4 oz)	150	2	2	600
Soft Taco	1 (2.8 oz)	160	8	20	330
Soft Taco Chicken	1 (3.3 oz)	210	12	30	520
Taco	1 (2.2 oz)	160	10	20	150
Taco Big Fat	1 (5.4 oz)	320	11	35	680
Taco Big Fat Chicken	1 (5.4 oz)	340	13	45	840
Taco Big Fat Steak	1 (5.4 oz)	390	19	45	960
Taco Salad Deluxe	1 (18.8 oz)	760	37	70	2010
Tostada Salad	1 (4.5 oz)	210	9	15	640
DENNY'S					
breakfast selections					
All American Slam	1 serv (15 oz)	1028	87	724	1942
Applesauce	1 serv (3 oz)	60	0	0	13
Bacon	4 strips (1 oz)	162	18	36	640
Bagel Dry	1 (3 oz)	235	1	0	495
Banana	1 (4 oz)	110	0	0	0
Banana Strawberry Medley	1 serv (4 oz)	108	1	0	6
Biscuit Plain	1 (3 oz)	375	22	0	750
Biscuit w/ Sausage Gravy	1 serv (7 oz)	570	38	24	1475
Blueberry Topping	1 serv (3 oz)	106	0	0	15
Canadian Bacon	1 serv (3 oz)	110	5	43	1039
Cantaloup	1 serv (3 oz)	32	0	0	16
Cheddar Cheese Omelette	1 serv (13 oz)	770	62	675	1133
Cherry Topping	1 serv (3 oz)	86	0	0	5
Chicken Fried Steak & Eggs	1 serv (14 oz)	723	56	452	1505

FOOD	PORTION	CALS	FAT	CHOL	SOD
Country Scramble	1 serv (16 oz)	795	50	409	1819
Cream Cheese	1 oz	100	10	31	6
Egg	1 (2 oz)	134	12	205	61
Egg Beaters	1 serv (2.3 oz)	71	5	1	138
Eggs Benedict	1 serv (19 oz)	860	56	525	1943
English Muffin Dry	1 (4 oz)	125	1	0	198
Farmer's Omelette	1 serv (18 oz)	912	69	633	1816
French Slam	1 serv (14 oz)	1029	71	777	1428
French Toast	2 pieces (8 oz)	510	25	317	413
Fresh Fruit Mix	1 serv (3 oz)	36	0	0	16
Grapefruit	1/2 (5 oz)	60	0	0	0
Grapes	1 serv (3 oz)	55	1	0	0
Grits	1 serv (4 oz)	80	0	0	520
Ham	1 serv (3 oz)	94	3	23	761
Ham'n'Cheddar Omelette	1 serv (14 oz)	743	55	657	1518
Hashed Browns	1 serv (4 oz)	218	14	0	424
Hashed Browns Covered	1 serv (6 oz)	318	23	30	604
Hashed Browns Covered & Smothered	1 serv (8 oz)	359	26	30	790
Honeydew	1 serv (3 oz)	31	0	0	22
Junior Meals Basic Breakfast	1 serv (9 oz)	558	39	230	1103
Junior Meals Junior French Slam	1 serv (7 oz)	461	35	386	663
Junior Meals Junior Grand Slam	1 serv (5 oz)	397	25	230	1118
Junior Meals Junior Waffle Supreme	1 serv (4 oz)	190	11	73	102
Meat Lover's Sampler	1 serv (14 oz)	806	62	481	2211
Moon Over My Hammy	1 serv (12 oz)	807	48	430	2247
Muffin Blueberry	1 (3 oz)	309	14	0	190
Oatmeal	1 serv (4 oz)	100	2	0	175
Original Grand Slam	1 serv (10 oz)	795	50	460	2237
Pancakes	3 (5 oz)	491	7	0	1818
Pork Chop & Eggs	1 serv (12 oz)	555	36	469	968
Porterhouse Steak & Eggs	1 serv (18 oz)	1223	95	570	1369
Ready To Eat Cereal	1 serv (1 oz)	100	0	0	276
Sausage	4 links (3 oz)	354	32	64	944
Sausage Cheddar Omelette	1 serv (16 oz)	1036	86	721	1841
Scram Slam	1 serv (18 oz)	974	80	694	1750
Senior Belgian Waffle Slam	1 serv (6 oz)	399	33	302	612
Senior Omelette	1 serv (12 oz)	623	47	439	1194
Senior Starter	1 serv (7 oz)	336	24	205	541
Senior Triple Play	1 serv (8 oz)	537	25	409	1445
Sirloin Steak & Eggs	1 serv (13 oz)	808	64	474	952
Slim Slam	1 serv (14 oz)	638	12	34	1772
Southern Slam	1 serv (13 oz)	1065	84	484	2449
Strawberries w/ Sugar	1 serv (3 oz)	115	1	0	12
Strawberry Topping	1 serv (3 oz)	115	1	0	12

FOOD	PORTION	CALS	FAT	CHOL	SOD
Sunshine Slam	1 serv (8 oz)	537	25	409	1445
Super Play It Again Slam	1 serv (15 oz)	1192	75	690	3555
Syrup	3 tbsp (1.5 oz)	143	0	0	26
Syrup Reduced Calorie	1 serv (1.5 oz)	25	0	0	96
T-Bone Steak & Eggs	1 serv (16 oz)	1045	82	530	1191
Toast Dry	1 slice (1 oz)	92	1	0	166
Ultimate Omelette	1 serv (17 oz)	780	62	639	1360
Vegggie Cheese Omelette	1 serv (16 oz)	714	53	644	955
Waffle	1 (6 oz)	304	21	146	200
Whipped Margarine	1 serv (0.5 oz)	87	10	0	117
Whipped Cream	1 serv (2 oz)	23	2	7	3
desserts					
Apple Pie	1 serv (7 oz)	430	20	<5	390
Apple Pie w/ Equal	1 serv (7 oz)	370	20	<5	360
Banana Split	1 serv (19 oz)	894	43	78	177
Blueberry Topping	1 serv (3 oz)	106	0	0	15
Cheesecake Pie	1 serv (4 oz)	470	27	90	280
Cherry Topping	1 serv (3 oz)	86	0	0	5
Cherry Pie	1 serv (7 oz)	540	21	<5	430
Chocolate Topping	1 serv (2 oz)	317	25	0	83
Chocolate Cake	1 serv (4 oz)	370	17	29	374
Chocolate Pecan Pie	1 serv (6 oz)	790	37	70	460
Chocolate Shake	1 serv (10 oz)	579	27	108	278
Coconut Cream Pie	1 serv (7 oz)	480	26	15	440
Double Scoop Sundae	1 serv (6 oz)	375	27	74	86
Dutch Apple Pie	1 serv (7 oz)	440	19	0	290
French Silk Pie	1 serv (6 oz)	650	43	165	220
Fudge Topping	1 serv (2 oz)	201	10	3	96
German Chocolate Pie	1 serv (7 oz)	580	33	15	460
Hot Fudge Cake Sundae	1 serv (8 oz)	687	38	62	486
Ice Cream Float	1 serv (12 oz)	280	10	39	109
Key Lime Pie	1 serv (6 oz)	600	27	35	300
Lemon Meringue Pie	1 serv (7 oz)	460	17	95	310
Pecan Pie	1 serv (6 oz)	600	28	50	430
Single Scoop Sundae	1 serv (3 oz)	188	14	37	43
Strawberry Topping	1 serv (3 oz)	115	1	0	12
Vanilla Shake	1 serv (11 oz)	581	27	108	236
main menu selections					
BBQ Sauce	1 serv (1.5 oz)	47	1	0	595
Bacon Cheddar Burger	1 (14 oz)	935	63	164	1732
Bacon Lettuce & Tomato Sandwich	1 (6 oz)	634	46	54	1116
Baked Potato Plain	1 (6 oz)	186	0	0	14
Battered Cod Dinner w/ Tartar Sauce	1 serv (9 oz)	732	47	105	1335
Broccoli In Butter Sauce	2 serv (4 oz)	50	2	5	280
Brown Gravy	1 serv (1 oz)	13	0	0	184

FOOD	PORTION	CALS	FAT	CHOL	SOD
Buffalo Chicken Strips	1 serv (10 oz)	734	42	96	1673
Buffalo Wings	12 pieces (15 oz)	856	54	500	5552
Carrots In Honey Glaze	2 serv (4 oz)	80	3	0	220
Charleston Chicken Sandwich	1 (11 oz)	632	32	81	1967
Chicken Quesadilla	1 serv (16 oz)	827	55	181	1982
Chicken Fried Chicken	1 serv (6 oz)	327	18	65	993
Chicken Fried Steak w/ Gravy	1 serv (4 oz)	265	17	27	668
Chicken Gravy	1 serv (1 oz)	14	1	2	139
Chicken Melt Sandwich	1 (7 oz)	520	29	39	1096
Chicken Strip w/ Dressing	1 serv (10 oz)	635	25	95	1510
Chicken Strips	5 pieces (10 oz)	720	33	95	1666
Classic Burger	1 (11 oz)	673	40	106	1142
Classic Burger w/ Cheese	1 (13 oz)	836	53	137	1595
Corn In Butter Sauce	2 serv (4 oz)	120	4	5	260
Cornbread Stuffing Plain	1 serv (2 oz)	182	9	0	405
Cottage Cheese	1 serv (3 oz)	72	3	10	281
Country Gravy	1 serv (1 oz)	17	1	0	93
Delidinger Sandwich	1 (14 oz)	852	45	80	3142
Deluxe Grilled Cheese Sandwich	1 (7 oz)	482	26	1	1135
Dinner Roll	1 (1.5 oz)	132	2	0	265
French Fries Unsalted	1 serv (4 oz)	323	14	0	130
Fried Fish Sandwich	1 (11 oz)	905	56	69	1704
Gardenburger Patty	1 patty (3.4 oz)	160	3	10	390
Gardenburger Patty w/ Bun & Fat Free Honey Mustard Dressing	1 serv (11.1 oz)	653	32	26	1017
Green Beans w/ Bacon	2 serv (4 oz)	60	4	5	390
Green Peas In Butter Sauce	2 serv (4 oz)	100	2	5	360
Grilled Mushrooms	1 serv (2 oz)	14	0	0	0
Grilled Alaskan Salmon	1 serv (7 oz)	296	14	102	257
Grilled Chicken Breast	1 serv (4 oz)	130	4	67	566
Grilled Chicken Dinner	1 serv (4 oz)	130	4	67	560
Grilled Chicken Sandwich	1 (11 oz)	509	19	83	1809
Grilled Chopped Steak w/ Gravy	1 serv (10 oz)	400	26	91	447
Ham & Swiss On Rye	1 (9 oz)	533	31	36	1638
Hashed Browns	1 serv (4 oz)	218	14	0	424
Herb Toast	1 serv (2 oz)	200	11	0	372
Horseradish Sauce	1 serv (1.5 oz)	170	20	43	227
Junior Meals Junior Burger	1 serv (3 oz)	261	15	41	115
Junior Meals Junior Chicken Strips	1 serv (5 oz)	318	12	48	755
Junior Meals Junior Fried Fish	1 serv (5 oz)	465	34	68	743
Junior Meals Junior Grilled Cheese	1 serv (4 oz)	375	22	1	811
Junior Meals Junior Shrimp Basket	1 serv (4 oz)	291	16	60	774

FOOD	PORTION	CALS	FAT	CHOL	SOD
Lunch Basket Charleston Chicken Ranch Melt	1 serv (14 oz)	975	59	96	2479
Lunch Basket Chicken Strips	1 serv (8 oz)	568	26	70	1239
Lunch Basket Classic Burger	1 serv (12 oz)	674	39	121	1161
Lunch Basket Delidinger	1 serv (14 oz)	852	45	80	3142
Lunch Basket Five Star Philly	1 serv (10 oz)	657	29	97	652
Lunch Basket Patty Melt	1 serv (8 oz)	696	42	129	1026
Mashed Potatoes Plain	1 serv (6 oz)	105	1	0	378
Mayonnaise	2 tbsp (1 oz)	200	22	16	159
Mozzarella Sticks w/ Sauce	8 pieces (10 oz)	756	43	48	5423
Onion Ring Basket	1 serv (5 oz)	439	27	7	1158
Onion Rings	1 serv (3 oz)	264	16	4	695
Patty Melt Sandwich	1 (8 oz)	695	44	114	1007
Pork Chop Dinner w/ Gravy	1 serv (8 oz)	386	24	121	844
Porterhouse Steak	1 (14 oz)	708	54	161	713
Pot Roast Dinner w/ Gravy	1 serv (7 oz)	260	11	140	1085
Rice Pilaf	1 serv (3 oz)	112	2	0	328
Roast Turkey & Stuffing	1 serv (12 oz)	701	27	100	2346
Sampler	1 serv (15 oz)	1120	59	69	3430
Seasoned Fries	1 serv (4 oz)	261	12	0	556
Senior Battered Cod	1 serv (5 oz)	465	34	68	743
Senior Chicken Fried Steak	1 serv (8 oz)	341	18	27	943
Senior Grilled Chicken Breast	1 serv (6 oz)	219	6	67	880
Senior Liver w/ Bacon & Onions	1 serv (8 oz)	322	19	270	643
Senior Pork Chop	1 serv (4 oz)	193	12	60	422
Senior Pot Roast	1 serv (5 oz)	149	6	71	818
Senior Roast Turkey & Stuffing	1 serv (8 oz)	596	25	51	1750
Senior Sandwich Ham & Swiss	1 serv (9 oz)	497	30	36	1537
Shrimp Dinner	1 serv (8 oz)	558	32	135	1114
Sirloin Steak Dinner	1 serv (5.5 oz)	271	21	62	273
Sliced Tomatoes	3 slices (2 oz)	13	0	0	6
Sour Cream	1 serv (1.5 oz)	91	9	19	23
Steak & Shrimp Dinner w/ Gravy	1 serv (9 oz)	645	42	150	1143
Super Bird Sandwich	1 (9 oz)	620	32	60	1880
T-Bone Steak Dinner	1 serv (10 oz)	530	40	121	534
Turkey Breast On Multigrain	1 (9 oz)	476	26	57	1107
salad dressings					
Bleu Cheese	1 oz	124	12	18	405
Caesar	1 oz	142	15	2	340
Creamy Italian	1 oz	106	10	0	306
Fat Free Honey Mustard	1 oz	38	0	0	121
French	1 oz	106	10	7	274
Oriental Peanut Dressing	1 serv (1 oz)	106	8	0	399
Ranch	1 oz	101	11	8	215
Reduced Calorie French	1 oz	76	5	0	265
Reduced Calorie Italian	1 oz	32	1	0	515
Thousand Island	1 oz	104	10	21	208

FOOD	PORTION	CALS	FAT	CHOL	SOD
salads and salad bars					
Buffalo Chicken Salad	1 serv (17 oz)	615	37	88	1258
Fried Chicken Salad	1 serv (13 oz)	506	31	94	1174
Garden Chicken Delight Salad	1 serv (16 oz)	277	5	67	785
Grilled Chicken Caesar Salad w/ Dressing	1 serv (13 oz)	655	47	86	1728
Oriental Chicken Salad w/ Dressing	1 serv (20 oz)	568	26	67	1656
Side Caesar w/ Dressing	1 serv (6 oz)	338	25	7	725
Side Garden Salad w/ Dressing	1 serv (7 oz)	113	4	0	147
soups					
Cheese	1 serv (8 oz)	293	23	19	895
Chicken Noodle	1 serv (8 oz)	60	2	10	640
Clam Chowder	1 serv (8 oz)	214	11	5	903
Cream Of Broccoli	1 serv (8 oz)	193	12	0	818
Cream of Potato	1 serv (8 oz)	222	12	0	761
Split Pea	1 serv (8 oz)	146	6	5	819
Vegetable Beef	1 serv (8 oz)	79	1	5	820
DOMINO'S PIZZA					
12 inch medium pizzas					
Add A Topping Anchovies	1 topping serv	23	1	9	395
Add A Topping Bacon	1 topping serv	81	7	12	226
Add A Topping Canned Mushrooms	1 topping serv	4	tr	0	75
Add A Topping Cheddar Cheese	1 topping serv	57	5	15	88
Add A Topping Cooked Beef	1 topping serv	56	5	11	154
Add A Topping Extra Cheese	1 topping serv	48	4	7	150
Add A Topping Fresh Mushrooms	1 topping serv	4	tr	0	1
Add A Topping Green Olives	1 topping serv	12	1	0	255
Add A Topping Green Peppers	1 topping serv	3	tr	0	tr
Add A Topping Ham	1 topping serv	18	1	7	162
Add A Topping Italian Sausage	1 topping serv	55	4	11	171
Add A Topping Onion	1 topping serv	4	tr	0	tr
Add A Topping Pepperoni	1 topping serv	62	6	13	199
Add A Topping Pineapple Tidbits	1 topping serv	10	0	0	1
Add A Topping Ripe Olives	1 topping serv	14	1	0	71
Deep Dish Cheese	2 slices (6.3 oz)	477	22	19	1085
Hand Tossed Cheese	2 slices (5.2 oz)	347	11	15	723
Thin Crust Cheese	1/4 pie (3.7 oz)	271	12	15	809
14 inch large pizzas					
Add A Topping Anchovies	1 topping serv	23	1	9	395
Add A Topping Bacon	1 topping serv	75	6	11	207
Add A Topping Canned Mushrooms	1 topping serv	3	tr	0	50

FOOD	PORTION	CALS	FAT	CHOL	SOD
Add A Topping Cheddar Cheese	1 topping serv	48	4	12	73
Add A Topping Cooked Beef	1 topping serv	44	4	8	123
Add A Topping Extra Cheese	1 topping serv	45	4	7	140
Add A Topping Fresh Mushrooms	1 topping serv	3	tr	0	tr
Add A Topping Green Olives	1 topping serv	11	1	0	63
Add A Topping Green Peppers	1 topping serv	2	tr	0	tr
Add A Topping Ham	1 topping serv	17	1	7	156
Add A Topping Italian Sausage	1 topping serv	44	3	9	137
Add A Topping Onion	1 topping serv	3	tr	0	tr
Add A Topping Pepperoni	1 topping serv	55	5	12	177
Add A Topping Pineapple Tidbits	1 topping serv	8	0	0	1
Add A Topping Ripe Olives	1 topping serv	12	1	0	63
Deep Dish Cheese	2 slices (6.1 oz)	455	20	18	1029
Hand-Tossed Cheese	2 slices (4.8 oz)	317	10	14	669
Thin Crust Cheese	1/6 pie (3.5 oz)	253	11	14	757
6 inch deep dish pizzas					
Add A Topping Anchovies	1 topping serv	45	2	18	790
Add A Topping Bacon	1 topping serv	82	7	12	226
Add A Topping Canned Mushrooms	1 topping serv	2	tr	0	36
Add A Topping Cheddar Cheese	1 topping serv	86	7	22	132
Add A Topping Cooked Beef	1 topping serv	44	4	8	122
Add A Topping Extra Cheese	1 topping serv	57	5	9	180
Add A Topping Fresh Mushrooms	1 topping serv	2	tr	0	tr
Add A Topping Green Olives	1 topping serv	10	1	0	204
Add A Topping Green Peppers	1 topping serv	2	tr	0	tr
Add A Topping Ham	1 topping serv	17	1	7	156
Add A Topping Italian Sausage	1 topping serv	44	3	9	137
Add A Topping Onion	1 topping serv	3	tr	0	tr
Add A Topping Pepperoni	1 topping serv	50	5	10	159
Add A Topping Pineapple Tidbits	1 topping serv	5	0	0	tr
Add A Topping Ripe Olives	1 topping serv	11	1	0	57
Cheese	1 pie (7.6 oz)	595	27	23	1300
main menu selections					
Breadstick	1 (0.8 oz)	78	3	0	158
Buffalo Wings Barbeque	1 piece (0.9 oz)	50	2	26	175
Buffalo Wings Hot	1 piece (0.9 oz)	45	2	26	354
Cheesy Bread	1 piece (1 oz)	103	5	5	187
Garden Salad	1 lg (7.7 oz)	39	tr	0	26
Garden Salad	1 sm (4.3 oz)	22	tr	0	14

FOOD	PORTION	CALS	FAT	CHOL	SOD
salad dressings					
Marzetti Blue Cheese	1 serv (1.5 oz)	220	24	40	440
Marzetti Creamy Caesar	1 serv (1.5 oz)	200	22	10	470
Marzetti Fat Free Ranch	1 serv (1.5 oz)	40	0	0	560
Marzetti Honey French	1 serv (1.5 oz)	210	18	0	300
Marzetti House Italian	1 serv (1.5 oz)	220	24	0	440
Marzetti Light Italian	1 serv (1.5 oz)	20	1	0	780
Marzetti Ranch	1 serv (1.5 oz)	260	29	5	380
Marzetti Thousand Island	1 serv (1.5 oz)	200	20	25	320
DUNKIN' DONUTS					
bagels and cream cheese					
Bagel Blueberry	1	340	1	0	670
Bagel Cinnamon Raisin	1	340	1	0	480
Bagel Egg	1	350	2	25	610
Bagel Everything	1	360	2	0	710
Bagel Garlic	1	360	1	0	720
Bagel Onion	1	330	1	0	660
Bagel Plain	1	340	1	0	710
Bagel Poppyseed	1	360	3	0	710
Bagel Pumpernickel	1	350	2	0	560
Bagel Salt	1	340	1	0	3030
Bagel Sesame	1	380	5	0	720
Bagel Wheat	1	330	2	0	670
Cream Cheese Chive	1 pkg	190	19	55	220
Cream Cheese Garden Vegetable	1 pkg	180	17	45	310
Cream Cheese Lite	1 pkg	130	11	30	250
Cream Cheese Plain	1 pkg	200	19	60	230
Cream Cheese Salmon	1 pkg	180	17	50	150
baked selections					
Bow Tie Donut	1	300	17	0	340
Cake Donut Blueberry	1	290	16	10	400
Cake Donut Butternut	1	300	16	0	360
Cake Donut Chocolate Coconut	1	300	19	0	370
Cake Donut Chocolate Frosted	1	300	16	0	370
Cake Donut Chocolate Glazed	1	290	16	0	370
Cake Donut Cinnamon	1	270	15	0	360
Cake Donut Coconut	1	290	17	0	360
Cake Donut Double Chocolate	1	310	17	0	370
Cake Donut Glazed	1	270	15	0	360
Cake Donut Old Fashioned	1	250	15	0	360
Cake Donut Powdered	1	270	15	0	350
Cake Donut Toasted Coconut	1	300	17	0	370
Cake Donut Whole Wheat Glazed	1	310	19	0	380

FOOD	PORTION	CALS	FAT	CHOL	SOD
Chocolate Frosted Donut	1	200	9	0	260
Chocolate Kreme Filled Donut	1	270	13	0	260
Cinnamon Bun	1	510	15	10	420
Coffee Roll	1	270	14	0	340
Coffee Roll Chocolate Frosted	1	290	15	0	340
Coffee Roll Maple Frosted	1	290	14	0	340
Coffee Roll Vanilla Frosted	1	290	14	0	340
Cookie Chocolate Chocolate Chunk	1	210	11	35	110
Cookie Chocolate Chunk	1	220	11	35	105
Cookie Chocolate Chunk w/ Nut	1	230	12	35	110
Cookie Chocolate White Chocolate Chunk	1	230	12	35	160
Cookie Oatmeal Raisin Pecan	1	220	10	30	110
Cookie Peanut Butter Chocolate Chunk w/ Nuts	1	240	14	25	125
Cookie Peanut Butter w/ Nuts	1	240	14	30	150
Croissant Almond	1	350	22	5	270
Croissant Chocolate	1	400	25	5	240
Croissant Plain	1	290	18	5	270
Cruller Plain	1	240	15	0	340
Cruller Powdered	1	270	15	0	340
Cruller Sugar	1	250	15	0	340
Crullers Glazed Chocolate	1	280	15	0	360
Crullers Glazed	1	290	15	0	350
Donut Apple Crumb	1	230	10	0	270
Donut Apple N' Spice	1	200	8	0	270
Donut Bavarian Kreme	1	210	9	0	270
Donut Black Raspberry	1	210	8	0	280
Donut Blueberry Crumb	1	240	10	0	260
Donut Boston Kreme	1	240	9	0	280
Donut Chocolate Iced Bismark	1	340	15	0	290
Dunkin' Donut	1	240	15	0	340
Eclair Donut	1	270	11	0	290
Fritter Glazed	1	260	14	0	330
Glazed Donut	1	180	8	0	250
Jelly Filled Donut	1	210	8	0	280
Jelly Stick	1	290	12	0	390
Lemon Donut	1	200	9	0	270
Maple Frosted Donut	1	210	9	0	260
Marble Frosted Donut	1	200	9	0	260
Muffin Apple Cinnamon Pecan	1	510	21	70	590
Muffin Apple N'Spice	1	350	12	35	390
Muffin Banana Nut	1	360	15	35	490
Muffin Blueberry	1 (6 oz)	490	17	75	610
Muffin Blueberry	1 (4 oz)	320	12	35	480

FOOD	PORTION	CALS	FAT	CHOL	SOD
Muffin Bran	1	390	12	20	620
Muffin Cherry	1	340	12	40	510
Muffin Chocolate Hazelnut	1	610	26	70	610
Muffin Chocolate Chip	1 (4 oz)	400	17	35	440
Muffin Chocolate Chip	1 (6 oz)	590	24	75	560
Muffin Corn	1 (4 oz)	390	15	55	590
Muffin Corn	1 (6 oz)	500	16	80	920
Muffin Cranberry Orange	1	470	15	75	600
Muffin Cranberry Orange Nut	1	350	15	35	500
Muffin Lemon Poppyseed	1	360	13	35	530
Muffin Oat Bran	1	370	13	20	620
Muffin Lowfat Apple & Spice	1	240	2	0	460
Muffin Lowfat Banana	1	250	2	0	430
Muffin Lowfat Blueberry	1	250	2	0	430
Muffin Lowfat Bran	1	240	1	0	430
Muffin Lowfat Cherry	1	250	2	0	430
Muffin Lowfat Chocolate	1	250	3	0	470
Muffin Lowfat Corn	1	240	3	45	480
Muffin Lowfat Cranberry Orange	1	240	2	0	430
Muffin Reduced Fat Blueberry	1	450	12	65	590
Muffin Reduced Fat Corn	1	460	11	75	900
Munchkins Chocolate Cake Glazed	3	200	10	0	250
Munchkins Cake Butternut	3	200	11	0	240
Munchkins Cake Cinnamon	4	250	14	0	350
Munchkins Cake Coconut	3	200	12	0	240
Munchkins Cake Glazed	3	200	10	0	250
Munchkins Cake Plain	4	220	14	0	310
Munchkins Cake Powdered	4	250	14	0	310
Munchkins Cake Sugared	4	240	14	0	310
Munchkins Yeast Glazed	5	200	9	0	220
Munchkins Yeast Jelly Filled	5	210	9	0	240
Munchkins Yeast Lemon Filled	4	170	8	0	190
Munchkins Yeast Sugar Raised	7	220	12	0	290
Strawberry Frosted Donut	1	210	9	0	260
Strawberry Donut	1	210	8	0	260
Sugar Raised Donut	1	170	8	0	250
Sugared Cake Donut	1	250	15	0	350
Vanilla Frosted Donut	1	210	9	0	260
Vanilla Kreme Filled Donut	1	270	13	0	250
beverages					
Coffee Coolatta w/ 2% Milk	1 (16 oz)	240	2	10	80
Coffee Coolatta w/ Cream	1 (16 oz)	410	22	75	65
Coffee Coolatta w/ Milk	1 (16 oz)	260	4	15	75
Coffee Coolatta w/ Skim Milk	1 (16 oz)	230	0		80
Collatta Orange Mango Fruit	1 (16 oz)	290	0	0	30

FOOD	PORTION	CALS	FAT	CHOL	SOD
Collatta Pink Lemonade Fruit	1 (16 oz)	350	0	0	30
Collatta Raspberry Lemonade	1 (16 oz)	280	0	0	35
Collatta Vanilla	1 (16 oz)	450	7	0	170
Coolatta Strawberry Fruit	1 (16 oz)	280	0	0	30
Dark Roast Coffee	1 serv (10 oz)	5	0	0	5
Decaf	1 serv (10 oz)	0	0	0	0
Dunkaccino	1 (10 oz)	250	11	10	240
French Vanilla Coffee	1 serv (10 oz)	5	0	0	5
Hazelnut Coffee	1 serv (10 oz)	5	0	0	10
Hot Cocoa	1 (10 oz)	230	8	0	310
Regular Coffee	1 serv (10 oz)	5	0	0	5
sandwiches					
Breakfast Sandwich Ham Egg Cheese	1	320	12	195	1340
Omwich Bagel Bacon Cheddar	1	600	21	295	1630
Omwich Bagel Spanish Cheese	1	570	18	280	1370
Omwich Bagel Three Cheese	1	610	22	305	1630
Omwich Croissant Spanish Cheese	1	530	36	285	930
Omwich Croissant Bacon Cheddar	1	560	38	295	1190
Omwich Croissant Three Cheese	1	560	39	305	1200
Omwich English Muffin Bacon Cheddar	1	400	21	295	1440
Omwich English Muffin Spanish Cheese	1	370	18	280	1180
Omwich English Muffin Three Cheese	1	400	22	305	1450
EINSTEIN BROS BAGELS					
bagels					
Bagel Chips Cinnamon Raisin Swirl	1 serv (1 oz)	90	1	0	120
Bagel Chips Plain	1 serv (1 oz)	90	0	0	14
Bagel Chips Sourdough Dill	1 serv (1 oz)	90	1	0	120
Bagel Chips Sun Dried Tomato	1 serv (1 oz)	90	1	0	130
Bagel Chips Sunflower	1 serv (1 oz)	100	2	0	190
Bagel Chips Wild Blueberry	1 serv (1 oz)	90	1	0	105
Chocolate Chip	1 (4 oz)	380	3	0	480
Chopped Garlic	1 (4.2 oz)	377	4	0	593
Chopped Onion	1 (4 oz)	340	3	0	500
Cinnamon Raisin Swirl	1 (4 oz)	360	1	0	480
Cinnamon Sugar	1	330	0	0	510
Dark Pumpernickel	1 (3.8 oz)	330	1	0	710
Everything	1 (4 oz)	342	2	0	653
Honey 8 Grain	1 (4 oz)	320	1	0	500

FOOD	PORTION	CALS	FAT	CHOL	SOD
Nutty Banana	1 (4 oz)	370	3	0	500
Plain	1 (3.7 oz)	330	1	0	520
Poppy Dip'd	1 (3.9 oz)	346	2	0	520
Salt	1 (3.9 oz)	330	1	0	1626
Sesame Dip'd	1 (4.1 oz)	381	5	0	523
Spinach Herb	1 (3.8 oz)	320	1	0	510
Sun Dried Tomato	1 (3.8 oz)	320	1	0	520
Veggie Confetti	1 (3.8 oz)	330	1	0	480
Wild Blueberry	1 (4 oz)	360	1	0	510
sandwiches and fillings					
Butter & Margarine Blend	1 serv (0.4 oz)	60	7	0	75
Capers	1 tbsp	0	0	0	320
Cheddar Cheese	1 serv (0.75 oz)	110	9	30	180
Classic New York Lox & Bagel	1 (11.4 oz)	560	24	75	1120
Cream Cheese Cheddarpeno	1 serv (1 oz)	90	8	30	150
Cream Cheese Chive	1 serv (1 oz)	90	9	35	125
Cream Cheese Maple Walnut Raisin	1 serv (1 oz)	100	8	25	95
Cream Cheese Plain	1 serv (1 oz)	100	9	35	130
Cream Cheese Smoked Salmon	1 serv (1 oz)	90	8	35	130
Cream Cheese Strawberry	1 serv (1 oz)	90	8	30	105
Cream Cheese Sun Dried Tomato	1 serv (1 oz)	90	8	35	160
Cucumbers	1 serv (1 oz)	0	0	0	0
Fruit Spreads	1 tbsp	40	0	0	10
Ham	1 serv (2.5 oz)	75	2	20	560
Ham & Cheese Sandwich	1 (9.9 oz)	520	15	70	1280
Honey	1 tbsp	64	0	0	1
Hummus	2 tbsp	60	3	0	105
Hummus Sandwich	1 (6 oz)	440	7	0	590
Lettuce	1 leaf	0	0	0	0
Lite Cream Cheese Plain	1 serv (1 oz)	60	5	20	150
Lite Cream Cheese Spinach Dill	1 serv (1 oz)	60	5	20	150
Lite Cream Cheese Veggie	1 serv (1 oz)	60	5	20	170
Lite Cream Cheese Wildberry	1 serv (1 oz)	70	4	15	85
Lowfat Chicken Salad Sandwich	1 (11.6 oz)	440	9	45	940
Lowfat Tuna Salad Sandwich	1 (11.6 oz)	440	8	30	970
Marshall's Loz	1 serv (2 oz)	90	4	10	400
Mayonnaise Lite Reduced Calorie	1 serv (0.5 oz)	50	5	5	115
Peanut Butter	1 serv (1.1 oz)	190	16	0	140
Peanut Butter & Jelly Sandwich	1 (6 oz)	595	17	0	663
Scrambled Egg Sandwich	1 (7.7 oz)	480	17	385	630

FOOD	PORTION	CALS	FAT	CHOL	SOD
Scrambled Egg Sandwich w/ Meat & Cheese	1 (8.9 oz)	520	31	8	1000
Smoked Turkey	1 serv (2.5 oz)	75	1	20	550
Smoked Turkey Sandwich	1 (9.9 oz)	480	14	45	1180
Sprouts Alfalfa	1 serv (0.5 oz)	0	0	0	10
Sweet Onions	1 serv (1 oz)	0	0	0	0
Swiss Cheese	1 serv (0.75 oz)	100	8	25	60
Tasty Turkey Sandwich	1 (10 oz)	530	22	90	1210
Tomato	1 serv (1.5 oz)	0	0	0	0
Turkey Pastrami 99% Fat Free	1 serv (2.5 oz)	75	6	0	510
Veg Out Sandwich	1 (8.9 oz)	350	17	3	570
Whitefish Salad Sandwich	1 (9.2 oz)	630	23	45	1020

EL POLLO LOCO
main menu selections

FOOD	PORTION	CALS	FAT	CHOL	SOD
Broccoli Slaw	1 serv (5 oz)	203	17	0	365
Burrito BRC	1 (9.3 oz)	482	15	15	1250
Burrito Classic Chicken	1 (9.3 oz)	556	22	117	1499
Burrito Grilled Steak	1 (11.3 oz)	705	32	77	1689
Burrito Loco Grande	1 (13.1 oz)	632	26	129	1649
Burrito Smokey Black Bean	1 (9.3 oz)	566	22	22	1337
Burrito Spicy Hot Chicken	1 (9.8 oz)	559	22	117	1503
Burrito Whole Wheat Chicken	1 (10.8 oz)	592	26	146	1199
Chicken Breast	1 piece (3 oz)	160	6	110	390
Chicken Leg	1 piece (1.75 oz)	90	5	75	150
Chicken Soft Taco	1 (4 oz)	224	12	66	585
Chicken Thigh	1 piece (2 oz)	180	12	130	230
Chicken Wing	1 (1.5 oz)	110	6	80	220
Chicken Tamale	1 (3.5 oz)	190	8	10	480
Cole Slaw	1 serv (5 oz)	206	16	11	358
Corn-On-Cob	1 ear (5.5 oz)	146	2	0	18
Cornbread Stuffing	1 serv (6 oz)	281	12	0	832
Crispy Green Beans	1 serv (5 oz)	41	2	0	667
Cucumber Salad	1 serv (4.2 oz)	34	0	0	11
Fiesta Corn	1 serv (5 oz)	152	6	0	397
Flame Broiled Chicken Salad	1 serv (14.9 oz)	167	5	56	765
French Fries	1 serv (4.4 oz)	323	14	0	330
Garden Salad	1 serv (6.4 oz)	29	0	0	20
Gravy	1 serv (1 oz)	14	0	2	139
Honey Glazed Carrots	1 serv (5 oz)	104	6	0	403
Lime Parfait	1 serv (5 oz)	125	3	0	107
Macaroni & Cheese	1 serv (6 oz)	238	12	31	919
Mashed Potatoes	1 serv (5 oz)	97	1	0	369
Pinto Beans	1 serv (6 oz)	185	4	0	744
Polo Bowl	1 serv (19 oz)	504	13	56	2068
Potato Salad	1 serv (6 oz)	256	14	15	527
Rainbow Pasta Salad	1 serv (5 oz)	157	1	0	533
Salad Shell	1 (5.6 oz)	440	27	0	610
Smokey Black Beans	1 serv (5 oz)	255	13	11	609

FOOD	PORTION	CALS	FAT	CHOL	SOD
Southwest Cole Slaw	1 serv (5 oz)	178	13	8	267
Spanish Rice	1 serv (4 oz)	130	3	0	397
Spiced Apples	1 serv (5 oz)	146	0	0	139
Steak Bowl	1 serv (15.2 oz)	616	26	68	1743
Taco Al Carbon Chicken	1 serv (4.4 oz)	265	12	28	223
Taco Al Carbon Steak	1 (4.4 oz)	394	22	46	473
Taquito	1 serv (5 oz)	370	17	25	690
Tortilla Corn	1 (1.1 oz)	70	1	0	35
Tortilla Flour	1 (1 oz)	90	3	0	224
Tortilla Wrap Chicken Caesar	1 (10.47 oz)	518	19	48	1709
Tortilla Wrap Southwest	1 (11.97 oz)	632	27	61	1792
Tostada Salad Chicken	1 serv (14.7 oz)	332	14	80	1280
Tostado Salad Steak	1 serv (13.2 oz)	525	31	100	1206
salad dressings					
Blue Cheese	1 serv (2 oz)	300	32	50	590
Light Italian	1 serv (2 oz)	25	1	0	990
Ranch	1 serv (2 oz)	350	39	5	500
Thousand Island	1 serv (2 oz)	270	27	30	460
FOSTERS FREEZE					
Soft Serve Vanilla	1 serv (4 oz)	152	4	9	100
GODFATHER'S PIZZA					
Golden Crust Cheese	1/8 med (3.1 oz)	212	8	12	311
Golden Crust Cheese	1/10 lg (3.5 oz)	242	9	14	363
Golden Crust Combo	1/10 lg (4.9 oz)	305	14	25	674
Golden Crust Combo	1/8 med (4.4 oz)	271	12	22	562
Original Crust Cheese	1/8 med (3.5 oz)	231	5	14	338
Original Crust Cheese	1/10 jumbo (5.8 oz)	382	9	27	580
Original Crust Cheese	1/4 mini (1.9 oz)	131	3	8	183
Original Crust Cheese	1/10 lg (4 oz)	258	6	18	396
Original Crust Combo	1/10 lg (5.6 oz)	338	12	31	740
Original Crust Combo	1/10 jumbo (8.3 oz)	503	18	47	1096
Original Crust Combo	1/8 med (5.1 oz)	306	11	27	660
Original Crust Combo	1/4 mini (2.9 oz)	176	7	16	382
HARDEE'S					
breakfast selections					
Apple Cinnamon 'N' Raisin Biscuit	1 (2.18 oz)	200	8	0	350
Bacon & Egg Biscuit	1 (5.5 oz)	570	33	275	1400
Bacon Egg & Cheese Biscuit	1 (5.9 oz)	610	37	280	1630
Big Country Breakfast Bacon	1 serv (9.4 oz)	820	49	535	1870
Big Country Breakfast Sausage	1 serv (11.4 oz)	1000	66	570	3210
Biscuit 'N' Gravy	1 (7.8 oz)	510	28	15	1500
Country Ham Biscuit	1 (3.8 oz)	430	22	25	1930
Frisco Breakfast Sandwich Ham	1 (7.4 oz)	500	25	290	1370
Ham Biscuit	1 (4 oz)	400	20	15	1340
Ham Egg & Cheese Biscuit	1 (6.5 oz)	540	30	285	1660
Hash Rounds	1 serv (2.8 oz)	230	14	0	560
Jelly Biscuit	1 (3.5 oz)	440	21	0	1000

FOOD	PORTION	CALS	FAT	CHOL	SOD
Rise 'N' Shine Biscuit	1 (2.9 oz)	390	21	0	1000
Sausage Biscuit	1 (4.1 oz)	510	31	25	1360
Sausage & Egg Biscuit	1 (6.3 oz)	630	40	285	1480
Three Pancakes	1 serv (4.8 oz)	280	2	15	890
Ultimate Omelet Biscuit	1 (5.8 oz)	570	33	120	1370
desserts					
Big Cookie	1 (2.0 oz)	280	12	15	150
Cone Chocolate	1 (4.1 oz)	180	2	15	110
Cone Vanilla	1 (4.1 oz)	170	2	10	130
Cool Twist Cone Vanilla/ Chocolate	1 (4.1 oz)	180	2	10	120
Peach Cobbler	1 serv (6 oz)	310	7	0	360
Sundae Hot Fudge	1 (5.5 oz)	290	6	20	310
Sundae Strawberry	1 (5.8 oz)	210	2	10	140
main menu selections					
Baked Beans	1 serv (5 oz)	170	1	0	600
Big Roast Beef Sandwich	1 (6.5 oz)	460	24	70	1230
Cheeseburger	1 (4.3 oz)	310	14	40	890
Chicken Fillet Sandwich	1 (7.5 oz)	480	18	55	1280
Cole Slaw	1 serv (4 oz)	240	20	10	340
Cravin' Bacon Cheeseburger	1 (8.1 oz)	690	46	95	1150
Fisherman's Fillet	1 (8.3 oz)	560	27	65	1330
French Fries	1 lg (6 oz)	430	18	0	190
French Fries	1 sm (3.4 oz)	240	10	0	100
French Fries	1 med (5 oz)	350	15	0	150
Fried Chicken Breast	1 piece (5.2 oz)	370	15	75	1190
Fried Chicken Leg	1 piece (2.4 oz)	170	7	45	570
Fried Chicken Thigh	1 piece (4.2 oz)	330	15	60	1000
Fried Chicken Wing	1 piece (2.3 oz)	200	8	30	740
Frisco Burger	1 (8.1 oz)	720	46	95	1340
Gravy	1 serv (1.5 oz)	20	tr	0	260
Grilled Chicken Sandwich	1 (7.1 oz)	350	11	65	950
Hamburger	1 (3.9 oz)	270	11	35	670
Hot Ham 'N' Cheese	1 (5.1 oz)	310	12	50	1410
Mashed Potatoes	1 serv (4 oz)	70	tr	0	330
Mesquite Bacon Cheeseburger	1 (4.5 oz)	370	18	45	970
Mushroom 'N' Swiss Burger	1 (6.8 oz)	490	25	80	1100
Quarter Pound Double Cheeseburger	1 (6 oz)	470	27	80	1290
Regular Roast Beef	1 (4.3 oz)	320	16	43	820
The Boss	1 (7 oz)	570	33	85	910
The Works Burger	1 (8.1 oz)	530	30	80	1030
salad dressings					
French Fat Free	1 serv (2 oz)	70	0	0	300
Ranch	1 serv (2 oz)	290	29	25	510
Thousand Island	1 serv (2 oz)	250	23	35	540

FOOD	PORTION	CALS	FAT	CHOL	SOD
salads and salad bars					
Garden Salad	1 (10.2 oz)	220	13	40	350
Grilled Chicken Salad	1 (11.5 oz)	150	3	60	610
Side Salad	1 (4.6 oz)	25	tr	0	45
HOT SAM'S PRETZELS					
Bavarian	1 lg (5.1 oz)	390	0	0	780
Bavarian	1 reg (2.5 oz)	200	0	0	390
Bavarian Stix	10 (5 oz)	390	0	0	780
Sweet Dough	1 (4.5 oz)	360	3	0	780
Sweet Dough Blueberry	1 (4.5 oz)	400	4	0	610
JACK IN THE BOX					
breakfast selections					
Breakfast Jack	1 (4.2 oz)	300	12	185	890
Country Crock Spread	1 pat (5 g)	25	3	0	40
Grape Jelly	1 serv (0.5 oz)	40	0	0	5
Pancake Syrup	1 serv (1.5 oz)	120	0	0	5
Pancakes w/ Bacon	1 serv (5.6 oz)	400	12	30	980
Sausage Croissant	1 (6.4 oz)	670	48	250	940
Sourdough Breakfast Sandwich	1 (5.2 oz)	380	21	355	1120
Supreme Croissant	1 (6 oz)	570	20	235	1240
Ultimate Breakfast Sandwich	1 (8.5 oz)	620	36	245	1800
desserts					
Carrot Cake	1 serv (3.5 oz)	370	16	35	340
Cheesecake	1 serv (3.5 oz)	310	18	65	210
Double Fudge Cake	1 serv (3 oz)	300	10	50	320
Hot Apple Turnover	1 (3.8 oz)	340	18	0	510
main menu selections					
1/4 lb Burger	1 (6 oz)	510	27	65	1080
American Cheese	1 slice (0.4 oz)	45	4	10	200
Bacon & Cheddar Potato Wedges	1 serv (9.3 oz)	800	58	55	1470
Bacon Ultimate Cheeseburger	1 (10.4 oz)	1150	89	230	1770
Barbeque Dipping Sauce	1 serv (1 oz)	45	0	0	300
Cheeseburger	1 (4 oz)	330	15	60	760
Chicken & Fries	1 serv (9.3 oz)	730	34	65	1690
Chicken Caesar Sandwich	1 (8.3 oz)	520	26	55	1050
Chicken Fajita Pita	1 (6.6 oz)	280	9	75	840
Chicken Sandwich	1 (5.9 oz)	450	26	45	1030
Chicken Strips Breaded	5 pieces (5.3 oz)	360	17	80	970
Chicken Supreme Sandwich	1 (8.2 oz)	680	45	85	1500
Chili Cheese Curly Fries	1 serv (8.1 oz)	650	41	25	1640
Double Cheeseburger	1 (5.3 oz)	450	24	75	970
Egg Rolls	5 pieces (10 oz)	730	41	60	1700
Egg Rolls	3 pieces (6 oz)	440	24	35	1020
Fish & Chips	1 serv (9 oz)	720	35	35	1580
French Fries	1 reg (4.1 oz)	360	17	0	740
Grilled Chicken Fillet Sandwich	1 (8.1 oz)	520	26	140	1240
Hamburger	1 (3.6 oz)	280	12	45	560

FOOD	PORTION	CALS	FAT	CHOL	SOD
Jumbo Fries	1 serv (5 oz)	430	20	0	890
Jumbo Jack	1 (7.8 oz)	560	36	80	680
Jumbo Jack w/ Cheese	1 (8.6 oz)	650	43	105	1090
Ketchup	1 pkg (0.3 oz)	10	0	0	100
Monster Taco	1 (4 oz)	290	18	40	550
Onion Rings	1 serv (4.2 oz)	460	25	0	780
Philly Cheesesteak Sandwich	1 (7.6 oz)	520	25	155	1980
Salsa	1 serv (1 oz)	10	0	0	200
Seasoned Curly Fries	1 serv (4.5 oz)	420	24	0	1030
Sour Cream	1 serv (1 oz)	60	6	20	30
Sourdough Jack	1 (7.8 oz)	670	43	110	1180
Soy Sauce	1 serv (0.3 oz)	5	0	0	480
Spicy Crispy Chicken Sandwich	1 (7.9 oz)	560	27	50	1020
Stuffed Jalapenos	7 pieces (5.3 oz)	470	28	50	1560
Stuffed Jalapenos	10 pieces (7.6 oz)	680	40	75	2220
Super Scoop French Fries	1 serv (7 oz)	610	28	0	1250
Sweet & Sour Dipping Sauce	1 serv (1 oz)	40	0	0	160
Swiss-Style Cheese	1 slice (0.4 oz)	40	3	10	190
Taco	1 (2.7 oz)	190	11	20	410
Tartar Dipping Sauce	1 pkg (1.5 oz)	220	23	20	240
Teriyaki Bowl Chicken	1 serv (17.6 oz)	670	4	15	1620
Ultimate Cheeseburger	1 (9.8 oz)	1030	79	205	1200
salad dressings					
Blue Cheese	1 serv (2 oz)	210	18	15	750
Buttermilk House	1 serv (2 oz)	290	30	20	560
Buttermilk House Dipping Sauce	1 serv (0.9 oz)	130	13	10	240
Low Calorie Italian	1 serv (2 oz)	25	2	0	670
Thousand Island	1 serv (2 oz)	250	24	20	570
salads and salad bars					
Croutons	1 serv (0.4 oz)	50	2	0	105
Garden Chicken Salad	1 serv (8.9 oz)	200	9	65	420
Side Salad	1 (3 oz)	50	3	10	75
KFC					
BBQ Baked Beans	1 serv (5.5 oz)	190	3	5	760
Biscuit	1 (2 oz)	180	10	0	560
Chicken Pot Pie	1 (13 oz)	770	42	70	2160
Chicken Twister	1 (8.7 oz)	550	32	85	980
Cole Slaw	1 serv (5 oz)	180	9	5	280
Corn On The Cob	1 ear (5.7 oz)	150	2	0	20
Cornbread	1 (2 oz)	228	13	42	194
Crispy Strips Colonel's	3 (3.25 oz)	261	16	40	658
Crispy Strips Spicy Buffalo	3 (4.2 oz)	350	19	35	1110
Extra Tasty Crispy Breast	1 (5.9 oz)	470	28	80	930
Extra Tasty Crispy Drumstick	1 (2.4 oz)	190	11	60	260
Extra Tasty Crispy Thigh	1 (4.2 oz)	370	25	70	540
Extra Tasty Crispy Whole Wing	1 (1.9 oz)	200	13	45	290

FOOD	PORTION	CALS	FAT	CHOL	SOD
Green Beans	1 serv (4.7 oz)	45	2	5	730
Hot & Spicy Breast	1 (6.5 oz)	530	35	110	1110
Hot & Spicy Drumstick	1 (2.3 oz)	190	11	50	300
Hot & Spicy Thigh	1 (3.8 oz)	370	27	90	570
Hot & Spicy Whole Wing	1 (1.9 oz)	210	15	50	340
Hot Wings	6 (4.8 oz)	471	33	150	1230
Macaroni & Cheese	1 serv (5.4 oz)	180	8	10	860
Mashed Potatoes With Gravy	1 serv (4.8 oz)	120	6	tr	440
Mean Greens	1 serv (5.4 oz)	70	3	10	650
Original Recipe Breast	1 (5.4 oz)	400	24	135	1116
Original Recipe Chicken Sandwich	1 (7.3 oz)	497	22	52	1213
Original Recipe Drumstick	1 (2.2 oz)	140	9	75	422
Original Recipe Thigh	1 (3.2 oz)	250	18	95	747
Original Recipe Whole Wing	1 (1.6 oz)	140	10	55	414
Potato Salad	1 serv (5.6 oz)	230	14	15	540
Potato Wedges	1 serv (4.8 oz)	280	13	5	750
Tender Roast Breast w/ Skin	1 (4.9 oz)	251	11	151	830
Tender Roast Breast w/o Skin	1 (4.2 oz)	169	4	112	797
Tender Roast Drumstick w/ Skin	1 (1.9 oz)	97	4	85	271
Tender Roast Drumstick w/o Skin	1 (1.2 oz)	67	2	63	259
Tender Roast Thigh w/ Skin	1 (3.2 oz)	207	12	120	504
Tender Roast Thigh w/o Skin	1 (2.1 oz)	106	6	84	312
Tender Roast Wing w/ Skin	1 (1.8 oz)	121	8	74	331
Value BBQ Chicken Sandwich	1 (5.3 oz)	256	8	57	782
KRISPY KREME					
Chocolate Iced	1 (2 oz)	260	14	<5	105
Chocolate Iced Cake	1 (2 oz)	230	12	15	280
Chocolate Iced Creme Filled	1 (2.3 oz)	270	14	<5	150
Chocolate Iced Cruller	1 (1.7 oz)	240	14	10	160
Chocolate Iced Custard Filled	1 (2.7 oz)	250	9	5	150
Chocolated Iced w/ Sprinkles	1 (2 oz)	220	10	<5	95
Cinnamon Apple Filled	1 (2.3 oz)	210	9	<5	150
Cinnamon Bun	1 (2.1 oz)	220	11	0	160
Glazed Blueberry	1 (2.4 oz)	300	15	5	200
Glazed Creme Filled	1 (2.3 oz)	270	14	<5	150
Glazed Cruller	1 (1.5 oz)	220	14	10	150
Glazed Devil's Food	1 (1.9 oz)	240	13	10	180
Lemon Filled	1 (2.2 oz)	210	10	5	150
Maple Iced	1 (1.8 oz)	200	9	0	100
Original Glazed	1 (1.3 oz)	180	10	<5	95
Powdered Blueberry Filled	1 (2.1 oz)	200	9	5	160
Powdered Cake	1 (1.8 oz)	220	11	15	250
Raspberry Filled	1 (2 oz)	210	10	<5	160
Traditional Cake	1 (1.7 oz)	200	11	15	280

FOOD	PORTION	CALS	FAT	CHOL	SOD
LONG JOHN SILVER'S					
main menu selections					
Batter-Dipped Fish	1 piece (3 oz)	170	11	30	470
Breaded Chicken Strips	1 piece (1.15 oz)	100	5	10	360
Breaded Clams	1 serv (3 oz)	300	17	40	670
Breaded Fish	1 piece (1.6 oz)	110	5	20	340
Cheese Sticks	1 serv (1.6 oz)	160	9	10	360
Chicken Salsa	1 reg (11 oz)	690	32	20	1690
Corn Cobbette w/ Butter	1 piece (3.3 oz)	140	8	0	0
Corn Cobbette w/o Butter	1 (3.1 oz)	80	1	0	0
Fish Cajun	1 lg (23 oz)	1450	70	60	3630
Flavorbaked Chicken	1 piece (2.6 oz)	110	3	55	600
Flavorbaked Fish	1 piece (2.3 oz)	90	3	35	320
Fries	1 reg (3 oz)	250	15	0	500
Fries	1 lg (5 oz)	420	24	0	830
Honey Mustard Sauce	1 serv (0.4 oz)	20	0	0	60
Hushpuppy	1 (0.8 oz)	60	3	0	25
Ketchup	1 serv (.32 oz)	10	0	0	110
Popcorn Chicken Munchers	1 serv (4 oz)	380	23	35	1030
Popcorn Fish Munchers	1 serv (4 oz)	300	14	50	1220
Popcorn Shrimp Munchers	1 serv (4 oz)	320	15	85	1440
Rice	1 serv (3 oz)	140	3	0	210
Sandwich Batter Dipped Fish No Sauce	1 (5.4 oz)	320	13	30	800
Sandwich Flavorbaked Chicken	1 (5.8 oz)	290	10	60	970
Sandwich Flavorbaked Fish	1 (6 oz)	320	14	55	930
Sandwich Ultimate Fish	1 (6.4 oz)	430	21	35	1340
Shrimp Sauce	1 serv (0.4 oz)	15	0	0	180
Side Salad	1 (4.3 oz)	25	0	0	15
Slaw	1 serv (3.4 oz)	140	6	0	260
Sweet'N'Sour Sauce	1 serv (0.4 oz)	20	0	0	45
Tartar Sauce	1 serv (0.4 oz)	35	2	0	35
Wraps Chicken Cajun	1 reg (11 oz)	720	35	25	1860
Wraps Chicken Cajun	1 lg (22 oz)	1440	71	50	3730
Wraps Chicken Ranch	1 lg (22 oz)	1450	72	50	3620
Wraps Chicken Ranch	1 reg (11 oz)	730	36	25	1810
Wraps Chicken Salsa	1 lg (22 oz)	1370	64	35	3370
Wraps Chicken Tartar	1 lg (22 oz)	1450	72	45	3560
Wraps Chicken Tartar	1 reg (11 oz)	730	36	25	1780
Wraps Fish Cajun	1 reg (11.5 oz)	730	35	30	1820
Wraps Fish Ranch	1 lg (23 oz)	1460	72	60	3520
Wraps Fish Ranch	1 reg (11.5 oz)	730	36	30	1760
Wraps Fish Salsa	1 lg (23 oz)	1380	64	45	3280
Wraps Fish Salsa	1 reg (11.5 oz)	690	32	25	1640
Wraps Fish Tartar	1 reg (11.5 oz)	730	36	25	1730
Wraps Fish Tartar	1 lg (23 oz)	1470	72	55	3460
Wraps Popcorn Shrimp Cajun	1 reg (11 oz)	720	35	50	1830

FOOD	PORTION	CALS	FAT	CHOL	SOD
Wraps Popcorn Shrimp Cajun	1 lg (22 oz)	1450	71	95	3660
Wraps Popcorn Shrimp Ranch	1 reg (11 oz)	720	35	50	1830
Wraps Popcorn Shrimp Ranch	1 lg (22 oz)	1460	72	100	3560
Wraps Popcorn Shrimp Salsa	1 lg (22 oz)	1380	64	85	3310
Wraps Popcorn Shrimp Salsa	1 reg (11 oz)	690	32	40	1660
Wraps Popcorn Shrimp Tartar	1 reg (11 oz)	730	36	45	1750
Wraps Popcorn Shrimp Tartar	1 lg (22 oz)	1460	72	95	3500
salad dressings					
Fat-Free French	1 serv (1.5 oz)	50	0	0	360
Fat-Free Ranch	1 serv (1.5 oz)	50	0	0	380
Italian	1 serv (1 oz)	130	14	0	280
Malt Vinegar	1 serv (0.3 oz)	0	0	0	15
Ranch Dressing	1 serv (1 oz)	170	18	5	260
Thousand Island	1 serv (1 oz)	110	10	15	280
MANHATTAN BAGEL					
Blueberry	1 (4 oz)	260	tr	0	560
Cheddar Cheese	1 (4 oz)	270	4	10	560
Chocolate Chip	1 (4 oz)	290	3	0	530
Cinnamon Raisin	1 (4 oz)	280	tr	0	560
Egg	1 (4 oz)	270	2	0	710
Everything	1 (4 oz)	290	3	0	2000
Jalapeno Cheddar	1 (4 oz)	260	2	0	310
Marble	1 (4 oz)	260	tr	0	540
Oat Bran	1 (4 oz)	260	1	0	470
Oat Bran Raisin Walnut	1 (4 oz)	270	3	0	450
Onion	1 (4 oz)	270	tr	0	560
Plain	1 (4 oz)	260	tr	0	560
Poppy	1 (4 oz)	300	4	0	560
Pumpernickel	1 (4 oz)	250	1	0	530
Rye	1 (4 oz)	260	1	0	560
Salt	1 (4 oz)	260	tr	0	7100
Sesame	1 (4 oz)	310	5	0	560
Spinach	1 (4 oz)	270	tr	0	580
Sun-Dried Tomato	1 (4 oz)	260	1	0	340
Whole Wheat	1 (4 oz)	260	tr	0	470
MAX & IRMA'S					
Black Bean Roll Up	1 serv	401	8	13	534
Fat Free French	2 tbsp	126	tr	0	1034
Fat Free Honey Mustard	2 tbsp	60	0	0	280
Fruit Smoothie	1 serv	114	tr	0	3
Garden Grill	1 serv	467	7	12	911
Garlic Breadstick	1	156	6	0	293
Gourmet Garden Grill	1 serv	484	8	12	912
Hula Bowl w/ Fat Free Honey Mustard Dressing	1 serv	526	8	91	1309
Lo-Cal Ranch	2 tbsp	54	6	7	141
Tijuana Tortilla Wrap	1	692	15	54	1958

FOOD	PORTION	CALS	FAT	CHOL	SOD
MCDONALD'S					
baked selections					
Apple Pie Baked	1 (2.7 oz)	260	13	0	200
Chocolate Chip Cookie	1 (1.2 oz)	170	10	20	120
Cinnamon Roll	1	390	18	65	310
Danish Apple	1	340	15	20	340
Danish Cheese	1	400	21	40	400
Lowfat Muffin Apple Bran	1 (4 oz)	300	3	0	380
McDonaldland Cookies	1 pkg (1.5 oz)	180	5	0	190
breakfast selections					
Bacon Egg & Cheese Biscuit	1	540	34	250	1550
Bagel Ham & Egg Cheese	1	550	23	255	1490
Bagel Steak & Egg Cheese	1	660	31	285	1300
Biscuit	1 (2.9 oz)	290	15	0	780
Breakfast Burrito	1 (4.1 oz)	320	20	195	660
Egg McMuffin	1 (4.8 oz)	290	14	235	790
English Muffin	1 (1.9 oz)	140	2	0	210
Hash Browns	1 serv (1.9 oz)	130	8	0	330
Hotcakes Margarine & Syrup	2 serv	600	17	20	770
Hotcakes Plain	1 serv	340	8	20	630
Sausage	1 (1.5 oz)	170	16	35	290
Sausage Biscuit	1 (4.5 oz)	470	31	35	1080
Sausage Biscuit w/ Egg	1 (6.2 oz)	550	37	245	1160
Sausage McMuffin	1 (3.9 oz)	360	23	45	740
Sausage McMuffin w/ Egg	1 (5.7 oz)	440	28	255	890
Scrambled Eggs	2 (3.6 oz)	160	11	425	170
desserts					
McFlurry Butterfinger	1	620	22	70	260
McFlurry M&M	1	630	23	75	210
McFlurry Nestle Crunch	1	630	24	75	230
McFlurry Oreo	1	570	20	70	280
Nuts For Sundaes	1 serv (7 g)	40	4	0	55
Reduced Fat Ice Cream Cone Vanilla	1 (3.2 oz)	150	5	20	75
Sundae Hot Caramel	1 (6.4 oz)	360	10	35	180
Sundae Hot Fudge	1 (6.3 oz)	340	12	30	170
Sundae Strawberry	1 (6.2 oz)	290	7	30	95
main menu selections					
Bagel Spanish Omelet	1	690	38	275	1560
Barbeque Sauce	1 pkg (1 oz)	45	0	0	250
Big Mac	1	570	32	85	1100
Big Xtra!	1	710	46	95	1400
Big Xtra! w/ Cheese	1	810	55	120	1870
Cheeseburger	1 (4.2 oz)	320	13	40	830
Chicken McNuggets	6 pieces (3.7 oz)	290	17	55	540
Chicken McNuggets	4 pieces (2.5 oz)	190	11	35	360
Chicken McNuggets	9 pieces	430	25	80	810

FOOD	PORTION	CALS	FAT	CHOL	SOD
Crispy Chicken Deluxe	1 (7.8 oz)	500	25	55	1100
Filet-O-Fish	1	470	26	50	890
French Fries	1 sm (2.4 oz)	210	10	0	135
French Fries	1 lg	540	26	0	350
French Fries	1 med	450	22	0	290
French Fries	1 super	610	29	0	390
Grilled Chicken Deluxe	1 (7.8 oz)	440	20	60	1040
Grilled Chicken Deluxe Plain w/o Mayonnaise	1 (7.2 oz)	300	5	50	930
Grilled Chicken Salad Deluxe	1 serv (9 oz)	120	2	45	240
Hamburger	1	270	9	30	600
Honey	1 pkg (0.5 oz)	45	0	0	0
Honey Mustard	1 pkg (0.5 oz)	50	5	10	85
Hot Mustard	1 pkg (1 oz)	60	4	5	240
Light Mayonnaise	1 pkg (0.4 oz)	40	4	5	80
Quarter Pounder	1	430	21	70	840
Quarter Pounder w/ Cheese	1 (7 oz)	530	30	95	1310
Sweet 'N Sour Sauce	1 pkg (1 oz)	50	0	0	140
salad dressings					
Caesar	1 pkg (2.1 oz)	160	14	20	450
Fat Free Herb Vinaigrette	1 pkg (2.1 oz)	50	0	0	330
Ranch	1 pkg (2.1 oz)	230	21	20	550
Reduced Calorie Red French	1 pkg (2.1 oz)	160	8	0	490
salads and salad bars					
Croutons	1 pkg	50	1	0	105
Garden Salad	1 serv (6.2 oz)	35	0	0	20
MRS. FIELDS					
Brownie Double Fudge	1 (3.1 oz)	420	20	35	125
Brownie Fudge Walnut	1 (3.4 oz)	500	29	40	135
Brownie Pecan Fudge	1 (2.8 oz)	390	21	40	135
Brownie Pecan Pie	1 (3 oz)	400	21	55	160
Cookie Chewy Fudge	1 (1.7 oz)	230	12	25	100
Cookie Coconut Macadamia	1 (1.7 oz)	250	15	35	230
Cookie Milk Chocolate Chip	1 (1.7 oz)	240	12	35	210
Cookie Milk Chocolate Macadamia	1 (1.7 oz)	250	14	30	190
Cookie Milk Chocolate w/ Walnuts	1 (1.7 oz)	250	13	30	200
Cookie Oatmeal Raisin	1 (1.7 oz)	220	10	30	230
Cookie Peanut Butter	1 (1.7 oz)	240	13	40	280
Cookie Semi-Sweet Chocolate	1 (1.7 oz)	230	12	30	210
Cookie Semi-Sweet Chocolate w/ Walnuts	1 (1.8 oz)	240	13	30	190
Cookie Triple Chocolate	1 (1.7 oz)	230	12	30	210
Cookie White Chunk Macadamia	1 (1.7 oz)	260	15	30	190

FOOD	PORTION	CALS	FAT	CHOL	SOD
Muffin Banana Walnut	1 (3.9 oz)	460	24	45	390
Muffin Blueberry	1 (4 oz)	390	15	45	470
Muffin Chocolate Chip	1 (4 oz)	450	19	40	470
Muffin Mandarin Orange	1 (4 oz)	420	17	45	490
Peanut Butter Dream Bar	1 (5 oz)	750	40	40	270
Stokabunga Energy Cookie	1 (5 oz)	750	48	60	310
NEWPORT CREAMERY					
ice cream					
Reduced Fat No Sugar Added Chocolate	1/2 cup (2.6 oz)	110	3	0	80
Reduced Fat No Sugar Added Coffee	1/2 cup (2.6 oz)	100	4	15	70
OLIVE GARDEN					
Garden Fare Apple Carmellina	1 serv (12.2 oz)	560	2	5	190
Garden Fare Dinner Capellini Pomodoro	1 serv (21.1 oz)	610	16	5	940
Garden Fare Dinner Capellini Primavera	1 serv (20.1 oz)	400	7	15	950
Garden Fare Dinner Capellini Primavera w/ Chicken	1 serv (23.8 oz)	560	10	95	1030
Garden Fare Dinner Chicken Giardino	1 serv (20.6 oz)	550	11	85	1000
Garden Fare Dinner Linguine Alla Marinara	1 serv (16.3 oz)	500	9	0	160
Garden Fare Dinner Penne Fra Diavolo	1 serv (14.3 oz)	420	7	10	940
Garden Fare Dinner Shrimp Primavera	1 serv (28.4 oz)	740	15	290	1630
Garden Fare Lunch Capellini Pomodoro	1 serv (11.7 oz)	360	9	5	540
Garden Fare Lunch Capellini Primavera	1 serv (11.2 oz)	260	5	15	560
Garden Fare Lunch Capellini Primavera w/ Chicken	1 serv (14.9 oz)	420	8	90	640
Garden Fare Lunch Chicken Giardino	1 serv (12.8 oz)	360	9	50	900
Garden Fare Lunch Linguine Alla Marinara	1 serv (10.2 oz)	310	6	0	105
Garden Fare Lunch Penne Fra Diavolo	1 serv (10.2 oz)	300	5	10	640
Garden Fare Lunch Shrimp Primavera	1 serv (15.2 oz)	410	8	145	840
Minestrone Soup	1 serv (6 oz)	80	1	0	450
PANDA EXPRESS					
Mixed Vegetables	1 serv (5 oz)	80	3	0	450
Steamed Rice	1 serv (8 oz)	220	0	0	0
Sweet & Sour Sauce	1 serv (2 oz)	60	0	0	150

FOOD	PORTION	CALS	FAT	CHOL	SOD
PIZZA HUT					
main menu selections					
Bread Stick	1 (1.3 oz)	130	4	0	170
Bread Stick Dipping Sauce	1 serv (1.2 oz)	30	1	0	170
Cavatini Pasta	1 serv (12.5 oz)	480	14	25	1170
Cavatini Supreme Pasta	1 serv (13.9 oz)	560	19	30	1400
Garlic Bread	1 slice (1.3 oz)	150	8	0	240
Ham & Cheese Sandwich	1 (9.7 oz)	550	21	65	2150
Hot Buffalo Wings	4 pieces (2.1 oz)	210	12	130	900
Spaghetti Marinara	1 serv (16.6 oz)	490	6	0	730
Spaghetti Meat Sauce	1 serv (16.4 oz)	600	13	25	910
Spaghetti Meatballs	1 serv (18.8 oz)	850	24	50	1120
Supreme Sandwich	1 (10.2 oz)	640	28	85	2150
Wild Buffalo Wings	5 pieces (2.9 oz)	200	12	150	510
pizza					
Beef Topping Hand Tossed	1 slice (3.9 oz)	280	10	20	860
Beef Topping Pan	1 slice (3.9 oz)	310	14	20	720
Beef Topping Stuffed Crust	1 slice (5.6 oz)	410	14	30	1270
Beef Topping Thin 'N Crispy	1 slice (3.1 oz)	240	11	20	790
Cheese Hand Tossed	1 slice (3.9 oz)	280	10	25	770
Cheese Pan	1 slice (3.9 oz)	300	14	25	610
Cheese Stuffed Crust	1 slice (5.4 oz)	380	11	25	1160
Cheese Thin 'N Crispy	1 slice (2.6oz)	210	9	20	530
Chicken Supreme Pan	1 slice (4.1 oz)	280	11	25	570
Chicken Supreme Stuffed Crust	1 slice (6.4 oz)	390	13	40	1130
Chicken Supreme Thin 'N Crispy	1 slice (4.2 oz)	240	6	25	660
Dessert Apple	1 slice (2.8 oz)	250	5	0	230
Dessert Cherry	1 slice (2.8 oz)	250	5	0	220
Ham Hand Tossed	1 slice (3.4 oz)	230	6	25	710
Ham Pan	1 slice (3.4 oz)	250	9	10	590
Ham Stuffed Crust	1 slice (5.4 oz)	380	14	45	1250
Ham Thin 'N Crispy	1 slice (2.4 oz)	190	6	15	560
Italian Sausage Hand Tossed	1 slice (4 oz)	300	12	30	780
Italian Sausage Pan	1 slice (4.3 oz)	350	18	40	740
Italian Sausage Stuffed Crust	1 slice (5.7 oz)	430	19	35	1200
Italian Sausage Thin 'N Crispy	1 slice (3.4 oz)	300	16	35	740
Meat Lover's Hand Tossed	1 slice (3.9 oz)	290	11	35	820
Meat Lover's Pan	1 slice (4.4 oz)	360	19	40	870
Meat Lover's Stuffed Crust	1 slice (6.6 oz)	500	23	60	1510
Meat Lover's Thin 'N Crispy	1 slice (3.7 oz)	310	16	35	900
Pepperoni Hand Tossed	1 slice (3.4 oz)	260	9	30	750
Pepperoni Lover's Hand Tossed	1 slice (4 oz)	320	13	35	910
Pepperoni Lover's Pan	1 slice (4.1 oz)	350	17	20	800
Pepperoni Lover's Stuffed Crust	1 slice (6.1 oz)	480	22	60	1440
Pepperoni Lover's Thin 'N Crispy	1 slice (3.1 oz)	270	12	25	780
Pepperoni Pan	1 slice (3.4 oz)	280	12	20	640
Pepperoni Stuffed Crust	1 slice (5.3 oz)	410	17	40	1250

FOOD	PORTION	CALS	FAT	CHOL	SOD
Pepperoni Thin 'N Crispy	1 slice (2.3 oz)	220	9	20	610
Personal Pan Cheese	1 pie (8.1 oz)	630	24	45	1160
Personal Pan Pepperoni	1 pie (8.1 oz)	670	29	60	1250
Personal Pan Supreme	1 pie (9.5 oz)	710	31	60	1380
Pork Topping Hand Tossed	1 slice (3.9 oz)	290	11	25	850
Pork Topping Pan	1 slice (3.6 oz)	300	13	30	720
Pork Topping Stuffed Crust	1 slice (5.6 oz)	420	16	30	1290
Pork Topping Thin 'N Crispy	1 slice (3.2 oz)	270	13	25	780
Super Supreme Hand Tossed	1 slice (4.7 oz)	290	10	35	830
Super Supreme Pan	1 slice (4.6 oz)	340	16	30	790
Super Supreme Stuffed Crust	1 slice (7.2 oz)	470	20	50	1440
Super Supreme Thin 'N Crispy	1 slice (4 oz)	280	13	30	810
Supreme Hand Tossed	1 slice (3.9 oz)	270	9	25	760
Supreme Pan	1 slice (4 oz)	300	13	25	670
Supreme Stuffed Crust	1 slice (6.4 oz)	440	16	40	1380
Supreme Thin 'N Crispy	1 slice (3.4 oz)	250	11	20	710
Veggie Lover's Hand Tossed	1 slice (4 oz)	240	7	20	650
Veggie Lover's Pan	1 slice (3.9 oz)	240	9	10	480
Veggie Lover's Stuffed Crust	1 slice (5.9 oz)	390	14	25	1140
Veggie Lover's Thin 'N Crispy	1 slice (2.6 oz)	170	6	10	460
POPEYE'S					
Apple Pie	1 serv (3.1 oz)	290	16	10	820
Biscuit	1 serv (2.3 oz)	250	15	<5	430
Breast Mild	1 (3.7 oz)	270	16	60	660
Breast Spicy	1 (3.7 oz)	270	16	60	590
Cajun Rice	1 serv (3.9 oz)	150	5	25	1260
Cole Slaw	1 serv (4 oz)	149	11	3	271
Corn On The Cob	1 serv (5.2 oz)	127	3	0	20
French Fries	1 serv (3 oz)	240	12	10	610
Leg Mild	1 (1.7 oz)	120	7	40	240
Leg Spicy	1 (1.7 oz)	120	7	40	240
Nuggets	1 serv (4.2 oz)	410	32	55	660
Nuggets Mild Tender	1 (1.2 oz)	110	7	15	160
Nuggets Spicy Tender	1 (1.2 oz)	110	7	15	215
Onion Rings	1 serv (3.1 oz)	310	19	25	210
Potatoes & Gravy	1 serv (3.8 oz)	100	6	<5	460
Red Beans & Rice	1 serv (5.9 oz)	270	17	10	680
Shrimp	1 serv (2.8 oz)	250	16	110	650
Thigh Mild	1 (3.1 oz)	300	23	70	620
Thigh Spicy	1 (3.1 oz)	300	23	70	450
Wing Mild	1 (1.6 oz)	160	11	40	290
Wing Spicy	1 (1.6 oz)	160	11	40	290
QUINCY'S					
baked selections					
Banana Nut Bread	1 serv (2 oz)	165	7	5	195
Biscuit	1 (2.5 oz)	270	15	11	610
Cornbread	1 serv (2 oz)	140	5	0	340
Yeast Roll	1 (2 oz)	160	4	0	285

FOOD	PORTION	CALS	FAT	CHOL	SOD
breakfast selections					
Bacon	1 serv (0.25 oz)	35	3	5	100
Corned Beef Hash	1 serv (4.5 oz)	210	15	45	795
Country Ham	1 serv (1.5 oz)	90	6	35	1100
Escalloped Apples	1 serv (3.5 oz)	120	2	0	20
Oatmeal	1 serv (1 oz)	175	2	0	285
Pancakes	1 (1.5 oz)	95	3	30	250
Sausage Gravy	1 serv (4 oz)	70	6	10	150
Sausage Links	1 (2 oz)	225	22	20	390
Sausage Patties	1 (2 oz)	230	23	45	350
Scrambled Eggs	1 serv (2 oz)	95	7	215	270
Steak Fingers	1 serv (3.5 oz)	360	25	50	690
Syrup	1 oz	75	0	0	15
desserts					
Banana Pudding	1 serv (5 oz)	240	12	10	240
Brownie Pudding Cake	1 serv (4 oz)	310	5	0	395
Caramel Topping	1 serv (1 oz)	105	1	0	120
Chocolate Chip Cookies	1 (0.5 oz)	60	8	5	35
Cobbler Apple	1 serv (6 oz)	255	8	5	285
Cobbler Cherry	1 serv (6 oz)	410	8	5	185
Cobbler Peach	1 serv (6 oz)	305	8	5	190
Frozen Yogurt	1 serv (4 oz)	135	2	5	85
Fudge Topping	1 serv (1 oz)	105	4	0	75
Sugar Cookie	1 (0.5 oz)	60	3	5	30
main menu selections					
1/3 Pound Hamburger	1 serv (8 oz)	565	33	66	603
BBQ Beans	1 serv (4 oz)	114	1	0	604
Bacon Cheeseburger	1 (9 oz)	663	41	87	997
Baked Potato	1 (6 oz)	115	0	0	0
Broccoli	1 serv (4 oz)	34	0	0	50
Cheese Sauce	1 serv (1 oz)	58	5	11	212
Chopped Steak	1 serv (8 oz)	499	42	89	348
Cinnamon Apples	1 serv (4 oz)	172	5	0	149
Corn	1 serv (4 oz)	96	1	0	271
Country Steak w/ Gravy	1 serv (8 oz)	530	25	54	1161
Cowboy Steak	1 serv (14 oz)	580	33	176	1308
Filet w/ Bacon	1 serv (7 oz)	340	17	124	311
Green Beans	1 serv (4 oz)	61	4	0	796
Grilled Chicken	1 reg serv (5 oz)	120	2	55	540
Grilled Chicken Sandwich	1 (9 oz)	324	4	55	1183
Grilled Salmon	1 serv (7 oz)	228	4	109	112
Homestyle Chicken Fillet	1 serv (3 oz)	217	9	25	682
Junior Sirloin Steak	1 serv (5.5 oz)	194	10	69	199
Large Sirloin Steak	1 serv (10 oz)	368	20	119	390
Mashed Potatoes	1 serv (4 oz)	54	6	0	195
NY Strip Steak	1 serv (10 oz)	450	26	148	156
Philly Cheese Steak	1 serv (11 oz)	588	30	87	1684
Porterhouse Steak	1 serv (17 oz)	683	46	154	346

FOOD	PORTION	CALS	FAT	CHOL	SOD
Regular Sirloin Steak	1 serv (8 oz)	285	16	71	317
Ribeye Steak	1 serv (10 oz)	452	29	116	156
Rice Pilaf	1 serv (4 oz)	119	2	0	1283
Roasted BBQ Chicken	1 serv (14 oz)	941	65	340	1548
Roasted Herb Chicken	1 serv (14 oz)	875	65	340	1238
Sirloin Tips w/ Mushroom Gravy	1 serv (6 oz)	196	7	64	578
Sirloin Tips w/ Peppers & Onions	1 serv (5 oz)	203	8	63	793
Smothered Steak Sandwich	1 (9 oz)	429	15	69	846
Smothered Strip Steak	1 serv (10 oz)	622	41	148	239
Southern Breaded Shrimp	1 serv (7 oz)	546	31	135	821
Spicy BBQ Chicken Sandwich	1 (10 oz)	368	1	55	1608
Steak & Shrimp	1 serv (9 oz)	677	39	170	816
Steak Fries	1 serv (4 oz)	358	19	0	245
T-Bone Steak	1 serv (13 oz)	521	35	118	265
salad dressings					
Blue Cheese	1 serv (1 oz)	155	16	10	165
French	1 serv (1 oz)	125	12	0	500
Honey Mustard	1 serv (1 oz)	100	6	0	220
Italian	1 serv (1 oz)	135	14	0	230
Light Creamy Italian	1 serv (1 oz)	65	4	0	485
Light French	1 serv (1 oz)	85	4	0	285
Light Italian	1 serv (1 oz)	20	2	0	485
Light Thousand Island	1 serv (1 oz)	65	4	20	340
Parmesan Peppercorn	1 serv (1 oz)	150	14	0	280
Ranch	1 serv (1 oz)	110	11	10	195
soups					
Chili With Beans	1 serv (6 oz)	235	11	15	920
Clam Chowder	1 serv (6 oz)	180	9	0	835
Cream Of Broccoli	1 serv (6 oz)	170	10	0	770
Vegetable Beef	1 serv (6 oz)	90	2	0	325
RALLY'S					
main menu selections					
Big Buford	1	743	46	151	1860
Chicken Fillet Sandwich	1	399	15	42	790
Chili w/ Cheese & Onion	1 serv (7 oz)	360	22	74	1144
Chili w/ Cheese & Onion	1 serv (13 oz)	669	41	137	2125
French Fries	1 extra lg (8 oz)	423	21	13	585
French Fries	1 reg (4 oz)	211	11	7	293
French Fries	1 lg (6 oz)	317	16	10	439
Onion Rings	1 serv	210	2	0	855
Rallyburger	1	433	22	63	1176
Rallyburger w/ Cheese	1	488	35	27	1376
Spicy Chicken Sandwich	1	437	18	40	887
Super Barbecue Bacon	1	593	31	88	1709
Super Double Cheeseburger	1	762	48	154	1734

FOOD	PORTION	CALS	FAT	CHOL	SOD
RED LOBSTER					
children's menu selections					
Cheeseburger	1 serv	1040	56	130	720
Fried Chicken Fingers	1 serv	680	33	35	630
Fried Shrimp	1 serv	650	33	80	510
Grilled Chicken Tenders	1 serv	580	24	55	400
Hamburger	1 serv	920	47	100	550
Popcorn Shrimp	1 serv	650	35	120	480
Popcorn Shrimp & Cheesesticks	1 serv	750	41	125	680
Spaghetti & Cheesesticks	1 serv	830	39	5	950
desserts					
Fudge Overboard	1 serv	620	23	105	110
Ice Cream	1 serv (4.5 oz)	140	7	30	60
Sensational 7	1 serv	790	41	140	690
main menu selections					
Admiral's Feast	1 serv	1060	52	265	2400
Appetizer Calamari	1 serv	350	22	190	510
Appetizer Chicken Fingers	1 serv	390	18	65	770
Appetizer Chilled Shrimp In The Shell	1 serv (6 oz)	110	2	235	270
Appetizer Crab & Shrimp Cakes	1 serv	480	24	80	1550
Appetizer Crab Add-On	1 serv	60	1	55	160
Appetizer Fresh Fried Mushrooms	1 serv	790	51	<5	1280
Appetizer Lobster Quesadilla	1 serv	760	47	160	1300
Appetizer Lobster Stuffed Mushroom	1 serv	400	26	100	960
Appetizer Mozzarella Cheesesticks	1 serv	730	46	50	1570
Appetizer Parmesan Zucchini	1 serv	620	40	10	1200
Appetizer Shrimp Cocktail	1 serv	50	1	105	120
Appetizer Stuffed Mushrooms	1 serv	420	27	90	940
Applesauce	1 serv (4 oz)	90	0	0	5
Atlantic Cod	1 serv (8 oz)	200	2	105	150
Atlantic Cod	1 lunch serv (5 oz)	110	1	60	85
Atlantic Salmon	1 serv (8 oz)	340	15	135	105
Atlantic Salmon	1 lunch serv (5 oz)	200	9	80	60
Baked Atlantic Cod	1 serv	220	6	100	440
Baked Atlantic Haddock	1 serv	220	6	100	440
Baked Flounder	1 lunch serv	190	7	90	440
Baked Potato	1 (8 oz)	130	0	0	10
Broccoli	1 serv (3 oz)	25	0	0	10
Broiled Fisherman's Platter	1 serv	600	23	250	1660
Broiled Rock Lobster Tail	1 tail	190	6	110	750
Broiled Seafarer's Platter	1 serv	450	19	190	1100
Caesar Salad w/ Dressing	1 serv	240	21	15	490
Catfish	1 lunch serv (5 oz)	130	2	75	115

FOOD	PORTION	CALS	FAT	CHOL	SOD
Catfish	1 serv (8 oz)	220	3	130	200
Catfish Santa Fe	1 serv	340	9	165	890
Catfish Santa Fe	1 lunch serv	180	6	85	450
Chicken Fingers	1 lunch serv	390	18	64	770
Chicken Fresco	1 lunch serv	660	36	120	990
Chicken Fresco	1 serv	1320	73	240	1990
Clam Strips	1 serv	720	39	35	1820
Clam Strips	1 lunch serv	360	19	15	910
Cocktail Sauce	1 oz	30	0	0	380
Cole Slaw	1 serv (4 oz)	190	16	25	260
Crab Alfredo	1 lunch serv	590	33	135	980
Crab Alfredo	1 serv	1170	66	270	1970
Fish & Shrimp Combo	1 serv	730	35	230	1630
Fish Nuggets	1 lunch serv	320	14	95	760
Fish Seasoning Add On For Blackened Dinner	1 serv	70	5	0	410
Fish Seasoning Add On For Blackened Lunch	1 serv	50	4	0	280
Fish Seasoning Add On For Broiled Dinner	1 serv	45	5	0	300
Fish Seasoning Add On For Broiled Lunch	1 serv	35	4	0	240
Fish Seasoning Add On For Grilled Dinner	1 serv	35	4	0	30
Fish Seasoning Add On For Grilled Lunch	1 serv	25	3	0	25
Fish Seasoning Add On For Lemon Pepper Dinner	1 serv	35	4	0	80
Fish Seasoning Add On For Lemon Pepper Lunch	1 serv	30	3	0	65
Fish Seasoning Add On For Sante Fe Style Dinner	1 serv	60	4	0	330
Fish Seasoning Add On For Sante Fe Style Lunch	1 serv	40	3	0	260
Flounder	1 serv (8 oz)	220	3	130	200
Flounder	1 lunch serv (5 oz)	130	2	75	115
French Fries	1 serv (4 oz)	350	22	0	180
Fried Flounder	1 lunch serv	230	10	60	590
Fried Shrimp	12 lg	500	27	290	950
Fried Shrimp	1 lunch serv	270	15	115	460
Garden Salad w/o Dressing	1 serv	50	1	0	90
Garlic Cheese Biscuit	1	140	8	5	320
Grilled Cheeseburger	1	580	34	130	540
Grilled Chicken Breast	1 serv	230	7	105	280
Grilled Chicken Salad w/o Dressing	1 serv	320	10	70	910
Grouper	1 serv (8 oz)	220	3	90	100
Grouper	1 lunch serv (5 oz)	130	2	50	60

FOOD	PORTION	CALS	FAT	CHOL	SOD
Haddock	1 lunch serv (5 oz)	120	1	80	95
Haddock	1 serv (8 oz)	210	2	140	160
Halibut	1 serv (8 oz)	260	6	75	130
Halibut	1 lunch serv (5 oz)	150	4	45	75
King Salmon	1 serv (8 oz)	420	25	160	110
King Salmon	1 lunch serv (5 oz)	250	15	95	70
Lake Trout	1 serv (8 oz)	340	16	140	125
Lake Trout	1 lunch serv (5 oz)	200	9	80	75
Lemon Pepper Grilled Mahi Mahi	1 serv	240	7	130	280
Lobster Shrimp & Scallop Scampi	1 lunch serv	430	16	80	450
Lobster Shrimp & Scallop Scampi	1 serv	870	33	135	900
Mahi Mahi	1 lunch serv (5 oz)	130	2	75	115
Mahi Mahi	1 serv (8 oz)	220	3	130	200
Maine Lobster Steamed	1 serv (1.25 lb)	160	1	125	670
Maine Lobster Stuffed	1 serv (2 lb)	430	10	210	1610
Marinara Sauce	1 serv	50	4	0	220
Melted Butter	1 oz	200	22	60	240
Neptune's Feast	1 serv	1210	62	290	3050
New York Strip Steak	1 serv	560	34	180	530
Perch	1 lunch serv (5 oz)	130	2	75	120
Perch	1 serv (8 oz)	220	3	130	200
Pollock	1 lunch serv (5 oz)	120	2	100	120
Pollock	1 serv (8 oz)	120	2	100	120
Popcorn Shrimp	1 serv	580	37	360	880
Popcorn Shrimp	1 lunch serv	380	24	235	580
Red Rockfish	1 lunch serv (5 oz)	130	2	50	85
Red Rockfish	1 serv (8 oz)	230	4	85	140
Red Snapper	1 lunch serv (5 oz)	140	2	50	65
Red Snapper	1 serv (8 oz)	240	3	90	105
Rice Pilaf	1 serv (4 oz)	180	2	0	790
Roasted Vegetables	1 lunch serv (4 oz)	80	3	0	210
Roasted Vegetables	1 serv (6 oz)	120	4	0	310
Sailor's Platter	1 lunch serv	250	12	170	440
Sandwich Blackened Catfish	1	340	9	85	740
Sandwich Broiled Fish	1	300	8	80	690
Sandwich Cajun Grilled Chicken	1	370	14	55	740
Sandwich Classic Fish	1	520	23	90	1050
Sandwich Grilled Chicken	1	290	7	50	430
Sassy Sauce	1 oz	80	6	5	140
Seafood Broil	1 lunch serv	310	14	110	850
Shrimp & Chicken	1 serv	340	15	225	470
Shrimp Caesar Salad w/o Dressing	1 serv	240	11	110	580
Shrimp Carbonara	1 lunch serv	650	38	155	1060
Shrimp Carbonara	1 serv	1290	76	310	2130
Shrimp Combo	1 serv	380	23	210	610

FOOD	PORTION	CALS	FAT	CHOL	SOD
Shrimp Feast	1 serv	470	24	390	1040
Shrimp Milano	1 serv	1190	65	340	1970
Shrimp Milano	1 lunch serv	590	33	170	990
Shrimp Scampi	1 lunch serv	110	7	100	150
Smothered Chicken	1 serv	530	31	170	740
Snow Crab Legs	1 serv	110	2	115	320
Sockeye Salmon	1 lunch serv (5 oz)	240	12	95	75
Sockeye Salmon	1 serv (8 oz)	410	21	165	125
Sole	1 lunch serv (5 oz)	130	2	75	115
Sole	1 serv (8 oz)	220	3	130	200
Soup Bread Salad w/o Dressing	1 lunch serv	430	18	40	1960
Steak & Fried Shrimp	1 serv	780	46	340	770
Steak & Rock Lobster Tail	1 serv	570	31	220	880
Swordfish	1 serv (8 oz)	290	10	115	150
Swordfish	1 lunch serv (5 oz)	170	6	70	90
Tartar Sauce	1 oz	160	17	15	210
Teriyaki Grilled Chicken Breast	1 serv	240	7	105	660
Twice Baked Potato	1	430	23	60	1320
Walleye	1 lunch serv (5 oz)	120	2	120	70
Walleye	1 serv (8 oz)	210	3	205	120
Yellow Lake Perch	1 serv (8 oz)	220	3	130	200
Yellow Lake Perch	1 lunch serv (5 oz)	130	2	75	120
salad dressings					
Blue Cheese	1 serv	170	18	30	200
Buttermilk Ranch	1 serv	110	11	15	300
Caesar	1 serv	170	18	10	290
Dijon Honey Mustard	1 serv	140	13	20	180
Fat Free Ranch	1 serv	50	0	0	310
Lite Red Wine Vinaigrette	1 serv	50	3	0	270
soups					
Bayou Style Gumbo	1 serv (6 oz)	120	4	65	710
Broccoli Cheese	1 serv	160	9	25	800
Clam Chowder	1 serv (6 oz)	130	5	20	820
SBARRO					
Pizza Veggie Slice	1 serv (10 oz)	490	12	15	1350
SEE'S CANDIES					
Bridge Mix	14 pieces (1.4 oz)	200	12	10	45
Dark Chocolate Bordeaux	2 (1.4 oz)	170	27	25	40
Dark Chocolates	2 (1.2 oz)	160	10	10	35
Lollypop Butterscotch	1	90	3	10	75
Lollypop Cafe Latte	1	90	3	10	40
Lollypop Chocolate	1	90	5	5	40
Lollypop Peanut Butter	1	90	4	0	95
Marshmints	3 (1.4 oz)	140	4	0	10
Milk Chocolate Bordeaux	2 (1.4 oz)	170	8	15	45
Milk Chocolate Butter	2 (1.4 oz)	190	9	15	50
Milk Chocolate Buttercreams	2 (1.4 oz)	180	8	15	50

FOOD	PORTION	CALS	FAT	CHOL	SOD
Milk Chocolate California Brittle	2 (1.3 oz)	220	16	25	115
Milk Chocolate Nuts & Chews	3 (1.7 oz)	250	16	15	60
Milk Chocolate Peanuts	3 (1.5 oz)	230	17	5	90
Milk Chocolate Soft Centers	2 (1.4 oz)	170	9	15	40
Milk Chocolates	2 (1.2 oz)	160	9	10	40
Nuts & Chews	3 (1.6 oz)	240	16	10	50
P-Nut Crunch	2 (1.4 oz)	220	15	10	80
Peanut Brittle	1.5 oz	230	16	25	280
Pecan Buds	3 (1.7 oz)	270	21	10	30
Red Hot Swamp Goo	3 pieces (1.4 oz)	140	4	0	10
Soft Centers	2 (1.4 oz)	170	9	10	40
Truffles Black or Gold	2 (1.4 oz)	180	11	10	25
Truffles Mint	3 (1.6 oz)	200	11	15	30
Victoria Toffee	1.5 oz	250	19	20	115
SMOOTHIE KING					
Activator Banana	1 (20 oz)	429	1	2	260
Activator Chocolate	1 (20 oz)	429	1	2	260
Activator Strawberry	1 (20 oz)	559	1	2	260
Activator Vanilla	1 (20 oz)	429	1	2	260
Angel Food	1 (20 oz)	330	1	2	71
Blackberry Dream	1 (20 oz)	343	tr	0	39
Caribbean Way	1 (20 oz)	392	tr	0	18
Celestial Cherry High	1 (20 oz)	285	tr	0	22
Coconut Surprise	1 (20 oz)	457	6	3	126
Cranberry Supreme	1 (20 oz)	577	1	24	120
Cranberry Cooler	1 (20 oz)	538	tr	0	95
GoGuava	1 (20 oz)	300	0	0	50
Grape Expectations	1 (20 oz)	399	tr	0	24
Grape Expectations II	1 (20 oz)	529	tr	0	24
Hawaiian Cafe Au Lei	1 (20 oz)	286	tr	5	170
High Protein Almond Mocha	1 (20 oz)	402	13	17	245
High Protein Banana	1 (20 oz)	412	14	14	315
High Protein Chocolate	1 (20 oz)	401	13	17	244
High Protein Lemon	1 (20 oz)	390	13	12	177
High Protein Pineapple	1 (20 oz)	380	13	12	206
Hulk Chocolate	1 (20 oz)	846	29	102	626
Hulk Strawberry	1 (20 oz)	953	29	102	645
Hulk Vanilla	1 (20 oz)	846	29	102	646
Immune Builder	1 (20 oz)	333	1	24	47
Instant Vigor	1 (20 oz)	359	1	0	38
Island Treat	1 (20 oz)	334	1	0	29
Lemon Twist Banana	1 (20 oz)	339	tr	0	24
Lemon Twist Strawberry	1 (20 oz)	399	tr	0	23
Light & Fluffy	1 (20 oz)	389	tr	0	12
Malt	1 (20 oz)	887	41	166	370
Mangofest	1 (20 oz)	320	0	0	50
Mo'cuccino	1 (20 oz)	440	12	75	190

FOOD	PORTION	CALS	FAT	CHOL	SOD
Muscle Punch	1 (20 oz)	339	1	2	75
Muscle Punch Plus	1 (20 oz)	340	1	2	65
Peach Slice	1 (20 oz)	341	tr	2	93
Peach Slice Plus	1 (20 oz)	471	tr	2	93
Peanut Power	1 (20 oz)	502	21	2	88
Peanut Power Plus Grape	1 (20 oz)	703	21	2	87
Peanut Power Plus Strawberry	1 (20 oz)	632	21	2	87
Pep Upper	1 (20 oz)	334	1	0	39
Pineapple Pleasure	1 (20 oz)	313	tr	0	29
Power Punch	1 (20 oz)	430	1	2	91
Power Punch Plus	1 (20 oz)	499	2	2	91
Raspberry Sunrise	1 (20 oz)	335	1	0	39
Shake	1 (20 oz)	875	41	166	359
Slim & Trim Chocolate	1 (20 oz)	270	2	4	261
Slim & Trim Strawberry	1 (20 oz)	357	1	2	149
Slim & Trim Vanilla	1 (20 oz)	227	1	2	150
Super Punch	1 (20 oz)	425	tr	0	179
Super Punch Plus	1 (20 oz)	516	tr	0	195
Yogurt D'Lite	1 (20 oz)	341	4	14	183
Youth Fountain	1 (20 oz)	267	tr	0	40
STARBUCKS					
ice cream					
Biscotte Bliss	1/2 cup	240	12	55	70
Caffe Almond Fudge	1/2 cup	260	13	55	80
Caffe Almond Roast	1 bar	280	18	25	45
Dark Roast Expresso Swirl	1/2 cup	220	10	55	60
Frappuccino Coffee	1 bar	110	2	10	50
Italian Roast Coffee	1/2 cup	230	12	65	65
Javachip	1/2 cup	250	13	60	55
Low Fat Latte	1/2 cup	170	3	10	65
Low Fat Mocha Mambo	1/2 cup	170	3	10	75
Vanilla Mochachip	1/2 cup	270	16	75	60
snacks					
Crunchy Honey Bar	1 (1.06 oz)	150	7	0	40
Lively Lemon Bar	1 (1.23 oz)	140	4	0	70
Tangy Apple Bar	1 (1.23 oz)	140	4	0	80
SUBWAY					
cookies					
Brazil Nut	1 (1.7 oz)	215	10	14	153
Chocolate Chip	1 (1.8 oz)	214	10	12	144
Chocolate Chip M&M	1 (1.8 oz)	212	10	13	144
Chocolate Chunk	1 (1.8 oz)	215	10	13	144
Low Fat Oatmeal Raisin	1 (1.7 oz)	168	3	15	171
Macadamia Nut	1 (1.8 oz)	222	11	12	144
Oatmeal Raisin	1 (1.8 oz)	199	8	14	159
Peanut Butter	1 (1.8 oz)	223	12	0	214
Sugar	1 (1.8 oz)	225	12	18	180

FOOD	PORTION	CALS	FAT	CHOL	SOD
salad dressings					
Creamy Italian	1 tbsp	65	7	4	133
Fat Free French	1 tbsp	15	0	0	178
Fat Free Italian	1 tbsp	5	0	0	153
Fat Free Ranch	1 tbsp	18	0	0	98
French	1 tbsp	70	6	0	100
Ranch	1 tbsp	88	10	6	118
Thousand Island	1 tbsp	65	7	8	155
salads and salad bars					
Classic Italian BMT	1 serv (11.6 oz)	269	19	52	1305
Cold Cut Trio	1 serv (11.6 oz)	193	12	47	1162
Ham	1 serv (11.1 oz)	112	3	25	1068
Meatball	1 serv (12.1 oz)	232	13	35	751
Roast Beef	1 serv (11.1 oz)	115	3	20	654
Roasted Chicken Breast	1 serv (11.6 oz)	162	4	48	693
Steak & Cheese	1 serv (12 oz)	182	8	37	887
Subway Club	1 serv (11.6 oz)	123	3	26	965
Subway Melt	1 serv (11.8 oz)	190	9	41	1346
Subway Seafood & Crab w/ Light Mayonnaise	1 serv (11.6 oz)	157	7	14	761
Tuna w/ Light Mayonnaise	1 serv (11.6 oz)	198	12	32	669
Turkey & Ham	1 serv (11.1 oz)	107	2	23	982
Turkey Breast	1 serv (11.1 oz)	101	2	20	896
Veggie Delight	1 serv (9.1 oz)	51	1	0	308
sandwiches					
6 Inch Cold Sub Classic Italian BMT	1 (8.9 oz)	450	21	52	1579
6 Inch Cold Sub Cold Cut Trio	1 (8.9 oz)	374	14	47	1435
6 Inch Cold Sub Ham	1 (8.4 oz)	293	5	25	1342
6 Inch Cold Sub Roast Beef	1 (8.4 oz)	296	5	20	928
6 Inch Cold Sub Seafood & Crab w/ Light Mayonniase	1 (8.9 oz)	338	9	14	1034
6 Inch Cold Sub Subway Club	1 (8.9 oz)	304	5	26	1239
6 Inch Cold Sub Tuna w/ Light Mayonnaise	1 (8.9 oz)	378	14	32	942
6 Inch Cold Sub Turkey & Ham	1 (8.4 oz)	288	4	23	1256
6 Inch Cold Sub Turkey Breast	1 (8.4 oz)	282	4	20	1170
6 Inch Cold Sub Veggie Delight	1 (6.4 oz)	232	3	0	582
6 Inch Hot Sub Meatball	1 (9.4 oz)	413	15	35	1025
6 Inch Hot Sub Roasted Chicken Breast	1 (8.9 oz)	342	6	48	966
6 Inch Hot Sub Steak & Cheese	1	363	10	37	1160
6 Inch Hot Sub Subway Melt	1	370	11	41	1619
Bacon Slices	2 (0.3 oz)	42	3	9	160
Cheese Triangles	2 (0.4 oz)	41	3	10	204
Deli Stye Roll	1 (2.1 oz)	170	2	0	350
Deli Style Bologna	1	283	10	19	785

FOOD	PORTION	CALS	FAT	CHOL	SOD
Deli Style Ham	1	224	3	12	827
Deli Style Tuna w/ Light Mayonnaise	1	267	8	16	627
Deli Style Turkey Breast	1	227	3	13	839
Italian Bread	6 inch (2.5 oz)	190	1	0	420
Italian Bread	12 inch (5 oz)	380	2	0	840
Lettuce	1 serv (0.9 oz)	4	0	0	3
Mayonnaise	1 tsp (5 g)	37	4	3	27
Mayonnaise Light	1 tsp (5 g)	18	2	2	33
Mustard	2 tsp (0.3 oz)	0	0	0	115
Olive Oil Blend	1 tsp (5 g)	45	5	0	0
Olive Rings	2 (1 g)	2	tr	0	6
Onions	1 serv (0.6 oz)	5	0	0	0
Pepper Strips	2 (0.3 oz)	1	0	0	0
Pickle Chips	3 pieces (0.4 oz)	2	0	0	139
Super Subs Classic Italian BMT	1	668	39	104	2576
Super Subs Cold Cut Trio	1	517	24	93	2289
Super Subs Subway Club	1	377	7	52	1895
Tomato Slices	2 (1 oz)	6	0	0	2
Vinegar	1 tsp (5 g)	1	0	0	0
Wheat Sub	6 inch (2.6 oz)	210	3	0	430
Wheat Sub	12 inch (5.3 oz)	420	5	0	860
Wrap 10.5 Inches	1 (2.6 oz)	200	2	0	720
Wraps Chicken Parmesan Ranch	1 (9.4 oz)	333	5	45	1393
Wraps Steak & Cheese	1 (9.2 oz)	353	9	37	1450
Wraps Turkey Breast & Bacon	1 (9 oz)	355	10	39	1823
TACO BELL					
breakfast selections					
Breakfast Quesadilla Cheese	1 (5.5 oz)	380	21	280	1010
Breakfast Quesadilla w/ Bacon	1 (6 oz)	450	27	290	1200
Breakfast Quesadilla w/ Sausage	1 (6 oz)	430	25	285	1090
Country Breakfast Burrito	1 (4 oz)	270	14	195	690
Double Bacon & Egg Burrito	1 (6.25 oz)	480	27	405	1240
Fiesta Breakfast Burrito	1 (3.5 oz)	280	16	25	580
Grande Breakfast Burrito	1 (6.25 oz)	420	22	205	1050
Hash Brown Nuggets	1 serv (3.5 oz)	280	18	0	570
main menu selections					
7-Layer Burrito	1 (10 oz)	530	23	25	1280
BLT Soft Taco	1 (4.5 oz)	340	23	40	610
Bacon Cheeseburger Burrito	1 (8.5 oz)	570	31	70	1460
Bean Burrito	1 (7 oz)	380	12	10	1100
Big Beef Burrito Supreme	1 (10.5 oz)	520	23	55	1520
Big Beef MexiMelt	1 (4.75 oz)	290	15	45	850
Big Chicken Burrito Supreme	1 (9 oz)	510	24	95	1900
Border Sauce Fire	1 serv (0.3 oz)	0	0	0	110
Border Sauce Hot	1 serv (0.3 oz)	0	0	0	85

FOOD	PORTION	CALS	FAT	CHOL	SOD
Border Sauce Mild	1 serv (0.3 oz)	0	0	0	75
Burger Sauce	1 serv (0.5 oz)	60	5	5	110
Burrito Supreme	1 (9 oz)	440	19	35	1230
Cheddar Cheese	1 serv (0.25 oz)	30	2	5	45
Cheese Quesadilla	1 (4.25 oz)	350	18	50	860
Chicken Fajita Wrap	1 (8 oz)	470	22	60	1290
Chicken Fajita Wrap Supreme	1 (9 oz)	520	25	70	1300
Chicken Quesadilla	1 (6 oz)	410	21	90	1170
Chicken Club Burrito	1 (8 oz)	540	32	80	1250
Chili Cheese Burrito	1 (5 oz)	330	13	35	870
Choco Taco Ice Cream Dessert	1 serv (4 oz)	310	17	20	100
Cinnamon Twists	1 serv (1 oz)	140	6	0	190
Club Sauce	1 serv (0.5 oz)	80	8	10	105
Double Decker Taco	1 (5.75 oz)	340	15	25	750
Double Decker Taco Supreme	1 (7 oz)	390	19	35	760
Fajita Sauce	1 serv (0.5 oz)	70	7	5	130
Green Sauce	1 serv (1 oz)	5	0	0	150
Grilled Chicken Burrito	1 (7 oz)	410	15	55	1380
Grilled Chicken Soft Taco	1 (4.5 oz)	240	12	45	1110
Grilled Steak Soft Taco	1 (4.5 oz)	230	10	25	1020
Grilled Steak Soft Taco Supreme	1 (5.75 oz)	290	14	35	1040
Guacamole	1 serv (0.75 oz)	35	3	0	80
Mexican Pizza	1 serv (7.75 oz)	570	35	45	1040
Mexican Rice	1 serv (4.75 oz)	190	9	15	760
Nacho Cheese Sauce	2 serv (2 oz)	120	10	5	470
Nachos	1 serv (3.5 oz)	320	18	5	570
Nachos Beef Beef Supreme	1 serv (7 oz)	450	24	30	810
Nachos Bellgrande	1 serv (11 oz)	770	39	35	1310
Picante Sauce	1 serv (0.3 oz)	0	0	0	110
Pico De Gallo	1 serv (0.75 oz)	5	0	0	65
Pintos 'n Cheese	1 serv (4.5 oz)	190	9	15	650
Red Sauce	1 serv (1 oz)	10	0	0	320
Soft Taco	1 (3.5 oz)	220	10	25	580
Soft Taco Supreme	1 (5 oz)	260	14	35	590
Sour Cream	1 serv (0.75 oz)	40	4	10	10
Steak Fajita Wrap	1 (8 oz)	470	21	40	1190
Steak Fajita Wrap Supreme	1 (9 oz)	510	25	50	1200
Taco	1 (2.75 oz)	180	10	25	330
Taco Supreme	1 (4 oz)	220	14	35	350
Taco Salad w/ Salsa	1 (19 oz)	850	52	60	1780
Taco Salad w/ Salsa w/o Shell	1 (16.5 oz)	420	22	60	1520
Three Cheese Blend	1 serv (0.25 oz)	25	2	5	50
Tostada	1 (6.25 oz)	300	15	15	650
Veggie Fajita Wrap	1 (8 oz)	420	19	20	980
Veggie Fajita Wrap Supreme	1 (9 oz)	470	22	30	990

FOOD	PORTION	CALS	FAT	CHOL	SOD
TACO JOHN'S					
children's menu selections					
Kid's Meal Softshell Taco	1 serv (8.5 oz)	617	33	35	1037
Kid's Meal Crispy Taco	1 serv (8 oz)	579	34	35	789
desserts					
Choco Taco	1 serv (3.5 oz)	320	17	20	100
Churro	1 serv (1.5 oz)	147	8	4	160
Flauta Apple	1 serv (2 oz)	84	1	0	72
Flauta Cherry	1 serv (2 oz)	143	4	0	110
Flauta Cream Cheese	1 serv (2 oz)	181	8	10	135
Italian Ice	1 serv (4 oz)	80	0	0	5
main menu selections					
Bean Burrito	1 (6.5 oz)	387	11	18	866
Beans Refried	1 serv (9.5 oz)	357	9	17	1032
Beef Burrito	1 (6.5 oz)	449	20	52	863
Chicken Fajita Burrito	1 (6.25)	370	12	49	1536
Chicken Fajita Salad w/o Dressing	1 serv (12.25 oz)	557	33	56	1541
Chicken Fajita Softshell	1 (4.5 oz)	200	7	33	903
Chili	1 serv (9.25 oz)	350	21	56	865
Chimichanga Platter	1 serv (18 oz)	979	38	59	2341
Combination Burrito	1 (6.5 oz)	418	16	35	865
Crispy Tacos	1 serv (3.25 oz)	182	11	26	272
Double Enchilada Platter	1 serv (18.25 oz)	967	42	89	1921
Meat & Potato Burrito	1 (7.75 oz)	503	24	25	1341
Mexi Rolls w/ Nacho Cheese	1 serv (9.75 oz)	863	48	54	1392
Mexican Rice	1 serv (8 oz)	567	18	0	1293
Nachos	1 serv (3.5 oz)	333	21	0	611
Potato Oles Bravo	1 serv (8.88 oz)	579	38	7	1550
Ranch Burrito	1 (7 oz)	447	23	74	804
Sampler Platter	1 serv (25.5 oz)	1406	61	126	2875
Sierra Chicken Fillet Sandwich	1 (8.5 oz)	534	29	68	1406
Smothered Burrito Platter	1 serv (19.5 oz)	1031	40	70	2351
Softshell Tacos	1 serv (4.25 oz)	230	10	26	520
Super Burrito	1 (8.5 oz)	465	19	41	922
Super Nachos	1 serv (13 oz)	919	56	48	1484
Taco Bravo	1 serv (6.25 oz)	346	14	28	677
Taco Burger	1 (5 oz)	280	12	32	576
Taco Salad w/o Dressing	1 (12.4 oz)	584	38	46	766
TACOTIME					
Casita Burrito Meat	1 serv (12 oz)	647	31	89	1233
Cheddar Cheese	1 serv (0.75 oz)	86	7	22	132
Chicken	1 serv (2.5 oz)	109	6	33	402
Chips	1 serv (2 oz)	266	12	0	461
Crisp Burrito Bean	1 (5.25 oz)	427	18	12	453
Crisp Burrito Chicken	1 (4.75 oz)	422	25	54	795
Crisp Burrito Meat	1 (5.25 oz)	552	30	58	1000
Crisp Taco	1 (4 oz)	295	17	48	609

FOOD	PORTION	CALS	FAT	CHOL	SOD
Crustos	1 serv (3.5 oz)	373	15	0	86
Double Soft Bean Burrito	1 (9.5 oz)	506	12	22	860
Double Soft Combination Burrito	1 (9.5 oz)	617	23	63	1343
Double Soft Meat Burrito	1 serv (6.5 oz)	726	33	99	1809
Empanada Cherry	1 (4 oz)	250	9	0	46
Enchilada Sauce	1 serv (1 oz)	12	0	0	133
Flour Tortilla 10 in	1 (2.75 oz)	213	4	0	393
Flour Tortilla 7 in	1 (1.75 oz)	88	1	0	42
Flour Tortilla 8 in	1 (1.25 oz)	107	3	0	33
Fried Flour Tortilla 10 in	1 (2.75 oz)	318	16	0	315
Fried Flour Tortilla 8 in	1 (1.35 oz)	205	11	0	203
Guacamole	1 serv (1 oz)	29	2	0	94
Hot Sauce	1 serv (1 oz)	10	0	0	120
Lettuce	1 serv (0.5 oz)	2	0	0	1
Mexi Fries	1 reg (4 oz)	266	17	0	799
Mexi Fries	1 lg (8 oz)	532	34	0	1598
Mexican Rice	1 serv (4 oz)	159	2	0	530
Nachos	1 serv (10.5 oz)	680	38	78	1250
Nachos Deluxe	1 serv (15.25 oz)	1048	57	109	2252
Natural Super Taco Meat	1 (11.25 oz)	627	27	82	915
Olives	1 serv (0.50 oz)	16	2	0	124
Quesadilla Cheese	1 serv (3.25 oz)	205	11	30	255
Ranchero Salsa	1 serv (2 oz)	21	1	0	192
Refritos	1 serv (2.5 oz)	97	0	0	101
Refritos	1 serv (7 oz)	326	10	22	525
Rolled Soft Flour Taco	1 (7 oz)	512	23	63	1111
Soft Taco Chicken	1 (7 oz)	387	16	48	933
Sour Cream	1 serv (1 oz)	55	5	19	11
Sour Cream Dressing	1 serv (1.5 oz)	137	14	8	207
Super Shredded Beef Soft Taco	1 (8 oz)	368	11	22	556
Taco Cheeseburger	1 (7.5 oz)	633	36	66	1291
Taco Meat	1 serv (2.5 oz)	208	11	38	576
Taco Salad Chicken w/o Dressing	1 serv (9 oz)	370	21	48	861
Taco Salad w/o Dressing	1 serv (7.75 oz)	479	28	63	895
Taco Shell 6 inch	1 (1.25 oz)	110	6	0	48
Thousand Island Dressing	1 serv (1 oz)	160	16	10	270
Tomato	1 serv (0.5 oz)	3	0	0	1
Tostada Delight Salad Meat	1 (9.75 oz)	628	33	82	1004
Value Soft Bean Burrito	1 (6.75 oz)	380	10	15	715
Value Soft Meat Burrito	1 (6.75 oz)	491	21	56	1197
Value Soft Taco	1 (5.25 oz)	316	15	48	599
Veggie Burrito	1 (11 oz)	491	16	24	643
Wheat Tortilla 11 inch	1 (3.5 oz)	175	3	0	84
TCBY					
Hand Dipped All Flavors 96% Fat Free	1/2 cup (3 oz)	140	3	5	26

FOOD	PORTION	CALS	FAT	CHOL	SOD
Hand Dipped All Flavors Nonfat	1/2 cup (2.9 oz)	120	0	0	60
Lowfat Ice Cream All Flavors No Sugar Added	1/2 cup (2.6 oz)	110	3	10	60
Nonfat Ice Cream All Flavors	1/2 cup (2.9 oz)	120	0	0	55
Soft Serve All Flavors 96% Fat Free	1/2 cup (3.4 fl oz)	140	3	15	60
Soft Serve All Flavors No Sugar Added Nonfat	1/2 cup (2.8 oz)	80	0	<5	35
Soft Serve All Flavors Nonfat	1/2 cup (3.4 oz)	110	0	<5	60
Sorbet All Flavors Nonfat & Nondairy	1/2 cup (3.4 oz)	100	0	0	30

WENDY'S
children's menu selections

FOOD	PORTION	CALS	FAT	CHOL	SOD
French Fries Kid's Meal	1 serv (3.2 oz)	270	13	0	85
Kid's Meal Cheeseburger	1 (4.2 oz)	310	12	45	800
Kid's Meal Hamburger	1 (3.9 oz)	270	9	30	620
Kid's Meal Chicken Nuggets	4 pieces (2.1 oz)	190	13	25	380

main menu selections

FOOD	PORTION	CALS	FAT	CHOL	SOD
1/4 lb Hamburger Patty	1 (2.6 oz)	200	14	65	290
2 oz Hamburger Patty	1 (1.3 oz)	100	7	30	150
American Cheese	1 slice (0.6 oz)	70	6	15	260
American Cheese Jr.	1 slice (0.4 oz)	45	4	10	170
Bacon	1 strip (4 g)	20	2	5	90
Baked Potato Chili & Cheese	1 (15.4 oz)	630	24	40	770
Big Bacon Classic	1 (9.9 oz)	580	30	100	1460
Breaded Chicken Fillet	1 (3.5 oz)	230	11	50	390
Cheddar Cheese Shredded	2 tbsp (0.6 oz)	70	6	15	110
Cheddar Shredded	2 tbsp (0.6 oz)	70	6	15	110
Chicken Breast Fillet Sandwich	1 (7.3 oz)	430	16	56	750
Chicken Club Sandwich	1 (7.6 oz)	470	20	65	940
Chicken Nuggets	5 pieces (2.6 oz)	230	16	30	470
Chili	1 lg (12 oz)	310	10	45	1190
Chili	1 sm (8 oz)	210	7	30	800
Classic Single w/ Everything	1 (7.6 oz)	410	19	70	920
French Fries	1 Great Biggie (6.7 oz)	570	27	0	180
French Fries	1 med (5 oz)	420	20	0	130
French Fries	1 Biggie (5.6 oz)	470	23	0	150
Grilled Chicken Fillet	1 (2.9 oz)	110	3	55	400
Grilled Chicken Sandwich	1 (6.6 oz)	300	7	56	740
Honey Mustard Reduced Calorie	1 tsp (7 g)	25	2	0	40
Hot Stuffed Baked Potato Plain	1 (10 oz)	310	0	0	25
Hot Stuffed Baked Potato Bacon & Cheese	1 (12.6 oz)	530	18	25	820
Hot Stuffed Baked Potato Broccoli & Cheese	1 (14.4 oz)	470	14	5	470

FOOD	PORTION	CALS	FAT	CHOL	SOD
Jr. Bacon Cheeseburger	1 (5.8 oz)	380	19	55	870
Jr. Cheeseburger	1 (4.5 oz)	310	12	45	800
Jr. Cheeseburger Deluxe	1 (6.3 oz)	360	16	50	860
Kaiser Bun	1 (2.5 oz)	200	3	0	340
Ketchup	1 tsp (7 g)	10	0	0	80
Lettuce	1 leaf (0.5 oz)	0	0	0	0
Mayonnaise	1 1/2 tsp (9 g)	30	3	5	60
Mustard	1/2 tsp (5 g)	5	0	0	50
Nuggets Sauce Barbeque	1 pkg (1 oz)	45	0	0	160
Nuggets Sauce Honey Mustard	1 pkg (1 oz)	130	12	10	220
Nuggets Sauce Sweet & Sour	1 pkg (1 oz)	50	0	0	120
Onion	4 rings (0.5 oz)	5	0	0	0
Pickles	4 slices (0.4 oz)	0	0	0	140
Saltines	2 (0.2 oz)	25	1	0	80
Sandwich Bun	1 (2 oz)	160	2	0	300
Spicy Chicken Fillet	1 (3.6 oz)	210	9	60	920
Spicy Chicken Sandwich	1 (7.5 oz)	410	14	65	1280
Tomatoes	1 slice (0.9 oz)	5	0	0	0
Whipped Margarine	1 pkg (0.5 oz)	70	7	0	115
salad dressings					
Blue Cheese	1 pkg (2 oz)	360	36	30	350
French	1 pkg (2 oz)	250	21	0	670
Hidden Valley Ranch	1 pkg (2 oz)	200	20	25	410
Hidden Valley Ranch Reduced Fat Reduced Calorie	1 pkg (2 oz)	120	11	20	470
Italian Reduced Fat Reduced Calorie	1 pkg (2 oz)	80	7	0	690
Italian Caesar	1 pkg (1.5 oz)	230	24	25	350
Thousand Island	1 pkg (2 oz)	260	25	20	380
salads and salad bars					
Bacon Bits	2 tbsp (0.5 oz)	45	2	10	550
Ceasar Side Salad w/o Dressing	1 (3.2 oz)	110	5	15	360
Chicken Salad	2 tbsp (1.2 oz)	70	5	0	135
Deluxe Garden Salad w/o Dressing	1 (9.5 oz)	110	6	0	320
Grilled Chicken Salad w/o Dressing	1 (11.9 oz)	200	7	55	780
Side Salad w/o Dressing	1 (5.4 oz)	60	3	0	160
Soft Breadstick	1 (1.5 oz)	130	3	5	250
Taco Chips	15 (1.5 oz)	210	9	0	160
Taco Salad w/o Dressing	1 (16.4 oz)	380	19	65	1040
WHATABURGER					
baked selections					
Biscuit	1	280	13	3	509
Blueberry Muffin	1	239	8	0	538
Cinnamon Roll	1	320	16	10	190

FOOD	PORTION	CALS	FAT	CHOL	SOD
Cookie Chocolate Chunk	1	247	16	28	75
Cookie White Chocolate Macadamia Nut	1	269	16	34	80
Fried Apple Turnover	1	215	11	0	241
breakfast selections					
Biscuit w/ Bacon	1	359	20	15	730
Biscuit w/ Bacon Egg & Cheese	1	511	33	213	1010
Biscuit w/ Egg & Cheese	1	434	26	202	797
Biscuit w/ Sausage	1	446	29	37	794
Biscuit w/ Sausage Egg & Cheese	1	601	42	236	1081
Biscuit w/ Sausage Gravy	1	479	27	20	1253
Breakfast Platter w/ Bacon	1 serv	695	44	389	1162
Breakfast Platter w/ Sausage	1 serv	785	53	412	1234
Breakfast On A Bun w/ Bacon	1	365	19	210	815
Breakfast On A Bun w/ Sausage	1	455	28	232	886
Butter	1 pkg	36	4	11	42
Egg Omelette Sandwich	1	288	13	198	602
Grape Jelly	1 pkg	45	0	0	15
Hashbrown	1 serv	150	9	0	228
Honey	1 pkg	25	0	0	0
Margarine	1 pkg	25	3	0	40
Pancake Syrup	1 pkg	180	0	0	50
Pancakes	3	259	6	0	842
Pancakes w/ Bacon	1 serv	335	12	12	1074
Pancakes w/ Sausage	1 serv	426	21	34	1127
Srambled Eggs	2	189	15	374	211
Strawberry Jam	1 pkg	40	0	0	15
Taquito Bacon & Egg	1	335	16	286	761
main menu selections					
Bacon	1 slice	38	3	6	106
Cheese Slice	1 lg	89	7	22	338
Cheese Slice	1 sm	46	4	12	176
Chicken Strips	2	120	5	14	420
Club Crackers	1 pkg	30	2	0	75
Croutons	1 pkg	30	1	0	90
Fajita Beef	1	326	12	28	670
Fajita Grilled Chicken	1	272	7	33	691
French Fries	1 reg	332	18	0	208
French Fries	1 junior	221	12	0	139
French Fries	1 lg	442	24	0	227
Garden Salad	1	56	1	0	32
Grilled Chicken Salad	1 serv	150	1	49	434
Grilled Chicken Sandwich	1	442	14	66	1103
Grilled Chicken Sandwich w/o Bun Oil w/ Mustard	1	300	3	66	994
Grilled Chicken Sandwich w/o Bun Oil & Dressing	1	358	6	66	989

FOOD	PORTION	CALS	FAT	CHOL	SOD
Grilled Chicken Sandwich w/o Dressing	1	385	9	66	989
Jalapeno Pepper	1	3	tr	0	190
Justaburger	1	276	11	34	578
Ketchup	1 pkg	30	0	0	344
Onion Rings	1 reg	329	19	0	596
Onion Rings	1 lg	493	29	0	893
Peppered Gravy	1 serv (3 oz)	75	5	0	375
Picante Sauce	1 pkg	5	0	0	130
Taquito Potato & Egg	1	446	22	281	883
Taquito Sausage & Egg	1	443	26	315	790
Texas Toast	1 slice	147	5	0	250
Whataburger	1	598	26	84	1096
Whataburger Double Meat	1	823	42	168	1298
Whataburger Jr.	1	300	12	34	583
Whataburger w/o bun oil	1	407	19	84	839
Whatacatch Sandwich	1	467	25	33	636
Whatachick'n Sandwich	1	501	23	40	1122
salad dressings					
Low Fat Ranch	1 pkg	66	3	15	607
Low Fat Vinaigrette	1 pkg	37	2	0	896
Ranch	1 pkg	320	33	50	750
Thousand Island	1 pkg	160	12	15	470

Index

(q = quiz, t = table)

Visit the
Simon & Schuster Web site:
www.SimonSays.com

and sign up for our
mystery e-mail updates!

Keep up on the latest
new releases, author appearances,
news, chats, special offers, and more!
We'll deliver the information
right to your inbox — if it's new,
you'll know about it.

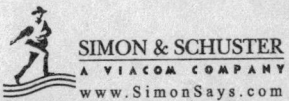

SIMON & SCHUSTER
A VIACOM COMPANY
www.SimonSays.com

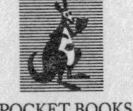

POCKET BOOKS

SONNET
BOOKS

2350